CULTURE & OCCUPATION

CULTURE & OCCUPATION

A Model of Empowerment in Occupational Therapy

Roxie M. Black, PhD, OTR/L, FAOTA
Shirley A. Wells, MPH, OTR, FAOTA

Foreword by Shirley J. Jackson, PhD, OTR

AOTA PRESS

The American
Occupational Therapy
Association, Inc.

Vision Statement
The American Occupational Therapy Association advances occupational therapy as the pre-eminent profession in promoting the health, productivity, and quality of life of individuals and society through the therapeutic application of occupation.

Mission Statement
The American Occupational Therapy Association advances the quality, availability, use, and support of occupational therapy through standard-setting, advocacy, education, and research on behalf of its members and the public.

American Occupational Therapy Association Centennial Vision
We envision that occupational therapy is a powerful, widely recognized, science-driven, and evidence-based profession with a globally connected and diverse workforce meeting society's occupational needs.

AOTA Staff
Frederick P. Somers, *Executive Director*
Christopher M. Bluhm, *Chief Operating Officer*

Chris Davis, *Director, AOTA Press*
Timothy Sniffin, *Production Editor*
Sarah E. Ely, *Book Production Coordinator*
Carrie Mercadante, *Editorial Assistant*
John Prudente, *Marketing Specialist*

Audrey Rothstein, *Director, Marketing and Communications*
Robert A. Sacheli, *Manager, Creative Services*

The American Occupational Therapy Association, Inc.
4720 Montgomery Lane
Bethesda, MD 20814
Phone: 301-652-AOTA (2682)
TDD: 800-377-8555
Fax: 301-652-7711
www.aota.org
To order: 1-877-404-AOTA (2682)

Disclaimers
This publication is designed to provide accurate and authoritative information in regard to the subject matter covered. It is sold or distributed with the understanding that the publisher is not engaged in rendering legal, accounting, or other professional service. If legal advice or other expert assistance is required, the services of a competent professional person should be sought.
—*From the Declaration of Principles jointly adopted by the American Bar Association and a Committee of Publishers and Associations*

It is the objective of the American Occupational Therapy Association to be a forum for free expression and interchange of ideas. The opinions expressed by the contributors to this work are their own and not necessarily those of the American Occupational Therapy Association.

ISBN 10: 1-56900-243-6

ISBN 13: 978-1-56900-243-8

Library of Congress Cataloging-in-Publication Data
Black, Roxie M.
    Culture and occupation : a model of empowerment in occupational therapy / Roxie M. Black, Shirley A. Wells.
        p. ; cm.
    Includes bibliographical references and index.
    ISBN-13: 978-1-56900-243-8 (pbk.)
    ISBN-10: 1-56900-243-6 (pbk.)
    1. Occupational therapy—United States. 2. Occupational therap—Politicala aspects—United States.
3. Occupational therapy—Social aspects—United States. 4. Transcultural medical care—United States.
I. Wells, Shirley A. II. Title.
    [DNLM: 1. Occupational Therapy—United States. 2. Cross-Cultural Comparison—United States. 3. Cultural Diversity—United States. 4. Prejudice—United States. 5. Socioeconomic Factors—United States. 6. Stereotyping—United States. WB 555 B627c 2007]
    RM735.B53 2007
    362.17'8—dc22   2007033153

Design by Sarah E. Ely
Cover art by Lynne Taetzsch, *Perennial.* Used with permission.
Composition by Cindy Stock, Silver Spring, MD
Printed by Versa Press, Inc., East Peoria, IL

Citation: Black, R. M., & Wells, S. A. (2007). *Culture and occupation: A model of empowerment in occupational therapy.* Bethesda, MD: AOTA Press.

Dedication

We dedicate this book to the children in our lives and in the world.

This book is dedicated to my wonderful grandchildren,
Caleb and Emma Litchfield, and to their brother, Micah, who was born
in the spring. They and the grandchildren of us all are the hope and
promise for a more peaceful and just world.

—ROXIE M. BLACK

I dedicate this book to my grandniece, Kyla Lewis.
May she grow up and live in a world without boundaries, prejudices,
and limitations because of her color, culture, or gender.

—SHIRLEY A. WELLS

Contents

Foreword

OCCUPATIONAL THERAPISTS ALWAYS HAVE TAKEN PRIDE in treating the total person. In today's global economy and health care arena, the total person seeking care is all too often from a different culture than that of the therapist. Two unfamiliar, dissimilar cultures interacting in a therapeutic context presents both obvious and not so obvious challenges, which can be quite substantial and can cause significant conflict in the worst of cases. To provide quality occupational therapy to all clients in an economy driven by results-based outcomes and dwindling health care dollars, occupational therapists must not settle for just becoming culturally aware. Indeed, therapists today must strive to become completely culturally competent.

With *Culture and Occupation: A Model of Empowerment for Occupational Therapy*, Roxie M. Black and Shirley A. Wells artfully demonstrate the significance of culture and cultural competence in the study and daily practice of occupational therapy, providing a compelling case for personal cultural awareness, knowledge, and proficiency in understanding one's own culture before learning to transcend a different culture. The authors cleverly illustrate the dynamic connection that exists between cultural exchanges and therapeutic outcomes. Essentially, occupational therapists practicing in the absence of cultural competence do not provide quality services to the total person without understanding and addressing many of the traits that make our clients who they are—their cultural interests, customs, patterns, values, and beliefs.

Throughout the book, Black and Wells use research, clinical findings, and thoughtful analysis to help therapists understand and achieve cultural competence. Much of the data and evidence is so bold and jarring that they prevent us from passively reading this text. Indeed, the text demands that we recognize the great disservice that would result if occupational therapists refuse to acknowledge and embrace the cultural differences that exist between them and their clients. As therapists daily encounter people from varied cultures in their clinics, communities, and walkways,

Black and Wells compel us to *run* and not *walk* to learn how to achieve cultural competence to more effectively serve the diverse communities in the United States.

The authors begin with the first important step in the cultural development process: understanding how culture influences and shapes behavior, values, and beliefs of them and their clients. Each individual's cultural landscape includes many complexities beyond ethnicity, including the person's age, sex, race, religion, and native language. Culture is at the heart of the person and often dictates choices, interests, and meaning in life. Thus, one of the essential lessons given by Black and Wells is that understanding the depths, facets, and implications of culture is complex, and stereotyping is not a fix to appreciating the effect each person's culture has on successful therapeutic interactions and outcomes.

Black and Wells masterfully analyze and advise how to bridge cultural divides in clinical practice, educational settings, and political arenas. They demonstrate how cross-cultural communication and language can be used as critical tools in effective treatment. Models, guidelines, case scenarios, a list of dos and don'ts, and clinical reasoning exercises provide excellent educational resources to teach cultural competence. Occupational therapists and students are challenged to use their power to become agents of political and social change. These concepts transcend theoretical approaches and educational curriculum to offer educators, researchers, and students an excellent multicultural teaching–learning model.

Data on health disparities show minority clients are disproportionally affected with the worst conditions at the most severe levels in greater proportions than any other cultural group. In addition, current health care trends highlight the worst of every health condition among minority cultures. They are portrayed in the worst light on every health care index, and access to certain levels of health care is routinely denied. As Black and Wells point out, many of these issues are promoted by unfair medical and political policies, practices, and procedures. Occupational therapists are challenged to use their power to become effective change agents and empower their culturally different clients.

In the end, *Culture and Occupation* equips occupational therapists to understand the relationship between culture and successful practice, providing them with a road map to empowerment and how to become culturally competent. Readers are given tools for developing cultural competence and to serve as agents for social change in reaching across the divides caused by cultural differences. With the instructive and practical guide this book offers, occupational therapists around the United States can embrace and transcend cultural differences and provide optimum quality service to the total person—which long has been a hallmark of occupational therapy practice.

Our goal as occupational therapists is to empower our clients to be able to safely and independently engage, participate, and perform their cultural occupation despite culture, age, injury, or disability. We do this by creating environments and using culturally aligned methods of assessment and intervention. This enlightening and comprehensive book compels us to acknowledge the importance of culture and to overcome cultural hurdles, not just tolerate people from other cultures. Black and Wells have invited us to develop our skills toward becoming culturally competent. We now need to give ourselves permission to begin that journey.

—**Shirley J. Jackson, PhD, OTR**
Department of Occupational Therapy
Howard University
Washington, DC

Preface

MUCH HAS CHANGED IN THE WORLD in the seven years since Shirley and I published our first book, *Cultural Competency for Health Professionals* (Wells & Black, 2000). The terrorist attacks of September 11, 2001, have resulted in increased suspicion in the United States and around the world of people of Arab descent. The Iraq war began in 2002, and people from many countries are being killed or seriously wounded, among them U.S. service members who are significantly challenging health care practitioners in the armed services and Veterans Administration hospitals across the country. Armed conflicts in other parts of the world are contributing to an increase in the number of refugees and immigrants entering the United States, and demographic data continue to indicate an inexorable increase in the numbers of people of color in the U.S. population. Technology has continued to improve, so we now easily interact with people and know about events around the world with the touch of a key, making us more and more aware of our culturally different global neighbors.

In the world of occupational therapy, Kronenberg, Algado, and Pollard (2005) published *Occupational Therapy Without Borders,* which introduced occupational therapists worldwide to the concepts of *occupational justice* and *community-based rehabilitation,* and the American Occupational Therapy Association (AOTA, 2005) established a task force to examine the issues of health disparities and cultural competence. AOTA published a *Centennial Vision* (AOTA, 2007) calling for a culturally diverse work force by 2017, and Iwama (2006) developed the first culturally sensitive practice model, the Kawa Model, which provides a culturally appropriate intervention option for Japanese clients.

Seven years ago, there was little in the occupational therapy literature about cultural competence, but interest in issues of culture and diversity has increased both in publications and in regional and national conferences. The events of the past seven years globally, nationally, and in our profession make the timing of this book optimal.

Culture and Occupation: A Model of Empowerment in Occupational Therapy is unapologetically political in the sense that Kronenberg spoke of—with a *little p* (Kronenberg & Pollard, 2005; F. Kronenberg, personal communication, November 1, 2005). We address the issue of power in several chapters, and power issues connote the political; we focus on inequities in the United States for disadvantaged people, inequities often held in place by institutionalized oppressive policies—again the political; and we write about the conflict many deal with in their daily lives, conflict that results in occupational injustices for so many who are sociopolitically disadvantaged. Occupational therapy can no longer provide services only in clinics, ignoring the larger contextual issues that continue to bring clients to our doors. We must recognize, as a profession and as educators and practitioners, the need to be social agents for change and to educate ourselves and our students about sociopolitical structures that maintain inequities and disparities in health and occupation. We must take action by getting involved in legislative issues and advocating for our clients, by empowering our clients to advocate for themselves in a participatory power model, and by becoming culturally competent so that we may interact effectively with all clients and their families. We must recognize the need to become more politically relevant (Duncan, Buchanan, & Lorenzo, 2005) and then act on this need. This book provides information, theories, and examples of how that may happen.

Contents of This Book

This book has been organized for clarity and with a focus on occupational therapy. Because this book focuses on occupational therapy, rather than addressing a more diverse health care audience, Part I emphasizes the role of culture and cultural competence in occupational therapy. Chapters 1–4 provide the foundation for cultural competence by discussing the need for and definitions of the concept. The final chapter in this part presents the Cultural Competency Model and how occupational therapists and occupational therapy assistants can use the model in providing culturally competent care.

Part II addresses the three major characteristics of cultural competence found in the Cultural Competency Model. Its three subsections address developing self-awareness and the concept of power, attaining cultural knowledge, and developing cross-cultural skills. This part incorporates 12 chapters and is the largest section in the book.

Section A of Part II contains four chapters that help readers think about and assess their own cultural self-knowledge. Chapter 5 discusses the importance of self-awareness in the development of cultural competence and emphasizes why we feel that self-awareness is the most important component of cultural competence. Chapter 6 introduces readers to the concepts of power and privilege and their impact on personal behaviors and professional practice, and Chapter 7 takes a closer look at White privilege and its implications. Chapter 8 helps readers examine what it means to be a professional and the inherent power within that role.

Section B focuses on cultural knowledge. Chapter 9 defines cultural knowledge and how one attains it. The other four chapters in this section provide examples of the kind of information one might gather while developing cultural knowledge: Chapters 10 and 11 give extensive information about health disparities and health status data; Chapter 12 offers an examination of one ethnic and cultural subgroup, Somali refugees in the United States, as an example of an in-depth look at a specific group; and Chapter 13 looks in detail at Shirley's hometown of Brownsville, Texas, and demonstrates how to gather important information about one's own community.

Section C addresses the development of cross-cultural skills. Chapter 14 emphasizes the importance of an attitude of willingness, analyzing this attitude through the double lens of the Model of Human Occupation (Kielhofner, 2002) and a research study on cultural competence (Black, 2000). Cross-cultural communication and language are the skills emphasized in Chapter 15, with particular emphasis on the power inherent in the words we use. Chapter 16, the final chapter of Part II, takes readers through the process of developing their own plan for acquiring cultural competence.

Applying the concept of cultural competence in a variety of venues is the focus of Part III. Chapter 17 focuses on the provision of culturally competent care within practice settings, and Chapter 18 examines how to educate for cultural competence, exploring multiple models of multicultural education and providing numerous pedagogical strategies and considerations. Community practice settings are the focus of Chapter 19, which provides numerous examples for the multiple approaches to community assessment. Chapter 20 introduces readers to the concept of *occupational justice* and its integration with cultural competence.

The final section of the book, Part IV, focuses on the evaluation of cultural competence. Chapter 21 provides provocative considerations in the development and implementation of research on culture, while Chapter 22 identifies research studies that inform the occupational therapy and other fields and can be used as evidence for aspects of cultural competence. The final chapter of the book, Chapter 23, presents the importance of ethical practice as a framework with which to evaluate our interactions with others. The appendixes include additional resources for readers interested in researching more about the information included in this book.

Accepting the Challenge

Not becoming culturally competent is no longer an option for occupational therapists and occupational therapy assistants. As we learn to interact as global citizens,
and as our client population and colleagues become more diverse, we must accept
the challenge of providing effective, client-centered, and culturally competent care
to individuals, communities, and populations. We stand at a critical crossroads: The
future of health care and the future of our profession are merging with the realities
of a changing world. We have the opportunity to become leaders as agents for
change so that all people, privileged and disadvantaged alike, have equal access to
health care, social and political resources, and meaningful occupation. It is vital that
we step forward to accept this challenge.

References

American Occupational Therapy Association. (2005). *AOTA Board Task Force on Health Disparities: Report to the Board of Directors.* Bethesda, MD: Author

American Occupational Therapy Association. (2007). Centennial vision. *American Journal
of Occupational Therapy, 61.*

Black, R. M. (2000). *The essence of cultural competence: Listening to the voices of occupational therapy students.* Unpublished doctoral dissertation, Lesley University, Cambridge, MA.

Duncan, M., Buchanan, H., & Lorenzo, T. (2005). Politics in occupational therapy education: A South African perspective. In F. Kronenberg, S. S. Algado, & N. Pollard (Eds.),
Occupational therapy without borders: Learning from the spirit of survivors (pp.
390–401). Edinburgh, Scotland: Elsevier/Churchill Livingstone.

Iwama, M. (2006). *The Kawa model: Culturally relevant occupational therapy.* Toronto,
Ontario: Elsevier/Churchill Livingstone.

Kielhofner, G. (2002). *A model of human occupation: Theory and application* (3rd ed.). Baltimore: Lippincott Williams & Wilkins.

Kronenberg, F., Algado, S. S., & Pollard, N. (Eds.). (2005). *Occupational therapy without borders:
Learning from the spirit of survivors.* Edinburgh, UK: Elsevier/Churchill Livingstone.

Kronenberg, F., & Pollard, N. (2005). Overcoming occupational apartheid: A preliminary
exploration of the political nature of occupational therapy. In F. Kronenberg, S. S.
Algado, & N. Pollard (Eds.), *Occupational therapy without borders: Learning from the
spirit of survivors* (pp. 58–86). Edinburgh, UK: Elsevier/Churchill Livingstone.

Wells, S. A., & Black, R. M. (2000). *Cultural competency for health professionals.* Bethesda,
MD: American Occupational Therapy Association.

Acknowledgments

ROXIE M. BLACK thanks all the students and colleagues who provided critical feedback on the first version of this book and appreciates their honesty and trust. She also thanks her research assistants, Katie Jewett and Sheila Glynn, without whom this book might never have been completed.

SHIRLEY A. WELLS thanks Vachinna, Earl, Sandy, Norma, John, and her town for sharing and for providing opportunities to learn, grow, and live with diversity.

Explanation of Terminology

THE TERMINOLOGY USED to describe racial and ethnic populations in the United States has changed over time. The self-reporting of ethnicity and race also has been found to change from year to year. In this book, we use the following descriptors:

- For research and statistical reports, we use the racial and ethnic categories defined by the Office of Management and Budget Directive No. 15 (see Chapter 21).
- For research and statistical studies, we use the terminology and descriptors that appear in the study.
- For general content, we use the following terms: *Native Americans, African Americans, Asian Americans and Pacific Islanders, White Americans,* and *Hispanics.*

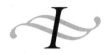

Occupational Therapy and Cultural Competence

Our maturity as a profession and ability to affect people's lives in powerfully positive ways hinges on a greater inclusion of diverse spheres of experience and meaning.

—IWAMA (2004, p. 1)

Objectives

The information in Part I will help readers

- Understand how culture affects each of our daily lives, including the lives of our clients, our students, our colleagues, and ourselves;

- Recognize the importance of understanding the impact of culture in occupational therapy practice;

- Define *cultural competence,* identify the skills and characteristics needed to be a culturally competent health care provider, and understand the need for culturally competent care in occupational therapy practice; and

- Understand the Cultural Competency Model and reflect on its application.

1

Cultural Aspects
of Occupation

Cultures are formed around the meanings people construct and share. Culture, in fact, is best understood as the processes of meaning-making within a given social group.

—LEWIS (2002, P. 3)

Key Points

- Culture affects the daily lives of all individuals.
- The concept of *culture* is complex and not easily defined.
- Culture influences occupational choice and performance.
- Cultural influences are derived from various levels, including global, societal, professional, and personal levels.
- Because of the importance of culture in each person's life, occupational therapists need to be culturally competent.

Culture

YESTERDAY WAS SATURDAY, and because I (R. B.) didn't have to go to work, I relaxed a bit in the morning, lying in bed a little longer than usual, reading a novel. When I arose, I made my bed, showered, walked my dog, and then fixed breakfast for myself. Later I finished a support letter for a colleague's tenure package and then mowed my lawn. The afternoon was spent with my mother watching a Boston Red Sox game, and then we both went to my daughter's home for dinner with her and her family.

Each activity was culturally influenced and meaningful to me. They were part of my daily occupations. If we are to believe Jeff Lewis's definition of culture presented on the previous page, then we must become aware of and recognize the importance of understanding the influence of culture on occupational choice and occupational performance. Every occupational activity in which we engage, whether for work, play, self-care, or rest, has social, cultural, and personal meaning for the actor.

Let me explain a little further. Because I am employed in a traditionally professional workplace, for our society I do not go to work on Saturdays and have more occupational choices on that day. One of my favorite leisure pastimes is reading, which was taught to me by my mother (family culture) and supported by the larger society—note the number of libraries and bookstores in most communities. I have a pet—again, a societally sanctioned activity—that needs to be exercised, which also gives me an opportunity for exercise—another cultural value. Family and societal values have taught me that breakfast is an important meal, as is cleanliness. My daily routine, therefore, includes a shower and a morning meal. I live in a middle-class neighborhood where the expectations are to maintain your property; hence, I keep my lawn mowed—another opportunity for physical exercise. Family visits and enjoying favorite activities or occupations together is another personal and cultural value. Because my 82-year-old mother is an avid Red Sox fan and because I enjoy spending time with her, we often watch the games together, and we both enjoy eating and sharing a meal with my grandchildren and their parents (see Figure 1.1).

Although this explanation may belabor the point, it emphasizes the influence of cultural values on everyday activities. Occupational therapists must be aware of the primacy of that interrelationship and its importance to effective practice.

Additional Definitions of *Culture*

Lewis's definition of culture certainly applies to occupational therapy theory and practice, but it also is important to examine additional definitions of culture. I agree with Michael Iwama (2004) when he describes *culture* as a "slippery concept, taking

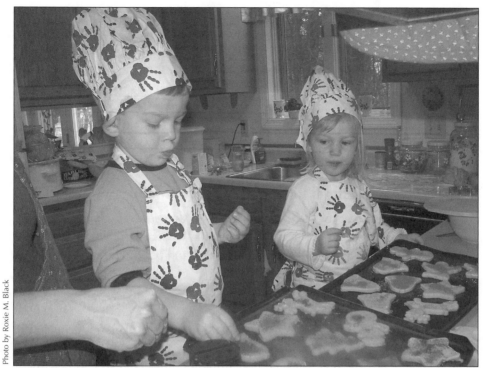

Photo by Roxie M. Black

Figure 1.1. Caleb and Emma making Christmas cookies at Nana's—everyone enjoying a favorite occupation together.

on a variety of definitions and meanings depending on how it has been socially situated and by whom" (p. 1); yet, for us all to have a beginning place for discussion, I'll offer some typical descriptors.

The *Merriam-Webster Dictionary* (1995) defines *culture* as "the customary beliefs, social forms, and material traits of a racial, religious, or social group" (p. 127). This general definition gives us a vague notion of the concept of culture, whereas others are more descriptive. In *Cultural Competency for Health Professionals* (the first iteration of this book; 2000), Shirley A. Wells and I defined *culture* as

> The sum total of a way of living, including values, beliefs, standards, linguistic expression, patterns of thinking, behavioral norms, and styles of communication that influence the behavior(s) of a group of people that is transmitted from generation to generation. It includes demographic variables such as age, gender, and place of residence; status variables such as social, educational, and economic levels; and affiliation variables. (p. 270)

Because culture is transmitted from one person or group to another, it is therefore learned.

Given the breadth of the above definition, the complexity of the concept becomes clear. Because of this complexity, people try to simplify it to make it understandable, and in doing so, compartmentalize their thinking in just one area. Perhaps this is why some folks think only of racial or ethnic difference when they consider "culture." The broader definition, however, makes us realize the influence of culture on each person's life. One's cultural orientation and beliefs help determine occupational choice, occupational behaviors, and occupational performance. As Iwama (2004) states, "Culture represents one of the most important issues facing occupational therapy today" (p. 1).

Levels of Cultural Influence and Occupational Choice

If culture is so important for each person, how does one begin to explore this complex topic? In this chapter, we begin by reviewing the multiple levels of cultural influence, considering global, societal, professional, and personal factors that affect people's perceptions (see Figure 1.2).

Global Considerations

Before the current technological age and the shift to a global economy, people were not as concerned about what happened in other parts of the world. They could focus their interests on their own family and community and sometimes might consider things of national concern. But with television, radio, and print media in most homes in developed countries, and with e-mail, instant messaging, and other technological advances in communication, people not only know what is going on in other parts of the world, but they know about it as it is happening.

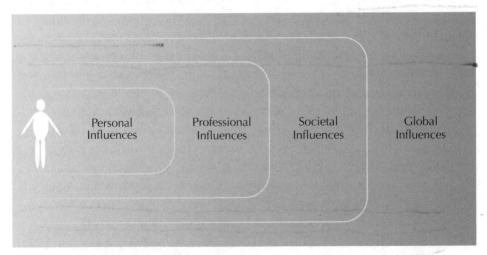

Figure 1.2. Cultural levels of influence.

As I wrote this chapter, Hurricane Katrina had just caused destruction to the U.S. Gulf Coast, and countries and citizens from around the world were lending support to the people and communities devastated by the storm by engaging in occupational activities, such as collecting items and sending them to the ravaged areas. People traveled to the United States to help as needed, while others helped manufacture necessary materials to send. At press time, still others are helping clear debris and rebuild homes in many communities. In other words, individuals, organizations, communities, and countries have shifted what they normally do to help. They have chosen atypical occupational activities for a time because of their own values regarding care and assistance.

World events also influence people's daily activities. After the terrorist attacks on the World Trade Center and Pentagon, Saddam Hussein's capture, the tsunami disaster in Indonesia and Sri Lanka, the subway attack in London, and the Israeli–Palestinian conflict in the Gaza Strip, how many people have increased their television viewing time, read the newspapers with more thoroughness, spend more time at work talking about these events, or have changed their travel plans because of an increased concern about the safety of flying? Perhaps the incidence of depression and other mental health issues have increased after these events (Proctor, 1998; Staudenmeier & Hill, 2002) and, if so, how has that influenced occupational performance and behaviors? How many more occupational therapists are now working in countries other than their own to provide help where needed (Kronenberg, Algado, & Pollard, 2005)? Increased awareness of world events affects everyone daily, often in ways we may not yet comprehend.

Societal Considerations

Being part of a culture is a social phenomenon. *Merriam-Webster's* definition addresses the social aspect of culture, and Lewis (2002) writes that "culture is constructed by humans in order to communicate and create community" (p. 13). A culture's beliefs, values, foods, artifacts, religion, and ways of communicating are all developed to share with like-minded people. Cultural members engage in activities sanctioned by others, but if they choose activities not sanctioned by society, they often are viewed as deviant (Becker, 1963; Erikson, 1966) and are somehow stigmatized or punished (Goffman, 1963). Members of the culture or society teach expected values, beliefs, and behaviors to the youngest or newest members of the group to enhance the group's cohesiveness and development. Occupational choices and behaviors are influenced by our values and beliefs and, therefore, are culturally constructed.

Sociologists have developed multiple concepts regarding cultural groups, including the terminology of dominant cultures, subaltern cultures, and subcultures

(Lewis, 2002). The *dominant culture* of the United States includes English-speaking, White, middle-class, heterosexual people who have become the "standard" by which others are measured. This group's beliefs and values dominate U.S. culture. The *U.S. Constitution* promises freedom, equality, and the pursuit of happiness to all people, yet most people recognize that members of the dominant group realize these promises more often than the nondominant members of society.

Subaltern cultures are marginalized by the dominant society (Lewis, 2002) and live on society's periphery, often struggling for equal access to goods and services. Lewis identifies some of these groups as "gays and lesbians, black Africans, Hispanic immigrants, [and] indigenous people" (p. 29). Although part of larger society and culture, members of the subaltern culture often develop their own cultural values, beliefs, traditions, and activities outside of the dominant culture. These characteristics enhance their identity as a specific cultural group but separate them from the larger sociocultural group, often resulting in conflict or lack of access to goods, services, and even civil rights.

Subcultures are those smaller groups within the larger culture to which a person belongs. These may include one's community or neighborhood; one's family; or one's church, temple, synagogue, mosque, or other organization. Not uncommonly, values and expectations of subgroups conflict with those of other subgroups or with the culture at large. The family of an occupational therapy student, for example, may expect her to be home often for family meals and outings, but the expectations from her occupational therapy program may cause her to spend an inordinate amount of time reading and studying at the library or with peers, affecting mealtime with her family. The expectations from these two subcultural groups conflict, and the student must make choices about what is most important to her at that time (values) and how she will respond (occupational choice). The decisions each person makes about what subcultures to be part of and what choices of activities to engage in contribute to her individuality and identity. While working with clients, it is imperative to understand the dominant and subcultural influences that affect their occupational choices and recognize the uniqueness of each person's choices and personality.

Professional Considerations

When a person decides to become an occupational therapist, he or she makes a decision to be part of a subculture of professionals. As with any other group, multiple influences guide occupational therapists' practice and behaviors. These influences derive from the larger health care arena, the discipline of occupational science, the American Occupational Therapy Association (AOTA), and the institution or agency where they work.

Health Care Influences

Although the profession of occupational therapy is moving slowly away from the medical model, currently more than 70% of occupational therapists continue to work in traditional medical centers such as hospitals, rehabilitation centers, outpatient programs, and skilled-nursing facilities (U.S. Department of Labor, 2005). With employment statistics like these, we cannot ignore the influence of the health care industry on the profession and its members.

Current laws and regulations determine the number of hours an occupational therapist must spend with patients or clients and how much documentation is required to meet those regulations. In addition, Shadley and Rexrode (2005) remind us that the movement toward evidence-based practice "has forced the health care industry to develop tools to measure quality improvement" (p. CE1). At a time when the occupational therapy profession is attempting to add quality time and meaning to its interventions, the pragmatic issues of tighter regulations and increased demands to meet productivity requirements affect the way an occupational therapist may choose to relate with her clients. Opacich (1997) raises the question of moral tensions and obligations of providing occupational therapy services within these constraints. Yet, if we are part of the current U.S. health care culture, we cannot escape these regulations. These external and very real demands on a therapist's time guide her or his occupational behavior and choices. These demands add stress and conflict to their daily work, and many therapists turn to areas of practice where the expectations are less regulated.

Occupational Science

The discipline of occupational science began in the late 20th century to "study humans as occupational beings" (Wilcock, 2003, p. 157) and to "generate knowledge about the form, the function, and the meaning of human occupation" (Zemke & Clark, 1996, p. vii). Occupational therapy educators at the University of Southern California developed it when they recognized the need for a scientific discipline to examine occupation and all its characteristics. Although conceived as a basic science, the developers of the discipline do perceive it as interlinked with occupational therapy practice. The birth of occupational science has contributed to and supported a paradigm shift from the medical model back to the study of occupation in the profession of occupational therapy.

Wilcock (2003) has identified four main beliefs of occupational scientists:

1. Occupation encompasses all human pursuits.
2. Occupation is fundamental to autonomy, health, well-being, and justice.
3. Occupational science generates knowledge about the rich diversity of human occupation.

4. Occupational science embraces a multidisciplinary, multiperspective approach to research, debate, and activism.

Although the practice of occupational therapy is not a scientific discipline itself, occupational science and its beliefs do influence occupational therapy practice, education, and research. If an occupational therapy practitioner subscribes to these beliefs, then the way she or he evaluates clients and develops interventions, teaches, or conducts research will reflect an occupation-centered approach. As professional occupational choices shift away from a more medical approach, the occupational therapist may choose to interact with clients in a different way.

Occupational Therapy Values and Beliefs

Practitioners, educators, students, and researchers of occupational therapy are all significantly influenced by the subculture of the profession. Occupational therapists and occupational therapy assistants are acculturated into the profession and encouraged to embrace the values and beliefs found in the *Occupational Therapy Code of Ethics (2005)* and the *Core Values and Attitudes of Occupational Therapy Practice* (AOTA, 1993, 2005). These include the ethical principles of beneficence (concern for the well-being of clients), non-maleficence (do no harm), autonomy, privacy, and confidentiality, as well as the concepts of altruism, equality, freedom, justice, dignity, truth, and prudence (AOTA, 2005). All these values guide our professional thinking and our practice (what we *do* in therapy, our occupational choices). Most occupational therapists can accept these values because they easily complement the values learned earlier in life. These common values often are what draw people into the occupational therapy field.

In addition to the previously listed concepts, many other valued beliefs in the profession guide our work, including the notions of holistic practice, the value of occupation in the development of health, client-centered care, and culturally competent care.

Holistic Practice. Many occupational therapists describe the holistic nature of practice when defining occupational therapy to others. Occupational therapists explain that they are not just concerned about the apparent physical disability of their client, for instance, but that they also are aware of and address social, cognitive, and mental health concerns. This belief was one of the premises of the profession seen in the earliest writings of its founders (Meyer, 1922; Pattison, 1922; Stevenson, 1932) and continues to be identified as important by contemporary writers (Burke, 2003; Hemphill-Pearson & Hunter, 1997; Nelson & Jepson-Thomas, 2003). Hemphill-Pearson and Hunter (1997) state, "one of the main premises of holistic care is that the patient's mind and body are inseparable" (p. 36). They went on to define *holism* "as the principle that the living organism is a whole that is more than the sum of its parts. The interdependence of all these parts determines the nature of the entire organism's existence" (p. 37).

In occupational therapy, "holism principles would be integrated into the ... treatment plan and shared with the patient or family, giving adequate attention to biological, psychological, social, and environmental factors" (Hemphill-Pearson & Hunter, 1997, p. 43). If a therapist subscribed to the premise of holistic care, he or she would undoubtedly choose a comprehensive evaluation and intervention plan. Believing in and applying holistic care would change that therapist's occupational performance.

Occupation and Its Necessity for Health. As the occupational therapy profession has returned to the paradigm of occupation (Schwartz, 2003), practitioners and educators have been reminded of the importance of meaningful occupation for a healthy life. The founders of the profession recognized that productive and meaningful activity were necessary for health, and with the emphasis once again on the importance of occupation, practitioners and researchers have begun again to examine the importance of meaning and occupational choice (Baker, Jacobs, & Tickle-Degnen, 2003; Hammell, 2004; Lazzarini, 2004).

The focus on activity in occupational therapy continued until the 1960s when the profession became enamored with the medical model and chose to focus on neurobehavioral and diagnostic categories. I remember being given a pin to wear in occupational therapy school in the mid-1960s that said "I don't do crafts." It was very clear to me at that time that the developing theory of sensory integration was more important and more highly valued than my craft classes!

> *The* Occupational Therapy Practice Framework *identifies culture as one of seven possible contextual features to evaluate when working with clients.*

A focus on occupation experienced a resurgence in the 1960s and 1970s, however, with Mary Reilly's theory of Occupational Behavior (Reilly, 1962, 1969), followed by the development of the Model of Human Occupation by her students Gary Kielhofner and Janet Burke (1980). This practice model was one of the first that intentionally identified the importance of a client's culture and its influence on occupational choice. Occupation-focused theoretical models developed thereafter (Christiansen & Baum, 1997; Dunn, Brown, & McGuigan, 1994; Law et al., 1996; Schkade & Schultz, 2003) also have identified culture as an important client characteristic to consider, and the new *Occupational Therapy Practice Framework: Domain and Process* (AOTA, 2002) identifies culture as one of seven possible contextual features to evaluate and be knowledgeable about when working with clients. This new knowledge has started to change the behaviors of occupational therapy practitioners and how they plan interventions with their clients—applying new theoretical constructs changes occupational choices and performance.

Many factors have shifted the way practitioners think and do business in occupational therapy. Educational programs have revised their curricula and courses to meet the ever-changing standards from the Accreditation Council for Occupational Therapy Education (2007), occupational therapy practitioners are focusing more on meaningful activities for their clients rather than emphasizing only exercise or less meaningful activities, and researchers are conducting studies to develop evidence for the effectiveness of occupation as intervention. Understanding the importance of occupation to the field of occupational therapy and to our practice significantly influences our own occupational choices as occupational therapy practitioners.

Client-Centered Care. A major tenet of occupational therapy that influences our performance as practitioners and educators is the concept of client-centered care. The roots of this concept come from the work of psychologist Carl Rogers (1951), who believed that a client was a partner in the therapeutic process and must take an active part in her or his intervention. Sumsion (1999) suggests it is important to try to imagine and understand the client's disability or illness through his or her eyes, not our own. The implications of this approach to practice are that the therapist must be willing to actively engage with the client, listen well to the client's story, be willing to share the therapist's authoritative power and expertise, and collaborate on goals and objectives to help the client reengage in meaningful activity in a way that supports his or her social roles (Black, 2005).

Because the concept of client-centered care is a strong component of the culture of occupational therapy, it moves us away from the model of the omniscient health care provider who makes all the decisions for practice in a very paternalistic fashion to that of a team player or a collaborator with the client. Client-centered practice changes how we perform evaluations, how we ask questions and listen to responses, the time we might spend with clients, and the choices of interventions used. In other words, client-centered practice is a culturally sanctioned approach to client care in occupational therapy, which affects our occupational performance.

Culturally Competent Care. Culturally competent care, the focus of this book, is an attitude and practice in which the practitioner exhibits skill in cross-cultural interactions with clients in a way that is knowledgeable of and sensitive to clients' unique beliefs and values regarding health care and collaboratively develops appropriate interventions that are meaningful to them. To provide excellent client-centered care, a practitioner also must provide culturally competent care (Black, 2005). The following chapters sufficiently describe culturally competent practice, but it is important to recognize that if an occupational therapy practitioner is culturally competent, his or her occupational performance during evaluation and intervention sessions will reflect that skill.

Personal Considerations

After this brief examination of the larger cultural influences that affect an occupational therapist's occupational choices and performance, we come now to the center of Figure 1.2—the occupational therapy practitioner. Individuals are significantly influenced by the cultural expectations with which they were raised and the expectations of the multiple subgroups to which they currently belong. Values, roles, habits, and abilities all influence occupational choice and performance (Kielhofner, 2002), and with the possible exception of natural abilities, all are culturally defined and constructed. As explained in the beginning of this chapter, individuals choose to do what is meaningful to them, and what is meaningful to them is influenced and often determined by cultural values and beliefs. One cannot escape the fact that all people are cultural beings.

Summary

At this point, it should be evident that occupational behavior and choice do not happen apart from cultural influences, which have many levels of influence. Occupational therapy practitioners, educators, and researchers enter every work setting viewing the world from their own cultural lenses and interact with clients who view the same world from their own unique perspectives. Often, these worldviews differ—sometimes minimally, sometimes considerably. If occupational therapists are to provide the best possible care during these interactions, including client-centered care, they cannot assume they know what each client needs. All occupational therapists must make an effort to know their clients and how the clients' beliefs and values affect the way they view health, their own illness, their belief in recovery, and their understanding of both their role and the occupational therapist's role in that process. This requires a beginning understanding of clients' cultural beliefs and behaviors and how they influence clients' lives. To be effective, occupational therapists must engage in culturally competent care. To achieve this, the occupational therapist must begin to move toward the development of cultural competence. The following chapters provide more information and strategies for accomplishing this goal.

Reflection

1. *Cultural Object Exercise.* Choose something in your life that means a lot to you. It might be a piece of jewelry, a picture, a memento, a religious icon, a recipe, or anything else that is special to you. Begin to analyze why this object is meaningful.

   a. Think of the people or person who is part of this experience.

   b. Think of what you do or did when engaged in the activities related to this object.

   c. Does the object reflect certain values or beliefs for you?

   d. Write a brief narrative about this experience.

   This exercise is one way to begin to look at your own culture. It often is effective
   when done in a group so that similarities and differences can be compared.

2. *Values Identification.* Our values often reflect our cultural beliefs. Make a list of
   your values. Try to be as comprehensive as possible. For each value listed, try to
   determine the following:

   a. Where you learned this from?

   b. Who influenced you to believe this way?

   c. What groups do you belong to that share this value?

   d. In what groups or situations is this value challenged?

   e. Has this value changed from the time you were a child?

References

Accreditation Council for Occupational Therapy Education. (2007). Accreditation Council
    for Occupational Therapy Education (ACOTE) standards and interpretive guidelines.
    American Journal of Occupational Therapy, 61.

American Occupational Therapy Association. (1993). Core values and attitudes of occupa-
    tional therapy practice. *American Journal of Occupational Therapy, 47,* 1085–1086.

American Occupational Therapy Association. (2002). Occupational therapy practice frame-
    work: Domain and process. *American Journal of Occupational Therapy, 56,* 609–639.

American Occupational Therapy Association. (2005). Occupational therapy code of ethics
    (2005). *American Journal of Occupational Therapy, 59,* 639–642.

Baker, N. A., Jacobs, K., & Tickle-Degnen, L. (2003). A methodology for developing evidence
    about meaning in occupation: Exploring the meaning of working. *OTJR: Occupation,
    Participation, and Health, 23*(2), 57–66.

Becker, H. S. (1963). *Outsiders: Studies in the sociology of deviance.* New York: Free Press.

Black, R. M. (2005). Intersections of care: An analysis of culturally competent care, client-
    centered care, and the feminist ethic of care. *WORK: A Journal of Prevention, Assess-
    ment, and Rehabilitation, 24,* 409–422.

Burke, J. P. (2003). Philosophical basis of human occupation. In P. Kramer, J. Hinojosa, & C.
    B. Royeen (Eds.), *Perspectives in human occupation: Participation in life* (pp. 32–44).
    Philadelphia: Lippincott Williams & Wilkins.

Christiansen, C., & Baum, C. (Eds.). (1997). *Occupational therapy: Enabling function and
    well-being* (2nd ed.). Thorofare, NJ: Slack.

Dunn, W., Brown, C., & McGuigan, A. (1994). The ecology of human performance: A
    framework for considering the effect of context. *American Journal of Occupational
    Therapy, 48,* 595–607.

Erikson, K. (1966). *Wayward Puritans: A study in the sociology of deviance.* New York:
    Macmillan.

Goffman, E. (1963). *Stigma: Notes on the management of spoiled identity.* New York: Simon & Schuster.

Hammell, K. W. (2004). Dimensions of meaning in the occupations of daily life. *Canadian Journal of Occupational Therapy, 71,* 296–305.

Hemphill-Pearson, B. J., & Hunter, M. (1997). Holism in mental health practice. *Occupational Therapy in Mental Health, 13*(2), 35–49.

Iwama, M. (2004). Meaning and inclusion: Revisiting culture in occupational therapy [Guest Editorial]. *Australian Occupational Therapy Journal, 51,* 1–2.

Kielhofner, G. (2002). *A model of human occupation: Theory and application* (3rd ed.). Baltimore: Lippincott Williams & Wilkins.

Kielhofner, G., & Burke, J. (1980). A model of human occupation, part one. Conceptual framework and content. *American Journal of Occupational Therapy, 34,* 572–581.

Kronenberg, F., Algado, S. S., & Pollard, N. (2005). *Occupational therapy without borders: Learning from the spirit of survivors.* Edinburgh, UK: Elsevier/Churchill Livingstone.

Law, M., Cooper, B., Strong, S., Stewart, D., Rigby, P., & Letts, L. (1996). The person–environment–occupation model: A transactive approach to occupational performance. *Canadian Journal of Occupational Therapy, 63,* 9–23.

Lazzarini, I. (2004). Neuro-occupation: The nonlinear dynamics of intention, meaning, and perception. *British Journal of Occupational Therapy, 67,* 342–352.

Lewis, J. (2002). *Cultural studies: The basics.* London: Sage.

Merriam-Webster Dictionary. (1995). Culture. Springfield, MA: Merriam-Webster.

Meyer, A. (1922). Philosophy of occupational therapy. *Archives of Occupational Therapy, 1,* 1–10.

Nelson, D. L., & Jepson-Thomas, J. (2003). Occupational form, occupational performance, and a conceptual framework for therapeutic occupation. In P. Kramer, J. Hinojosa, & C. B. Royeeen (Eds.), *Perspectives in human occupation: Participation in life* (pp. 87–155). Philadelphia: Lippincott Williams & Wilkins.

Opacich, K. J. (1997). Moral tensions and obligations of occupational therapy practitioners providing home care. *American Journal of Occupational Therapy, 51,* 430–435.

Pattison, H. (1922). The trend of occupational therapy for the tuberculous. *Archives of Occupational Therapy, 1,* 19–24.

Proctor, N. G. (1998). Violent ethnic wars and world-wide people movement: Implications for mental health nursing practice. *Contemporary Nurse, 7,* 148–151.

Reilly, M. (1962). Occupational therapy can be one of the great ideas of 20th-century medicine. *American Journal of Occupational Therapy, 16,* 1–9.

Reilly, M. (1969). The educational process. *American Journal of Occupational Therapy, 23,* 299–307.

Rogers, C. (1951). *Client-centered care.* Boston: Houghton-Mifflin.

Schkade, J. K., & Schultz, S. (2003). Occupational adaptation. In E. Crepeau, E. Cohn, & B.A.B. Schell (Eds.), *Willard and Spackman's occupational therapy* (10th ed., pp. 200–203). Philadelphia: Lippincott.

Schwartz, K. B. (2003). History of occupation. In P. Kramer, J. Hinojosa, & C. B. Royeen (Eds.), *Perspectives in human occupation: Participation in life* (pp. 18–31). Philadelphia: Lippincott Williams & Wilkins.

Shadley, T. S., & Rexrode, A. (2005). Home health: A journey to improve functional patient outcomes. *OT Practice, 10*(11, Suppl.), CE1.

Staudenmeier, J. J., & Hill, J. V. (2002). September 11th—Ripples across the ocean: Perspectives from Tripler Army Medical Center. *Military Medicine, 16*(9), 93–95.

Stevenson, G. (1932). The healing influence of work and play in a mental hospital. *Occupational Therapy and Rehabilitation, 11*, 85–89.

Sumsion, T. (Ed.). (1999). *Client-centered practice in occupational therapy: A guide to implementation.* New York: Churchill Livingstone.

U.S. Department of Labor, Bureau of Labor Statistics. (2005, May). *Occupational employment and wages* (29-1122 Occupational Therapists). Retrieved September 26, 2005, from www.bls.gov/oes/current/oes291122.htm

Wells, S. A., & Black, R. M. (2000). *Cultural competency for health professionals.* Bethesda, MD: American Occupational Therapy Association.

Wilcock, A. A. (2003). Occupational science: The study of humans as occupational beings. In P. Kramer, J. Hinojosa, & C. B. Royeen (Eds.), *Perspectives in human occupation: Participation in life* (pp. 156–180). Philadelphia: Lippincott Williams & Wilkins.

Zemke, R., & Clark, F. (1996). *Occupational science: The evolving discipline.* Philadelphia: F. A. Davis.

2

The Need for
Cultural Competence

It is not the eye that understands, but the mind.

—AFRICAN PROVERB (CITED IN JOHNSON, 1995, P. 287)

Key Points

- Western medicine is grounded in mainstream America and expounds a system in which individualization and independence are highly valued. It has evolved into one that emphasizes the individual as the focal point of problems and intervention.

- The political, social, and economic forces and events of society, both historically and currently, affect not only the lives of individuals but also institutions and health systems.

- A health care provider should constantly pursue cultural competence because of the social realities of a changing world; the influence of culture and ethnicity on human growth and development; the challenge of providing effective and quality health care to all people; the legislative, regulatory, and accreditation mandates; and marketplace edge.

- Cultural competency is key to success in a multicultural environment.

THE 21ST CENTURY HAS FOUND AMERICAN SOCIETY in uncharted waters. It is multiracial, multicultural, and multilingual. It may best be known as the time of the "cultural imperative" in the United States. Never before has the issue of race, ethnicity, and cultural differences had such saliency for so many Americans. The notions of *cultural competence, cultural diversity, multiculturalism, inclusivity, cultural pluralism,* and a host of other such terms dominate every aspect of our lives, including business, education, health care, and legislative policies.

The notion of cultural competence has critical and far-reaching implications for all institutions designed to provide health care and human services assistance. Health care providers are challenged to perform assessments and develop intervention plans and programs with consumers who may or may not share a common language with them; who may have differing beliefs, values, attitudes, and behaviors; and who may have a different understanding of the nature of health and wellness, work, leisure, and self-care. Cultural competence has even more urgency as the racial, socioeconomic, and gender disparities in health status increase. Changes in health care delivery models and reimbursement also are driving forces in moving toward culturally competent systems of care. By understanding and acknowledging other's customs, beliefs, and values, health care providers have a better chance to assess and produce effective outcomes.

Health care providers should constantly pursue cultural competence for several reasons:
- The social realities of a changing world,
- The influence of culture and ethnicity on human growth and development, and
- The challenge of providing effective and quality health care to all people.

To eliminate long-standing disparities in the health status of people of diverse racial, ethnic, and cultural backgrounds; to meet legislative, regulatory, and accreditation mandates; and to gain a competitive edge in the marketplace also are compelling arguments for pursing cultural competence. These reasons justify not only the need for cultural competency but also the knowledge and skills necessary to communicate and interact with people of any culture. Each reason plays an important and unique role in establishing the justifications, parameters, and directions for cultural competence.

Social Realities

Diversity is part of us—our neighborhoods, schools, workplaces, and communities. The United States is culturally pluralistic, socially stratified, and racially divided. Diversity of race, culture, ethnicity, social class, sexual identity, religion, language, and national origin is a fundamental feature of interpersonal interactions and community structures. Many societies in the past operated primarily within a monocultural and monolingual perspective. New individuals in the culture were expected to give up the values, norms, and beliefs of the society they were emigrating from in favor of new opportunities (Parrillo, 1997).

People today are unwilling to passively and submissively assimilate the way people in past generations may have. Many individuals and groups have stopped trying to deny their ethnicity for the sake of being accepted unconditionally into mainstream society. They now insist there is no inherent contradiction between allegiance to their own ethnic and cultural heritages and being an American. Instead, many view these dual identities as being complementary and believe both should be respected and promoted.

Barriers Regarding Culture and Ethnicity

Many people become unsettled and uneasy with increasing emphasis and focus on culture and ethnicity in this country. The legacies of racism, oppression, and discrimination are still unacceptable and untenable concepts that most Americans ignore or pretend do not exist. These issues evoke concepts and images that are in opposition of fundamental American values and ideals.

Individuals tend to personalize racism and oppression and cannot objectively view society and institutions from such perspectives. There is a natural American tendency to dismiss racial differences or cultural variations as key factors to be addressed by individuals or institutions. Several major precepts of American culture question the need for cultural competence (Cox & Blake, 1991; "The New Politics of Race," 1991). These include the following myths:

- The American value system supports the belief that an individual can overcome any condition (e.g., the old *pull oneself up by one's boot straps* or *mastery over nature* concept).
- The 1960s Civil Rights movement took care of any and all racial and ethnic problems.
- Cultural diversity is really a form of reverse discrimination.

Demographic Changes

Two major demographic changes in the United States that continue to shape the future are the increasing racial and ethnic diversity of the nation and the growth of the older population. From 1950 to 2004, the proportion of the population ages 75 years and older rose from 3% to 6%. It is projected to be 12% by 2050, with about 1 in 8 Americans ages 75 years or older (National Center for Health Statistics [NCHS], 2005).

The Hispanic and Asian populations have grown more rapidly than other racial and ethnic groups in the country. According to the U.S. Census Bureau (2004), roughly 41.3 million Hispanics live in the United States, representing more than 13% of the total population. Among this group, Mexicans rank as the largest cultural group at 66.9%, followed by Central and South Americans (14.3%), Puerto Ricans (8.6%), and Cubans (3.7%). The remaining 6.5% are of other Hispanic origins. States with the largest Hispanic populations are California, Texas, New York, Florida, and Illinois. In addition, 13.9 million Asian Americans live in the United States, accounting for 5% of the nation's population. States with the largest Asian American populations are California, New York, Texas, and New Jersey (Office of Minority Health [OMH], 2006; U.S. Census Bureau, 2004).

As the second largest minority population, African Americans account for 13% of the U.S. population (36 million people). The 10 states with the largest African American population are New York, California, Texas, Florida, Georgia, Illinois, North Carolina, Maryland, Michigan, and Louisiana. Among cities, Detroit has the largest proportion of African Americans (83%), followed by Philadelphia (44%) and Chicago (38%) (OMH, 2006; U.S. Census Bureau, 2003). Data from 2004 estimate 4 million people are classified as American Indian and Alaska Native, comprising 1.5% of the total U.S. population. Fifty-seven percent live in metropolitan areas and 538,300 live on reservations. Currently there are 569 federally recognized tribes (OMH, 2006; U.S. Census Bureau, 2002).

The number of immigrants who are documented, undocumented, and refugees are at an all-time high. Current waves of immigration consist primarily of Asians and Hispanic populations, as well as other visible racial and ethnic groups. Every 10th person in the United States is foreign-born, and this trend is expected to continue. Data from the 2002 U.S. Census reveal the number of people who speak a language other than English at home rose by 43%. Of these people, nearly 45% indicate they have trouble speaking English (Goode & Dunne, 2003). Unlike their early European counterparts, these two groups are not necessarily oriented toward assimilation. They often may prefer to retain their cultural heritage, accepting a bicultural status.

The implications associated with the dramatic increase of non-White populations are significant. These demographic changes have the following implications:

- Change is inevitable. The chances of working for a woman employer or supervisor at some point in a career are greater than ever before in our history; with baby boomers passing into middle and old age, the labor force will be older; and career mobility and success will belong to those who work well with people of all backgrounds.
- More and more differences in language and culture will be present in health care and human services systems.
- Intercultural experiences and knowledge of other languages will be important assets.
- Cultural competency will be a primary key to success in such a multicultural environment.

These changes have already transformed the United States and will continue to affect organizations, health care, government, communities, and society as a whole. They will alter the lives of those who live and work in America for the rest of the decade and beyond. The U.S. population's increasing demographic changes make cultural competency for all health care providers imperative.

Sociopolitical Reality

Many people in the United States still believe there is a single acceptable way to live, look, and behave as an American and a human being. Standards for determining what is appropriate are embedded in a Eurocentric orientation. Many are taught that European and American cultures, institutions, and lifestyles are superior to those of other groups (Gay, 1994; Jones & Carter, 1996). Any deviation from these standards is scorned, subjected to discrimination, or considered un-American. This leads to "denial of equal access to institutional opportunities, political rights, economic rewards, and respect for human dignity" (Gay, 1994, p. 5).

People of color—and others who do not meet this American "standard"—rarely operate or control the major institutions of American life, such as government, corporate, financial, media, and health care institutions, and their thoughts and beliefs do not become public opinion. Their views do not shape the actions of the major institutions, nor are their concerns or issues brought to public light as easily. The struggles of people from diverse backgrounds in the United States have been primarily for physical and cultural survival (Browser & Hunt, 1996).

Although laws exist to prohibit discrimination based on race, color, gender, age, creed, and disability, attitudes and behaviors that are derogatory to some and preferential to others continue to plague U.S. society. Unofficially, inequality flourishes, manifesting itself in racism, ethnocentrism, prejudices, favoritism, discrimination, cultural appropriation, and cultural hegemony. These inequalities and the power to change them—enlightened or otherwise—belong primarily to White Americans, not because they are the majority of the nation's population but because they have the status and associated power to maintain and advance their perceived interests (Browser & Hunt, 1996).

World views of both health care providers and clients are linked to the historical and current experiences of racism, heterosexism, classism, and oppression. Practitioner, clients, and the intervention process each are influenced by the state of discrimination and oppression in the larger society and by the cultural biases of their forebears. Health care providers must recognize that intervention does not occur in isolation from larger events in society. The political, social, and economic forces and events of society affect not only the lives of individuals but also institutions.

Cultural competency has the potential to correct these distortions and inequities. It is a way to help people perceive and understand the cultural diversity of the U.S. citizenry so that they may develop pride in their own cultural legacy, awaken to ideas embodied in the cultures of their neighbors, and develop an appreciation of the common humanity shared by all people of the earth.

Cultural Impact on Human Development

Culture influences and shapes our total way of living: our values, beliefs, linguistic expression, thinking patterns, behaviors, and attitudes. Human behaviors result from a process of socialization. Socialization occurs within a specific cultural environment and is passed on from generation to generation. Hence, humans are social beings that carry within them their individual biological and psychological traits as well as legacies of their ethnic group's historical background, collective heritage, and cultural experiences.

The influence of culture is established early and thoroughly in the process of human growth and development and prevails thereafter for the remainder of one's life. Some elements of culture can be modified over time and with experience, but the core features continue to be the mainstay of a person's sense of being and identity throughout life (Devore & Schleslinger, 1981; Gay, 1994). The stages of the life cycle are acted out in as many variations as there are groups. Major life events and stages—birth, childhood, adulthood, marriage, parenting, and late life—are perceived and carried out according to the norms of the group and culture. The movement to each stage of life may entail varying degrees of stress if the expected role tasks cannot be filled in a way that meets the standards of the individual or the group. During a celebratory baptism, for example, a Hispanic child becomes a member of a church; at the same time, *campadres* of the parents present themselves as caregivers, assuming responsibility, along with the parents, for continuity in the faith, as well as in the group. The giving of gifts celebrates entry into the social or cultural group. This ritual symbolizes its importance.

The marking of a Jewish male infant through circumcision is a *sign of union,* a permanent mark that incorporates him into the social group. Gifts that are given indicate acceptance and continuity. Hispanic and European female infants are marked by the ceremony of ear piercing. This act identifies them as female and needing protection. Whether children are viewed as small replicas of adults, or treated in another manner, is often a matter of culture and class perception. Viewing adolescence as the preparation period for the tasks of adulthood, as opposed to the beginning of adulthood, is a matter of historical and group perspective (Devore & Schleslinger, 1981).

Cultural and diverse groups do not all perceive gender roles in the same way. Some encourage equality of the sexes and some do not. Unequal treatment of the sexes begins early in life. Parents instill differences in subtle ways, including what they pack in children's lunch boxes. In Ecuador, girls between ages 16 and 20 cannot go out in public unaccompanied. Being seen outside the home without a chaperone would ruin their reputations. The varying requirements at each stage of development not only provide clues to the universal tasks to be achieved, but also indicate the cultural dispositions imposed on those tasks (Dresser, 1996).

Life cycle, life stage expectations, universal tasks, and cultural specificities are data, along with social class and other aspects of identity, that are essential for understanding the cultural perception and development of people. When individuals claim they treat all people the same—as human beings, regardless of ethnic identity, cultural backgrounds, sexual identity, or economic status—they are creating a false dichotomy. "A person's humanity cannot be isolated or divorced from his or her culture and ethnicity. One cannot be human without culture and ethnicity, and one cannot have culture and ethnicity without being human" (Gay, 1994, p. 7).

Responsible health care decision making cannot result if providers are not conscious of how culture shapes not only their own but also their clients' attitudes, values, behaviors, and beliefs. Understanding that everyone is a product of his or her own culture and that people live within given values and beliefs can free one from the effects of prejudicial interpretations. Knowing the influence of culture on human development ensures that one can recognize each person as an individual with his or her own identity, culture, background, and lifestyle.

Health Care

Western medicine is grounded in mainstream American cultural concepts. Its philosophy imbues institutional policies, practices, and power, and Anglo-centric and middle-class cultural values predominate (Gostin, 1995). The policies that govern access to parts of the health care system illustrate this bias. The ability to pay often is based on a person's occupation and insurance coverage, which in turn is based on one's cultural and class background. Another illustration of the predominance of Anglo-centric, middle-class culture is that people from this cultural background tend to hold significant power positions. Health care programs and systems are developed to meet a variety of needs identified by emissaries of the dominant society and culture. The negative implication is that the White culture is such a dominate norm, it acts as an invisible veil that prevents health care providers from seeing health services as potentially biased systems.

America's health care traditionally expounds a system in which individualization and independence are highly valued. In reality, it has evolved into a system that acknowledges and emphasizes individuals as the locus of problems and intervention (Gostin, 1995; Kavanagh & Kennedy, 1992). The health care process incorporates an intricate system of evaluation, diagnosis, and intervention. This approach assumes people are composed of parts to be examined for problems, which are then diagnosed and treated, and the client is then released. The role of the person seeking health services is to submit to the authority of the health care provider and follow the advice given (Reed & Sanderson, 1992). Many health care providers assume disease prevention is a matter of biological and chemical intervention, without consideration for the individual; the environment; or social, economic, or spiritual factors. One example of this approach is to provide training in the use of adaptive equipment and devices without considering the client's needs, culture, home environment, financial resources, and the lifestyle changes the equipment will bring.

Providing appropriate care to increasingly diverse consumer populations is a challenge. Despite similarities, fundamental differences exist among people because of nationality, ethnicity, culture, family background, and individual experiences. These differences affect the health beliefs and behaviors that both clients and providers have of each other.

There is an even greater need to eliminate practices and policies that require all consumers to adapt and conform to a limited set of norms and values in order to utilize resources. The influence of patterned culture characteristics, the symbolism and meaning attached to those characteristics, and the impact of those and other population-level factors have not been consistently incorporated into health care providers' knowledge bases (Kavanagh & Kennedy, 1992; Kreps & Kunimoto, 1994).

The delivery of high-quality health care services should be accessible, efficient, and cost-effective to improve health outcomes. It requires providers in a multicultural society to have a deeper understanding of the sociocultural background of clients, their families, and the environments in which they live. Culturally competent health services facilitate provider–client encounters with more favorable outcomes, enhancing the potential for more rewarding interpersonal experiences, and increasing the satisfaction not only of the person receiving the services (Goode & Dunne, 2003) but also of the health care provider.

Legislative and Regulatory Mandates

As a major purchaser of health care services, the federal government plays a pivotal role in ensuring culturally competent health care services. Title VI of the Civil Rights Act of 1964 (45 CFR Part 80) mandates that no person in the United States, on the grounds of race, color, or national origin, be excluded from participation in, be denied the benefits of, or be subjected to discrimination under any program or activity receiving federal financial assistance. Recipients of federal financial assistance include hospitals, nursing homes, home health agencies, managed care organizations, physicians, dentists, and hospital social workers, as well as occupational and physical therapists (Office for Civil Rights [OCR], 2006). These organizations and programs are responsible for complying with federal, state, and local regulations for the delivery of health services.

Healthy People 2010 objectives include an emphasis on cultural competency as an integral component of health service delivery (U.S. Department of Health and Human Services [DHHS], 2000). The National Health Promotion and Disease Prevention objectives accentuate cultural competence as a vital component of the delivery of health and nutrition services. The Bureau of Primary Health Care, in a policy information notice, acknowledges that health centers that serve culturally and linguistically diverse communities must respect and respond to the cultural diversity of the communities and clients they serve. These health centers should develop systems that ensure participation of the diverse cultures in their community, including participation of persons with limited English-speaking ability. They also should hire culturally and linguistically appropriate staff (DHHS, 2000). According to the Goode, Sockalingam, Brown, and Jones (2003), both the Joint Commission on the Accreditation of Healthcare Organizations, which accredits hospitals and other health care institutions, and the National Committee for Quality Assurance, which accredits managed care organizations and behavioral health managed care organizations, support standards that require cultural and linguistic competence in health care.

The American Occupational Therapy Association's *Code of Ethics* (2005) says that

> Occupational therapy personnel shall provide services in a fair and equitable manner. They shall recognize and appreciate the cultural components of economics, geography, race, ethnicity, religious and political factors, marital status, sexual orientation, and disability of all recipients of their services. (p. 6)

The *Guidelines to the AOTA Code of Ethics* (AOTA, 2006) state that "Occupational therapy personnel shall develop an understanding and appreciation for different cultures in order to be able to provide culturally competent service" (p. 18). AOTA also says that to provide ethical and sound decision making, practitioners need to recognize, respect, and be responsive to differences. If practitioners cannot provide culturally competent services, they will be out of compliance with their own code of ethics.

The Accreditation Council for Occupational Therapy Education (ACOTE, 2007) standards for occupational therapists also recognizes the importance of cultural diversity factors as part of the foundation requirements for occupational therapy education. Two standards that address this requirement are as follows:

- B.1.7. Demonstrate knowledge and appreciation of the role of sociocultural, socioeconomic, and diversity factors and lifestyle choices in contemporary society. Course content must include, but is not limited to, introductory psychology, abnormal psychology, and introductory sociology or introductory anthropology.

- B.4.7. Consider factors that might bias assessment results, such as culture, disability status, and situational variables related to the individual and content.

Adequate preparation of health care professionals is essential for good health care. In making a diagnosis as well as choosing a culturally appropriate intervention, occupational therapists must understand the beliefs that shape a person's approach to health and illness. Knowledge of customs and healing traditions are indispensable to the design of treatment and interventions. Health care services must be received and accepted to be successful.

Marketplace Edge

The economic survival of any health care facility lies in its ability to increase retention and access to care, expand recruitment, and increase the satisfaction of individuals seeking health care services. To reach these outcomes and gain a competitive edge in the health care marketplace, health care facilities must incorporate culturally competent policies, structures, and practices to provide services for people from diverse ethnic, racial, religious, cultural, and linguistic backgrounds. Entrenched attitudes and practices will yield obsolescence (Goode & Dunne, 2003).

Understanding the needs and preferences of the changing consumer base and responding to them in more effective ways is important for growth. Organizations whose workforce mirrors the composition of society at large are in a better position to understand and reach out to a pluralistic marketplace. These facilities often have the empathy and sensitivity not only to relate to consumers of different groups but also to anticipate needs and suggest ways to reach new market segments. Health care facilities that meet the challenges and capitalize on the opportunity to serve a diverse population will show bottom-line results and a significant edge over the competition (Gardenswartz & Rowe, 1993).

Liability or Malpractice Claims

Lack of awareness about cultural differences may result in liability or malpractice claims under tort principles. Health providers may be liable for damages due to discrimination, whether intentional or unintentional. Excluding people, denying them benefits, or otherwise discriminating against them because of their race or some other prohibited reason is discrimination. The question to ask is, Did the health care provider treat this group of patients or patient differently because of race, color, ethnicity, age, class, religion, gender, or sexual identity?

Despite legislation such as Title VI of the Civil Rights Act of 1964, many cultural communities maintain a legacy of distrust and reluctance to seek care because of past discrimination in health care. Health care organizations and programs face potential claims over their failure to understand clients' health beliefs and practices and provider behavior breaching professional standards of care. Beliefs or attitudes alone are not discriminatory acts, but if beliefs can be shown to affect the way people are treated, the treatment may be considered discriminatory (OCR, 2006).

The ability to communicate well with care recipients can effectively reduce the likelihood of malpractice claims. A study in the *Physicians Risk Management Update* (Physicians Insurance Exchange, 1995) indicated that patients of physicians who are frequently sued have the most complaints about a lack of commu- *The ability to communicate* nication. Physicians who had never been sued *well with care recipients* often were described as concerned, accessible, and *can effectively reduce the* willing to communicate. Effective communication *likelihood of malpractice* between providers and clients may be even more *claims.* challenging when there are cultural and linguistic barriers. Health care organizations and programs must address linguistic competence to ensure accurate communication of information in languages other than English (Goode et al., 2003).

Summary

Cultural diversity is a normative description of U.S. society. Culture and its various characteristics are influential variables in shaping individual identity and behavior. They influence and shape human behavior, values, and beliefs. Cultural socialization is ingrained early and deeply in the human personality, and persists thereafter. Because many people in the United States live in ethnic and cultural enclaves, they have only tangential interactions with and superficial knowledge of people who are culturally different from them. Regardless of whether differences are in age, culture, health status and condition, life experience, gender, ethnicity, sexual identity, or race, they all impact individuals and the health system.

Culturally competent providers allow the consumer to receive interventions reflective of both the dominant culture of the health care system and the individual. Culturally competent care is a form of holistic practice that interweaves the cultures of the consumer, health care system, provider, and traditional health practices.

Change is very frightening and difficult, but it has been far easier for society to ignore culture and ethnic diversity rather than confront it. For various reasons, American society is at a point where it can no longer ignore the issue. Americans cannot hope that the issues of cultural competence will go away. Many forces shape the present focus on ethnicity, culture, and other individual characteristics that require the nation to face and address the cultural imperative if it is to maintain its leadership position in the world.

The rationale for being culturally competent is complex and includes recognition of the changing demography; eliminating health disparities; improving quality of health services and outcomes; meeting legislative, regulatory, and accreditation mandates; avoiding liability and malpractice claims; and gaining a marketplace edge—just to name a few. Failure to understand social and cultural differences will have significant consequences on the interventions and health outcome of clients. Being knowledgeable of cultural influences on human development ensures each client is treated as an individual with his or her own identity, culture, background, and lifestyle. A practitioner who is knowledgeable of his or her own attitudes, values, behaviors, and beliefs and their effects on others helps free himself or herself of prejudicial interpretations.

Reflection

1. What are the cultural demographics in your community and health care facilities?

   a. Consider how you would begin to explore this information.

   b. Who would you contact? What databases would you use?

   c. What questions would you ask?

2. Develop a survey that identifies the need for culturally competent care in your community or within a particular health care facility.

   a. To whom will you give the survey?

   b. What primary questions will you ask?

   c. Can you use another method, other than survey, to gather this information?

   d. How will you use the survey's data?

3. Using the health care facility identified above, explore the guidelines, rules, regulations, and policies in place to ascertain culturally competent service provision.

References

Accreditation Council for Occupational Therapy Education. (2007). Accreditation Council for Occupational Therapy Education (ACOTE) standards and interpretive guidelines. *American Journal of Occupational Therapy, 61.*

American Occupational Therapy Association. (2005). Occupational therapy code of ethics (2005). *American Journal of Occupational Therapy, 59,* 639–642.

American Occupational Therapy Association. (2006). Guidelines to the occupational therapy code of ethics. *American Journal of Occupational Therapy, 52,* 663–667.

Browser, B. P., & Hunt, R. G. (1996). *Impacts of racism on White Americans.* Thousand Oaks,
CA: Sage.

Cox, T. H., & Blake, S. (1991). Managing cultural diversity: Implications for organizational
competitiveness. *Academy of Management Executive, 5*(3), 45–54.

Devore, W., & Schleslinger, E. (1981). *Ethnic-sensitive social work practice.* St. Louis, MO:
Mosby.

Dresser, N. (1996). *Multicultural manners: New rules of etiquette for a changing society.* New
York: Wiley.

Gardenswartz, L., & Rowe, A. (1993). *Managing diversity: A complete desk reference and planning guide.* Chicago: Irwin/Pfeiffer & Co.

Gay, G. (1994). A synthesis of scholarship in multicultural education. [Urban Education
Monograph Series.] Oak Brook, IL: North Central Regional Educational Laboratory.

Goode, T. D., & Dunne, C. (2003). *Policy Brief 1: Rationale for cultural competence in primary
care.* Washington, DC: National Center for Cultural Competence, Georgetown University, Center for Child and Human Development.

Goode, T., Sockalingam, S., Brown, M., & Jones, W. (2003). *Policy Brief 2: Linguistic competence in primary health care delivery systems: Implications for policy makers.* Washington, DC: National Center for Cultural Competence, Georgetown University, Center
for Child and Human Development.

Gostin, L. O. (1995). Informed consent, cultural sensitivity, and respect for persons. *Journal
of the American Medical Association, 274,* 844–845.

Johnson, V. (1995). *Heart full of grace: A thousand years of Black wisdom.* New York: Simon
& Schuster.

Jones, J. M., & Carter, R. T. (1996). Racism and White racial identity: Merging realities. In
B. P. Browser & R. G. Hunt (Eds.), *Impacts of racism on White Americans* (2nd ed., pp.
1–23). Thousand Oaks, CA: Sage.

Kavanagh, K. H., & Kennedy, P. H. (1992). *Promoting cultural diversity: Strategies for health
care professionals.* Newbury Park, CA: Sage.

Kreps, G. L., & Kunimoto, E. N. (1994). *Effective communication in multicultural health care
settings.* Thousand Oaks, CA: Sage.

National Center for Health Statistics. (2005). *Health, United States, 2005 with chartbook on
trends in the health of Americans.* Hyattsville, MD: Author.

The new politics of race. (1991, May 6). *Newsweek,* pp. 22–31.

Office for Civil Rights. (2006). *Racial and ethnic health disparities and the HHS Office for
Civil Rights.* Retrieved May 31, 2006, from www.hhs.gov/ocr

Office of Minority Health. (2006). *Minority populations.* Retrieved May 31, 2006, from
http://www.omhrc.gov

Parrillo, V. N. (1997). *Strangers to these shores: Race and ethnic relations in the United States*
(5th ed.). Boston: Allyn & Bacon.

Physicians Insurance Exchange. (1995). Poor communication with patients can get you sued. *Physicians Risk Management Update, 6*(1), 1.

Reed, L., & Sanderson, S. N. (1992). *Concepts of occupational therapy* (3rd ed.). Baltimore: Lippincott Williams & Wilkins.

U.S. Census Bureau. (2002). *The American Indian and Alaska Native population: 2000.* Washington, DC: Author.

U.S. Census Bureau. (2003). *The Black population in the United States: 2002.* Washington, DC: Author.

U.S. Census Bureau. (2004). *We the people: Hispanics in the United States.* Washington, DC: Author.

U.S. Department of Health and Human Services. (1998). *The initiative to eliminate racial and ethnic disparities in health* [Policy Statement]. Washington, DC: Author, Bureau of Primary Health Care.

U.S. Department of Health and Human Services. (2000). *Healthy people 2010.* Available online at www.healthypeople.gov/publications

3

Defining Cultural Competency

What should it matter that one bowl is dark and the other pale if each is of good design and serves its purpose well?

—HOPI PROVERB (CITED IN ZONA, 1994, P. 76)

Key Points

- Cultural competency is a journey rather than an end. It is a lifelong process designed to foster understanding, acceptance, knowledge, and constructive relations between people of various cultures and differences. It is an evolving and developing process that depends on self-exploration, knowledge, and skills.

- As an individual moves toward cultural competence, attitudes become less ethnocentric and biased; behaviors become more open, spontaneous, and flexible; and perceptions become more neutral and appreciative of all people.

- As a system moves toward cultural competence, policies become more flexible and culturally impartial, and the practice becomes more congruent with the culture of their clients.

AS THE U.S. POPULATION STEADILY BECOMES MORE DIVERSE, health care providers and institutions from small rural towns to large urban centers need to respond to individuals' varied perspectives, values, and behaviors about health and well-being. Every day, occupational therapists must manage complex differences in communication styles, attitudes, expectations, and worldwide views. Failure to understand and manage social and cultural differences may have significant health consequences. The great challenge of our time, therefore, is to view diversity and cultural competency as a resource and not a problem.

Occupational therapists may take many approaches to bridge barriers to communication and understanding that stem from racial, ethnic, cultural, and linguistic differences. The notion of cultural competence has come to encompass both interpersonal and organizational interventions and strategies that seek to facilitate the achievement of clinical and public health goals when cultural differences come into play. Cultural competence also has emerged as a strategy to reduce disparities in access to and quality of health care.

There have been many attempts to describe and quantify cultural competence in health care. The concept of cultural competence has appeared in the literature with increasing frequency since 1989 (Kavanagh & Kennedy, 1992; Davidhizar, Bechtel, & Giger, 1998; Cross, Bazron, Dennis, & Isaacs, 1989; Majumdar, Browne, Roberts, & Carpio, 2004). Efforts to define and implement the principles of cultural competence are ongoing. But what does cultural competence actually mean? Does it make a difference for clients, the health and human services delivery system, and health outcomes? Providing a framework for discussion, this chapter evaluates the current definition of cultural competence and identifies benefits to the health care system. It also provides models of culturally competent care and key components of cultural competence.

Defining *Cultural Competency*

Many conceptual definitions of *cultural competence* exist. Central to most are the ideas of culture and competence. *Culture,* as put forth by Linton (1945), is the configuration of learned behavior whose components and elements are shared and transmitted by the members of a particular society. It is the common patterns of interaction and perception shared by a group of people (Hecht, Collier, & Ribeau, 1993). Culture implies the integrated pattern of human behaviors that includes thoughts; communications; actions; customs; beliefs; values; and institutions of a racial, ethnic, religious, or social group (Cross et al., 1989). It is the sum total of ways of living developed by a group of human beings and transmitted from one generation to another. Anthropologists Daniel Bates and Fred Plog (1991) offer a widely cited definition of a culture: "A system of shared beliefs, values, customs, behaviors, and artifacts that the members of a society use to cope with their world and with one another, and that are transmitted from generation to generation through learning" (cited in Eddey & Robey, 2005, p. 706).

Competence refers to having suitable and sufficient skills, knowledge, and experience for some purpose (*Merriam-Webster Dictionary,* 1995). It applies to having the capacity to function in a particular way, within the realm of culturally integrated patterns of human behaviors, as defined by the group (Cross et al., 1989). Hence, *cultural competence* is the capacity to respond to the needs of populations whose cultures are different from what might be called *dominant* or *mainstream.* It is "a set of congruent behaviors, attitudes, and policies that come together in a system, agency, or among professionals and enable that system, agency, or those professionals to work effectively in cross-cultural situations" (Cross et al., 1989, p. 13). Cultural competence is the process of actively developing and practicing appropriate, relevant, and sensitive strategies and skills in interacting with culturally different people (American Occupational Therapy Association, Multicultural Task Force, 1995).

According to Walker (1991), *cultural competence* is the ability of people to see beyond the boundaries of their own cultural interpretations, to be able to maintain objectivity when faced with individuals from cultures different from their own, and to interpret and understand the behaviors and intentions of people from other cultures nonjudgmentally and without bias. Cultural competence refers to a program's ability to honor and respect the beliefs, interpersonal styles, attitudes, and behaviors of both the families who are clients and the multicultural staff who are providing services (Roberts, 1990).

Cultural competence is a broad term that includes cultural awareness and cultural knowledge (cognitive domain), cultural skills (behavioral domain), cultural sensitivity (affective domain), and cultural encounter (environment domain) (Callister, 2005). It is dynamic and develops over time. It incorporates layers of

- Self-awareness and reflection;
- Culture-generic knowledge and skills applicable across different cultural, ethnic, and racial groups;
- Culture-specific knowledge and skill relating to a specific cultural, ethnic, or racial group;
- Cross-cultural communication; and
- Appropriate effective interactions with others.

Cultural competency does not refer to the establishment or maintenance of diversity, per se. It is not related to numbers or equal representation, either in clients or in service providers. It is more about folkways, mores, traditions, customs, formal and informal helping networks, rituals, dialects, and so forth. It is an evolving and developmental process that depends on having the self-awareness, knowledge, skills, and attitude to make sound, ethical, and culturally appropriate decisions. It is an ongoing process that assumes that its goal of creating a multicultural environment will never be completed. Developing cultural competence is a lifelong process, designed to foster understanding, acceptance, knowledge, and constructive relations between people of various cultures and differences.

Cultural Competence in Health Care

Many health care professionals agree that cultural competence is a critical factor in providing relevant services to the nation's growing culturally and ethnically diverse patient population. In health care, cultural competency describes the ability of systems to provide care to patients with diverse values, beliefs, and behaviors and includes tailoring delivery to meet the social, cultural, and linguistic needs of the people with whom we work. It is a vehicle to increase access to quality care for all patient populations, to eliminate health disparities and, as a business strategy, to attract new patients and market share (Edwards, 2003; Goode & Dunne, 2003). In health care, cultural competency supports the integration and transformation of knowledge, information, and data about individuals and groups of people into specific standards, skills, service approaches, techniques, and marketing programs that match the individual's culture and increase the quality and appropriateness of health care and outcomes. It helps integrate and transform knowledge about individuals and groups of people into specific standards, policies, practices, and attitudes used in appropriate cultural settings to increase the quality of services, thereby producing better outcomes (Saldana, 2001).

The literature provides health care professionals with several definitions of cultural competence, ways of thinking about cultural competence, and numerous methods for providing culturally competent care. Cross and colleagues (1989) provide a theoretical approach in which cultural competence is seen as a process or continuum whereby an individual's view of other cultures transforms from destructive to proficient. Campinha-Bacote (2002) also views cultural competence as a process, not an end point, in which health professionals continually strive to work within the cultural context of the patient. Leininger (1993) believes that the Western medical model fails to explore cultural patterns of illness. She suggests that the worldview and social structure of the client are important areas to investigate and explore. Health care providers should base their selection of an intervention approach or combination of approaches on information gathered from their cultural assessment.

Occupational therapy practitioners must develop the skills, knowledge, and patience to explore and validate what their patients say and do. The various approaches to conceptualizing and operationalizing cultural competence that are identified in the literature stress the importance of viewing cultural competence as a dynamic process involving continual progression and involvement of all levels of the health care system. Competence in practice means using new patterns of behaviors and effectively applying them in appropriate settings. These practices may include

- Involving the extended family in the intervention process,
- Addressing elderly people more formally (by their last name and title) than younger clients,
- Acknowledging and working with traditional or faith healers,
- Being cautious about touching,
- Engaging in small talk at the beginning of a session that will be considered good manners and keeps one from appearing too rushed,
- Conducting the session in the preferred language of the client or arranging for a professional interpreter, and
- Adding culturally related questions during the evaluation process.

Cultural competence is vital for effective therapeutic interactions and outcomes. It implies a heightened consciousness of how clients experience their uniqueness and deal with their differences and similarities within a larger social context. It enhances the occupational therapy provider's knowledge of the relationship between sociocultural factors and health beliefs and behaviors. It equips therapists with the tools and skills to manage these factors appropriately, with quality occupational therapy delivery as the gold standard. A culturally competent occupational therapist is self-aware, has mastered the knowledge and developed the skills necessary to feel comfortable and communicate effectively with people of any culture encountered, and is able to effectively bridge differences.

Outcomes of Cultural Competence

Cultural competence has become imperative in health care delivery for a variety of reasons:

- The importance of eliminating health disparities
- Shifting demographic characteristics of the U.S. population
- Competition in the health care market
- Federal regulations against discrimination
- Legislative, regulatory, and accreditation requirements
- Concerns about liability for litigation (Bazaldue & Silas, 2004; deChesnay, Wharton, & Pamp, 2005).

For health professionals, the reasons for cultural competence include improving communication and rapport between client and provider, overcoming poor health outcomes for ethnically diverse patients, reducing the gap between the health status of the minority and White populations, and identifying and attempting to eliminate evidence of bias and prejudice among some health professionals (Callister, 2005; Taylor, 2005).

Each racial and ethnic community and linguistic group, with its own cultural traits and health profile, presents a challenge to the health care delivery service industry. The provider and the client each bring their individual learned patterns of language and culture to the health care experience, which must be transcended to achieve equal access and quality of care. The interaction of clients and practitioners embodies a form of multiculturalism in which several (sub)cultures, including the health care profession, institution, family, community, and traditional culture, are all merged. Every therapeutic interaction, therefore, is a cross-cultural interaction. This overlap and interaction of cultures can create conflicts and dilemmas in providing occupational therapy services, unless the practitioner is sensitive to and skilled in culturally competent care.

Culturally competent care generates a greater percentage of health care–seeking behaviors among cultural and ethnic groups and improves health status among

Every therapeutic interaction is a cross-cultural interaction.

vulnerable populations (Callister, 2005; Lynn-McHale & Deatrick, 2000; Majumdar et al., 2004). For health care organizations, culturally competent care can lead to increased quality and effectiveness of health care and decreased costs (Foriter & Bishop, 2004; Suh, 2004).

Simply put, health care services that are respectful of and responsive to the health beliefs and practices, as well as the culturally and linguistic needs, of diverse client populations may influence or improve

- Health, healing, and wellness belief systems;
- How illness, disease, and their causes are perceived, both by the client or consumer and the health care providers;
- The behaviors of clients or consumers who are seeking health care and their attitudes toward health care providers; and
- The delivery of services by the provider who views the world through his or her own personal and unique set of values, which can compromise access for patients from other cultures (Office of Minority Health [OMH], 2006).

Cultural appropriateness of occupational therapy services may be the most important factor in the accessibility of services. Developing culturally sensitive practices can help reduce barriers to effective treatment. Knowing whom the client perceives as a "natural helper" and whom he or she views as a traditional helper can facilitate the development of trust and enhance the individual's investment and continued participation in treatment. New approaches are needed in service delivery to address cultural differences among consumers (Saldana, 2001).

Although the need for cultural competency in health care is well established, integration is not yet a reality. Often well-intentioned health professionals, from their own cultural perspectives, fail to modify their approaches to be responsive to the needs of culturally diverse clients. They fail to recognize the ineffectiveness of their interventions (Sue & Sue, 2003). Many practice a one-size-fits-all approach with clients regardless of group differences. Without cultural competence, one can easily imagine the possible adverse consequences that can result when distrust, miscommunication, and misunderstanding interfere with the therapeutic relationship. The outcomes can range from frustration, confusion, or shame to anger by the client, family, and practitioner. Cultural incompetence can result in compromised quality of care, noncompliance by the client, inability to recognize differences, fear of the new or unknown, denial, and inability to look in-depth at the individual needs of the client and his or her family (Taylor, 2005).

Barriers to Cultural Competence

Many health care professionals struggle to become culturally competent. The literature shows that they often lack the awareness, knowledge, skills, and organizational support to be effective as culturally competent providers of care (American Occupational Therapy Association [AOTA], 2005; Crosson, Deng, Brazeau, Boyd, & Soto-Greene, 2004; Taylor, 2005). Studies have shown that many faculty members feel unprepared to teach cultural content within the curriculum, resulting in limited content in this area (Crosson et al., 2004; Majumdar et al., 2004; Wells, 2005). Faculty members cite a lack of time to handle the issues effectively, a lack of resources, a lack of educational preparation, and a lack of practical experiences with diverse clients as barriers to teaching cultural competence (Gonzalez, Gooden, & Porter, 2000).

Ethnocentrism and prejudice among health care professionals also have been mentioned as barriers to cultural competence. In these cases, the quality of the interaction between provider and patient is likely to be brief, less participatory, and less therapeutic (Cooper-Patrick et al., 1999). The lack of congruence among the health-related values, beliefs, and behaviors of the providers of care and those of the clients they serve has contributed to misunderstandings and ineffectiveness of intervention (Donnelly, 2003).

Individual cultural beliefs affect how occupational therapy practitioners approach, speak to, and measure outcomes with clients. Within a personal context, practitioners tend to make assumptions and judgments about individuals based on their own particular culture, ethnicity, race, religion, sexual orientation, language, disability, or life experiences, and that can lead to improper intervention. In the practice environment, the responsibility for making sound ethical decisions rests with the individual practitioner (Wells, 2005). Cultural competence requires occupational therapy practitioners enter into the therapeutic relationship with awareness about their own culture and cultural biases, knowledge about other cultures, and skills in cross-communication and intervention. Practitioners need a nonjudgmental attitude toward unfamiliar beliefs and health practices. Cultural competence requires occupational therapy practitioners detect and prevent exclusion or exploitation of diverse clients. This includes monitoring cultural competence among agencies, policies and procedures, and delivery systems (Exhibit 3.1).

Goals of Cultural Competence

The expected outcomes of cultural competency are embedded in its definitions, justifications, and assumptions. There are numerous goals and related objectives that vary only according to contextual factors such as audiences, timing, purposes, and perspectives. They tend to cover the domains of learning (cognitive, affective, and psychomotor) and incorporate both the intrinsic and instrumental values of cultural competence. These goals fall into several clusters—self-exploration, personal development, attitude and values, ethnic and cultural literacy, empowerment, basic skills proficiency, and social competence (Gay, 1994). The process of cultural competence involves the integration of cultural awareness, cultural desire, cultural knowledge, cultural skill, and cultural encounters (Campinha-Bacote, 2002; Taylor, 2005).

The range of skills needed to be culturally competent is as varied as there are people in the world (see Exhibit 3.2). Common to all these essential skills and characteristics is the requirement to *go beyond* learning tolerance and tact. Cultural competency addresses more than the problem of assimilating different perspectives and backgrounds and being aware of and sensitive to differences. It speaks to the nature of who people are, to the mainsprings of their energy, to the issue of motivation and creativity.

Institutions and health care systems also can address cultural competency. According to the Health Resources and Services Administration (2004), the literature identifies nine essential elements and conditions that must be present in health care systems to support cultural competence:

1. *Values* and *attitudes* refer to beliefs held by health care professionals and organizations that influence health care delivery.
2. *Cultural sensitivity* denotes providers' heightened sensitivity and can be a precursor to changing values, attitudes, and behaviors.
3. *Communication* encompasses the variety of ways information is exchanged among those involved in care delivery.
4. *Policies* and *procedures* consist of the programmatic and planning vehicles through which organizations can facilitate the provision of culturally competent care.
5. *Training* and *staff development* concentrate on providing professionals with the requisite knowledge and skills to supply culturally competent care.
6. *Facility characteristics, capacity,* and *infrastructure* focus on access and availability of care and the environment in which it is provided, including location, physical resources, and information systems.

(Text continued on p. 43)

Exhibit 3.1. Competency Guidelines for Occupational Therapy

The culturally competent practitioner is

- Aware of and sensitive to his or her own culture,
- Aware of and willing to explore his or her own biases and values,
- Respectful of and sensitive to diversity among individuals,
- Knowledgeable about another's culture, and
- Skilled in selecting and using culturally sensitive intervention strategies.

Characteristics of a culturally competent occupational therapist include

- Being willing to learn about another's culture;
- Acknowledging and valuing cultural diversity;
- Having specific and extensive knowledge of the language, values, and customs of a particular culture;
- Having a basic knowledge of human development as it relates to race, ethnicity, gender, disability, religion, sexual orientation, and lifestyle;
- Understanding the interaction of culture, gender, race or ethnicity, religion, disabling condition, and sexual orientation on behaviors and needs;
- Understanding the socioeconomic and political factors that significantly affect the psychosocial, political, and economic development of ethnic and culturally diverse groups;
- Understanding the effects of institutional and individual racism on the use of the health care system by ethnic and culturally diverse groups;
- Understanding the effects of institutional and individual racism on the therapist–client relationships and interactions;
- Understanding professional values and codes of conduct as they relate to cultural interaction;
- Understanding health-related values, perspectives, and behavioral patterns of diverse populations;
- Having the ability to decrease the degree of disparity among the cultures in clinical interaction;
- Having the ability to avoid applying a "cookbook approach" to all people associated with a population or diverse group;
- Having the ability to generate, modify, and adapt a variety of intervention strategies to accommodate the particular culture of the client;
- Having the ability to use, send, and interpret a variety of communication skills (verbal and nonverbal) to facilitate the therapist–client interaction;
- Being creative and resourceful in identifying and using cultural value systems on behalf of the client; and
- Helping clients understand, maintain, or resolve their own sociocultural identification.

Note. Data from *A multicultural education and resource guide for occupational therapy educators and practitioners,* by S. A. Wells, 1994, Bethesda, MD, American Occupational Therapy Association.

Exhibit 3.2. Literature Review of Skills and Characteristics for Cultural Competency

Saldana (2001). *Cultural competency: A practical guide for mental health service providers.* Austin: University of Texas at Austin, Hogg Foundation for Mental Health.

Essential Knowledge, Skills, and Attributes for Developing Cultural Competence
Ensuring the provision of culturally competent services to clients places a great deal of responsibility on the mental health professional. In particular, several generally expected levels of knowledge, skills, and attributes are essential to providing culturally competent mental health services.

Knowledge
- Of clients' culture (history, traditions, values, family systems, artistic expressions)
- Of the effects of racism and poverty on behavior, attitudes, values, and disabilities
- Of the help-seeking behaviors of ethnic-minority clients
- Of the roles of language, speech patterns, and communication styles in different communities
- Of the effects of social services policies on clients of color
- Of the resources (agencies, persons, informal helping networks, research) available for ethnic-minority clients and communities
- Of how professional values may either conflict with or accommodate the needs of clients from different cultures
- Of how power relationships within communities or institutions affect different cultures.

Professional Skills
Techniques for learning the cultures of ethnic-minority client groups.
- Ability to communicate accurate information on behalf of culturally different clients and their communities
- Ability to openly discuss racial and ethnic differences or issues and to respond to culturally based cues
- Ability to assess the meaning that ethnicity has for individual clients
- Ability to discern between the symptoms of intrapsychic stress and stress arising from the social structure
- Interviewing techniques that help the interviewer understand and accommodate the role of language in the client's culture
- Ability to use the concepts of empowerment on behalf of culturally different clients and communities
- Ability to use resources on behalf of ethnic-minority clients and their communities
- Ability to recognize and combat racism, racial stereotypes, and myths among individuals and institutions
- Ability to evaluate new techniques, research, and knowledge as to their validity and applicability in working with people of color.

Personal Attributes
- Personal qualities that reflect "genuineness, empathy, nonpossessiveness, warmth" and a capacity to respond flexibly to a range of possible solutions
- Acceptance of ethnic differences among people
- A willingness to work with clients of different ethnic backgrounds
- Articulation and clarification of the worker's personal values, stereotypes, and biases about his or her own and others' ethnicity and social class; also, recognizing ways that these views may accommodate or conflict with the needs of clients from different cultures.

Exhibit 3.2. Literature Review of Skills and Characteristics for Cultural Competency (*cont.*)

Dillard, Andonian, Flores, Lai, MacRae, and Sharkri (1992). Cultural competent occupational therapy in a diversely populated mental health setting. *American Journal of Occupational Therapy, 46,* 721–726.

A culturally competent therapist
- Has specific and extensive knowledge of the language, values, and customs of a particular culture;
- Possesses an acknowledgment and awareness of one's own cultural and willingness to explore one's own feelings and biases; and
- Reinforces the beauty of culture, incorporates it in the therapy, and is open to different ways of engaging the patient in treatment.

Fitzgerald (1992). Multicultural clinical interactions: Multiple cultures in rehabilitation. *Journal of Rehabilitation, 58,* 38–42.

- Acknowledge that multiple cultures are involved and that both the care providers and care receivers are bearers of culture.
- Decrease the degree of disparity among the cultures.
- Provide people with information about one another's cultures and medical systems (intercultural sensitivity training).
- Avoid a cookbook approach, compiling a list of information on the beliefs, values, attitudes, and behaviors characteristic of a society or population and then assuming this information applies to all people associated with that society or population, ignoring all the diversity within a population.
- Provide access to some basic information and then help people develop strategies for acquiring the necessary additional information.
- Decrease the number of cultures involved (train people in the community to provide them with the necessary technical knowledge and skills and then allow them to provide care in the most culturally acceptable manner).

Sue, Arredondo, and McDavis (1992). Multicultural counseling competencies and standards: A call to the profession. *Journal of Counseling and Development, 70,* 477–486.

Proposed multicultural counseling competencies and standards for the American Association for Counseling and Development:
- Awareness of own assumptions, values, and biases
- Understand the worldview of the culturally different client
- Develop appropriate intervention strategies and techniques.

Wells (1991). Clinical considerations in treating minority women who are disabled. *Occupational Therapy Practice, 2,* 13–22.

Occupational therapy intervention strategies for treating ethnic minority women with disabilities:
- Have basic knowledge of human development as it relates to ethnicity and race
- Understand the disabling conditions and the stigmas related to them
- Have self-awareness or knowledge of one's own ethnicity and values and their influence on practice
- Know and respect for the client's culture

(Continued)

Exhibit 3.2. Literature Review of Skills and Characteristics for Cultural Competency (*cont.*)

- Have ability to modify and adapt occupational therapy techniques in response to the client's culture
- Incorporate beliefs and values of the ethnic client into the assessment process and treatment plan.

Sayles-Folks and People (1990). Cultural sensitivity training for occupational therapists. *Physical Disabilities Special Interest Section Newsletter, 13*(3), 4–5.

Skills needed by the culturally skilled therapist to interact with diverse consumer population:
Cognitive Domain
1. Understanding of sociopolitical systems operating in the United States with respect to treatment of minorities
2. Specific knowledge about the similarities and differences among White people, African Americans, Hispanics, Native Americans, and other racial or ethnic groups
3. Awareness of the institutional barriers that prevent or discourage members of minority groups from using rehabilitation services.
Affective Domain
1. Awareness of and sensitivity to his or her own cultural heritage and sensitivity to the need to value and respect diversity
2. Awareness of his or her own values and biases and how they may affect the therapeutic relationship with minority consumers
3. Sensitivity to circumstances (e.g., socioeconomic factors, political factors, racism) that may dictate referral of the minority consumer to a minority therapist.
Psychomotor Domain
1. Ability to generate a wide variety of verbal and nonverbal responses that will facilitate the consumer's involvement
2. Ability to send and receive both verbal and nonverbal messages accurately and appropriately.

London and Devore (1988). Layers of understanding: Counseling ethnic-minority families. *Family Relations, 37,* 310–314.

Layers of understanding required of practitioners working with ethnic-minority families:
- Basic knowledge of human behavior
- Professional values
- Self-awareness
- Understanding the effect of ethnicity on the daily life of clients
- Modification and adaptation of skills in response to working with ethnic-minority families.

Green (1982). *Cultural awareness in the human services.* Englewood Cliffs, NJ: Prentice Hall.
- Awareness of one's own cultural limitation.
- Openness to cultural differences.
- Client-oriented, systematic learning style.

**Exhibit 3.2. Literature Review of Skills and
Characteristics for Cultural Competency (*cont.*)**

- Using cultural resources.
- Acknowledging cultural integrity.

Sue, Bernier, Durran, Feinberg, Pedersen, Smith, et al. (1982). Cross-cultural counseling competencies [Position Paper]. *Counseling Psychologist, 10*(2), 45–52.

Characteristics of culturally sensitive helping practitioners:
- Ability to generate a wide variety of verbal and nonverbal responses
- Ability to send and receive verbal and nonverbal messages "appropriately"
- Ability to exercise appropriate institutional intervention skills on behalf of the client.

Diversity Forum of the 1996 AOTA Annual Conference (Wells, 1996).

Clinicians, educators, and students outlined those skills and characteristics that they felt were necessary for a culturally competent occupational therapy practitioner. These include the following:
- Respect—Recognizing learning opportunities
- Willingness to share—Knowing yourself
- Willingness to risk—Being aware of ignorance
- Willingness to change—Having the attitude "Different is okay, not good or bad"
- Willingness to explore—Understanding the power of words, the power of action.

7. *Intervention* and *treatment model* features include evaluation, diagnosis, treatment, and referral and how culture-specific knowledge and sensitivity can enhance them.

8. *Family* and *communication participation* recognizes the role of the family and community in achieving quality health care.

9. *Monitoring, evaluation,* and *research* include activities to assess progress in cultural competence efforts, as well as to create and disseminate new knowledge.

Individuals who have mastered bridging cultural gaps can weave together tradition and culture. They bring together the various influences of their upbringing in a personal way, including a unique mixture of cultural influences and ideas and respect diverse values and approaches to life. These individuals are socially active, critically thinking members of society (Gorski, 1997). In health care, culturally competent providers have the ability to articulate problems from clients' perspectives, recognize and reduce resistance and defensiveness, and implement culturally appropriate intervention (Callister, 2005; Kavanagh & Kennedy, 1992; Wells, 1994).

Training can have a positive impact on health care providers' cultural competence. It can improve the communication across cultural and linguistic differences

(Webb, 2003) and attitudes about the importance of cultural assessment (Crosson et al., 2004). Training also can be effective in increasing knowledge and self-efficacy (Smith, 2001). The exploration of different cultures helps people learn new ways to interpret reality and increase their understanding of other people, their experiences, and the world in which they live. The demonstration of respect and interest in the cultural perspectives of others also serve as a foundation for developing supportive and cooperative relationships with people from different cultures. Cultural exploration can teach us a great deal and help us appreciate the great beauty in the different ways that cultures frame reality, establish social organization, and accomplish different goals (Kreps & Kunimoto, 1994).

Models for Development of Cultural Competence

Dealing with people whose cultures are different can be very pleasant or very painful. One major source of cultural misunderstanding and conflict lies in the clash of deeply rooted, conditioned perceptions of reality. As long as our way of perceiving the world—on which our communication styles and behavior patterns are based—is out of awareness, it is not accessible to being deliberately changed, managed, understood, or influenced (Pusch, 1979). This condition changes only as we become more aware and have more knowledge of the degree to which our own perceptions and behaviors are culturally conditioned. So how do we become culturally aware and competent?

Achieving cultural competence is not a simple process. Hoops (1979) states there is a natural inclination to resist being culturally competent because

- Everyone is vulnerable;
- Anything that probes the nature of our identities is threatening;
- We like to think of ourselves as autonomous and not subject, against our will, to forces buried within us by our cultural heritage; and
- Awareness is an emotional event derived from experience rather than an idea attained through an intellectual process.

The resistance to self-learning lies at an emotional, unconscious level. If one is to come to grips with cultural relativity and take significant steps toward cultural competence, as individuals, institutions, and systems, one must become fully engaged with his or her own perceptions, behaviors, and communication patterns.

Establishing a conceptual framework is important in defining the goals and strategies for training and success. The literature outside of the occupational therapy field provides several frameworks, models, and approaches for achieving cultural competency. Many have been developed over time and expound possible stages an individual or system may go through to be culturally competent. Several are described below.

Intercultural Learning Process

The *Intercultural Learning Process* focuses on learning another culture so as to be able to experience what it is like to be a part of it and to view the world from its point of view. The goal of learning in this way is to be able to function effectively and comfortably within a particular culture. This learning process takes place along a continuum, running from ethnocentrism at one end to some form of adaptation or integration at the other end (Hoops, 1979).

Cultural Competence Continuum

The *Cultural Competence Continuum* addresses systems, agencies, and practitioners. To better understand where one is in the process of becoming culturally competent, this model uses a continuum that ranges from cultural destructiveness to cultural proficiency. The six points along this continuum are as follows (Cross et al., 1989; Orlandi, 1992):

1. *Cultural destructiveness* includes a set of attitudes and practices that explicitly promotes one culture over another based on the notion of one being superior to the other. Hostility and active avoidance of knowledge about other cultures exist.
2. *Cultural incapacity* implicitly promotes one culture over another. There is a dislike of other cultures, people live separately but equal, and there is no knowledge of other cultures.
3. *Cultural blindness* is one perspective of being unbiased. There is ambivalence. Everyone is treated alike with little or no knowledge about other cultures.
4. *Cultural pre-competence (openness)* is the attitude of being receptive to different cultures and to actively learn about other cultures. It incorporates a curious attitude and culture awareness. It requires some knowledge of other cultures.
5. *Cultural competence* encompasses not only respect for other cultures, but people in this category also actively seek advice and consultation from members of the less dominant cultural group for suggestions on being culturally appropriate from their perspective. People show respect, tolerance, and cultural sensitivity. This level requires a fair amount of knowledge about other cultures.
6. *Cultural proficiency* involves not only proactively seeking knowledge and information about other cultures but also educating others about various cultures. Individuals at this level are fully comfortable, culturally attuned, and have extensive knowledge about other cultures.

Cross and colleagues (1989) describe several conditions that must exist for professionals to move along this continuum. Professionals must value diversity, understand their cultural biases, be conscious of the dynamics that occur when cultures interact, internalize cultural knowledge, and develop adaptations to diversity. Each condition set by Cross and his colleagues must function at every level of the health care system for that system to provide culturally competent care. At best, most human services agencies fall between cultural incapacity and cultural blindness on this continuum. Cross and colleagues suggest that agencies as well as individuals should assess where they fall along the continuum before any effective planning for achieving higher levels of cultural competence can occur.

Seven-Step Process (TSSP) of Cross-Cultural Understanding

The *TSSP Model* emphasizes basic rules about understanding people of a particular culture. This process moves the individual from the start of a cultural encounter, to the stage of getting acquainted, to the final stage of establishing trust and cooperation. The model indicates the process of cross-cultural understanding is not simple or clear cut. Very often individuals will go back and forth between the different stages and, at times, will start the whole process again (Kabagarama, 1993).

Model of Care

The *Model of Care* views cultural competence as a process, not an end point, in which health professionals continually strive to achieve the ability to effectively work within the cultural context of the client (individual, family, community). Campinha-Bacote (2002) outlines five constructs of cultural competence, similar to the five essential elements expounded by Cross and colleagues (1989):

1. *Cultural awareness* is the self-examination and exploration of one's own cultural and professional background.
2. *Cultural knowledge* is the process of seeking and obtaining a sound educational foundation about diverse cultural and ethnic groups.
3. *Cultural skill* is the ability to collect relevant cultural data regarding the client's problem, as well as accurately performing a culturally based physical assessment.
4. *Cultural encounter* is the process that encourages the health care provider to directly engage in cross-cultural interaction with clients from culturally diverse backgrounds.
5. *Cultural desire* is the motivation of the health care provider to *want* to, rather than *have* to, engage in the process of becoming culturally aware, culturally knowledgeable, culturally skillful, and familiar with cultural encounters.

The Model of Care is not a developmental model. Health care providers can work on any one of these constructs to improve the balance of all five, but all five constructs must be experienced and addressed. Campinha-Bacote explains that the intersection of these constructs represents the process of cultural competence, and as the area of intersection becomes bigger, health care providers internalize cultural constructs at a deeper level and provide higher quality care.

Purnell Model for Cultural Competence

The *Purnell Model for Cultural Competence* assumes that cultural competence is the adaptation of care in a manner that is consistent with the culture of the client. It is a conscious process and nonlinear in its acquisition. According to Purnell (2002), the model's 12 domains and their concepts flow from more general phenomena, to more specific phenomena. The order in which the care provider uses the domains can vary. These domains/concepts include overview/heritage, communication, family roles and organization, workforce, biocultural ecology, high-risk behaviors, nutrition, pregnancy and childbearing practices, death rituals, spirituality, health care practices, and health care practitioners. Purnell says that the global society, community, family, and individual all influence these domains. In this model, the individual will progress from being an *unconsciously incompetent* practitioner, to *consciously incompetent, consciously competent,* and *unconsciously competent.*

Sunrise Model

The *Sunrise Model* provides a method for assessing patients to provide comprehensive and culturally sensitive care. Leininger (1993) believes the Western medical model of care fails to explore cultural patterns of illness. This model suggests the worldview and social structure of the client are important areas to investigate and can be explored using seven dimensions:

1. Cultural values and life ways
2. Religious, philosophical, and spiritual beliefs
3. Economic factors
4. Educational factors
5. Kinship and social ties
6. Technological factors
7. Political and legal factors.

Once information is obtained for each dimension, health care professionals can provide more effective client interventions. According to the Sunrise Model, providers should base their selection of an intervention approach or combination of approaches on information gathered from the assessment. Leininger suggests that the client can be helped in a variety of ways: cultural care preservation or maintenance, cultural care accommodation or negotiation, and cultural care repat-terning or restructuring.

Transcultural Assessment Model

The *Transcultural Assessment Model* is a prototype to help health care professionals assess patients from diverse cultures. It focuses on six factors:

1. Communication
2. Space
3. Time
4. Social organization
5. Environmental control
6. Biological variations.

According to Davidhizar and colleagues (1998), health care professionals should receive training on how to use these factors to assess the health beliefs and practices of the patient and family, which may have a significant impact on how an individ-ual will respond to intervention and education. Using this assessment model will help health care professionals provide care that is sensitive and tailored to the needs of culturally diverse individuals.

Summary

The degree of cultural competence an individual, agency, or system achieves is not dependent on any one factor or method. As an individual moves toward cultural competence, attitudes change to become less ethnocentric and biased. Perceptions change to become more neutral and appreciative of the inner beauty of all people. Behaviors change to become more open, respectful, spontaneous, and flexible. To effectively interact with diverse populations, the field of occupational therapy must have culturally competent professionals. Therapists need education about evalua-tion, intervention, and disease prevention and wellness of cultural subgroups con-fronting a variety of disparities (AOTA, 2005).

Cultural competence is a basic reminder to all practitioners about their responsibility to protect the rights of clients and their families and to act as their advocates. Being culturally competent helps occupational therapy practitioners develop intervention approaches, health delivery systems, and health policies that fully recognize and include the effects of culture on health decisions. It helps prac-titioners integrate fair and equitable services for all people and the holistic, contex-tual, and need-centered nature of such services.

As a system moves toward cultural competence, policies change to become more flexible and culturally impartial. Practices become more congruent with the culture of the client, from initial contact through termination. Valuing differences, conducting self-assessment, understanding dynamics of relationship and communication, building cultural knowledge, and adapting to that knowledge are necessary to be culturally competent. Self-exploration, knowledge, and skills are three major areas where development and intervention can and must occur if an individual is to move toward competence.

Reflection

1. Individually or in a small group, compile a list of barriers and benefits to culturally competent care. Discuss how barriers can be eliminated and benefits enhanced to provide occupational therapy services to a specific population, for example, people with disabilities, African Americans, elderly people, or the homeless population.

2. Think of a specific occupational therapy practice setting with which you are familiar. Define "culturally competent care" for this practice area or setting. Include why cultural competency is important and what skills are needed to provide culturally competent services in this area.

References

American Occupational Therapy Association. (2006). AOTA's statement on health disparities. *American Journal of Occupational Therapy, 60,* 679.

American Occupational Therapy Association, Multicultural Task Force. (1995). *Definition and terms.* Bethesda, MD: Author.

Bazaldue, O. V., & Silas, J. (2004). Cultural competence: A pharmacy perspective. *Journal of Pharmacy Practice, 17,* 160–166.

Callister, L. C. (2005). What has the literature taught us about culturally competent care of women and children? *American Journal of Maternal/Child Nursing, 30,* 380–388.

Campinha-Bacote, J. (2002). The process of cultural competence in the delivery of healthcare services: A model of care. *Journal of Transcultural Nursing, 13,* 181–184.

Cooper-Patrick, L., Gallo, J. J., Gonzales, J. J., Vu, H. T., Powe, N. R., Nelson, C., et al. (1999). Race, gender, and partnership in the patient–physician relationship. *Journal of the American Medical Association, 282,* 583–589.

Cross, T. L., Bazron, B. J., Dennis, K. W., & Isaacs, M. R. (1989). *Towards a culturally competent system of care: A monograph on effective services for minority children who are severely emotionally disturbed.* Washington, DC: CASSP Technical Assistance Center, Georgetown University Child Development Center.

Crosson, J. C., Deng, W., Brazeau, C., Boyd, L., & Soto-Greene, M. (2004). Evaluating the effect of cultural competency training on medical students' attitudes. *Family Medicine, 36,* 199–203.

Davidhizar, R., Bechtel, G., & Giger, G. (1998). A model to enhance culturally competent care. *Hospital Topics Research Perspectives on Healthcare, 76*(2), 22–26.

deChesnay, M., Wharton, R., & Pamp, C. (2005). Cultural competence, resilience, and advocacy. In M. deChesnay (Ed.), *Caring for the vulnerable* (pp. 31–41). Boston: Jones &
Bartlett.

Dillard, M., Andonian, L., Flores, O., Lai, L., MacRae, A., & Shakir, M. (1992). Culturally
competent occupational therapy in a diversely populated mental health setting. *American Journal of Occupational Therapy, 46,* 721–726.

Donnelly, P. L. (2003). Ethics and cross-cultural nursing. *Journal of Transcultural Nursing,
11,* 119–126.

Eddey, G. E., & Robey, K. L. (2005). Considering the culture of disability in cultural competence education. *Academic Medicine, 80,* 706–712.

Edwards, K. (2003). Increasing cultural competence and decreasing disparities in health.
Journal of Cultural Diversity, 10, 111–112.

Fitzgerald, M. H. (1992). Multicultural clinical interaction: Multiple cultures in rehabilitation. *Journal of Rehabilitation, 58,* 38–42.

Fortier, J. P., & Bishop, D. (2004). *Setting the agenda for research on cultural competence in
health care, final report* (C. Brach, Ed.). Rockville, MD: U.S. Department of Health and
Human Services, Office of Minority Health, & Agency for Healthcare Research and
Quality. Retrieved June 10, 2006, from www.ahrq.gov/research/cultural.htm

Gay, G. (1994). A synthesis of scholarship in multicultural education. (*NCREL's Urban
Education Monograph Series*). Oak Brook, IL: North Central Regional Education
Laboratory.

Gonzalez, R., Gooden, M. B., & Porter. (2000). Eliminating racial and ethnic disparities in
health care. *American Journal of Nursing, 100,* 56–58.

Goode, T. D., & Dunne, C. (2003). *Policy Brief 1: Rationale for cultural competence in primary
care.* Washington, DC: National Center for Cultural Competence, Georgetown University Center for Child and Human Development. Retrieved May 6, 2006, from
www.gucchd.georgetown.edu/nccc/

Gorski, P. (1997). *A working definition. Initial thoughts on multicultural education.* Retrieved
July 2007 from http://curry.edschool.virginia.edu/go/multicultural/activityarch.html

Green, J. W. (1982). *Cultural awareness in the human services.* Englewood Cliffs, NJ: Prentice
Hall.

Health Resources and Services Administration. (2004). Section II: Conceptualizing cultural
competence. In *Study on measuring competence in health care delivery settings.*
Retrieved May 31, 2006, from www.hrsa.gov/culturalcompetence/measures/
sectionii.htm.

Hecht, M. L., Collier, M. J., & Ribeau, S. A. (1993). *African American communication: Ethnic
identity and cultural interpretation.* Newbury Park, CA: Sage.

Hoops, D. (1979). Intercultural communication concepts and the psychology of intercultural experiences. In M. Pusch (Ed.), *Multicultural education: A cross-cultural training
approach* (pp. 9–38). Yarmouth, ME: Intercultural Press.

Kabagarama, D. (1993). *Breaking the ice: A guide to understanding people from other cultures.*
Boston: Allyn & Bacon.

Kavanagh, K. H., & Kennedy, P. H. (1992). *Promoting cultural diversity: Strategies for health-care professionals.* Newbury Park, CA: Sage.

Kreps, G. L., & Kunimoto, E. N. (1994). *Effective communication in multicultural health care settings.* Thousand Oaks, CA: Sage.

Leininger, M. (1993). Toward conceptualization of transcultural health care systems: Concepts and a model. *Journal of Transcultural Nursing, 4*(2), 32–40.

Linton, R. (1945). *The science of man in world crisis.* New York: Columbia University.

London, H., & Devore, W. (1988). Layers of understanding: Counseling ethnic minority families. *Family Relations, 37,* 310–314.

Lynn-McHale, D. J., & Deatrick, J. A. (2000). Trust between family and health care providers. *Journal of Family Nursing, 6,* 210–230.

Majumdar, B., Browne, G., Roberts, J., & Carpio, B. (2004). Effects of cultural sensitivity training on health care provider attitudes and patient outcomes. *Journal of Nursing Scholarship, 36,* 161–166.

Merriam-Webster Dictionary. (1995). Competence. Springfield, MA: Merriam-Webster.

Office of Minority Health. (2006). *What is cultural competency?* Retrieved May 31, 2006, from www.omhrc.gov

Orlandi, M. A. (1992). Defining cultural competence: An organizing framework. In M. A. Orlandi, R. Weston, & L. G. Epstein (Eds.), *Cultural competence for evaluators: A guide for alcohol and other drug abuse prevention practitioners working with ethical/racial communities* (DHHS Publication ADM-92-1884, pp. 293–299). Washington, DC: U.S. Government Printing Office.

Purnell, L. (2002). The Purnell model for cultural competence. *Journal of Transcultural Nursing, 13,* 193–196.

Pusch, M. D. (1979). *Multicultural education: A cross-cultural approach.* Yarmouth, ME: Intercultural Press.

Roberts, R. (Ed.). (1990). *Workbook for developing culturally competent programs for families of children with special needs* (2nd ed.). Washington, DC: Georgetown University Child Development Center. (ERIC Reproduction Service No. ED 332 462)

Saldana, D. (2001). *Cultural competency: A practical guide for mental health service providers.* Austin: University of Texas at Austin, Hogg Foundation for Mental Health.

Sayles-Folks, S., & People, L. (1990). Cultural sensitivity training for occupational therapists. *Physical Disabilities Special Interest Section Newsletter, 13*(3), 4–5.

Smith, L. S. (2001). Evaluation of an educational intervention to increase cultural competence among registered nurses. *Journal of Cultural Diversity, 8*(2), 50–63.

Sue, D. W., Arredondo, P., & McDavis, R. J. (1992). Multicultural counseling competencies and standards: A call to the profession. *Journal of Counseling and Development, 70,* 477–486.

Sue, D. W., Bernier, J. E., Durran, A., Feinberg, L., Pedersen, P., Smith, E. J., et al. (1982). Cross-cultural counseling competencies [Position Paper]. *Counseling Psychologist, 10*(2), 45–52.

Sue, D. W., & Sue, D. (2003). *Counseling the culturally diverse: Theory and practice.* New York: Wiley.

Suh, E. E. (2004). The model of cultural competence through an evolutionary concept analysis. *Journal of Transcultural Nursing, 15,* 93–102.

Taylor, R. (2005). Addressing barriers to cultural competence. *Journal for Nurses in Staff Development, 21,* 135–142.

Walker, M. L. (1991). Rehabilitation service delivery to individuals with disabilities. . . A question of cultural competence. *OSERS News in Print, 4*(2).

Webb, E. (2003). Evaluation of cultural competence training in child health. *Journal of Interpersonal Care, 17,* 309–310.

Wells, S. A. (1991). Clinical considerations in treating minority women who are disabled. *Occupational Therapy Practice, 2,* 13–22.

Wells, S. A. (1994). *A multicultural education and resource guide for occupational therapy educators and practitioners.* Bethesda, MD: American Occupational Therapy Association.

Wells, S. A. (1996, April). *Diversity forum: Multicultural competency.* AOTA Annual Conference, Chicago.

Wells, S. A. (2005). An ethic of diversity. In R. B. Purtilo, G. M. Jensen, & C. B. Royeen (Eds.), *Educating for moral action: A sourcebook in health and rehabilitation ethics* (pp. 31–41). Philadelphia: F. A. Davis.

Zona, G. A. (1994). *The soul would have no rainbow if the eyes had no tears and other Native American proverbs.* New York: Simon & Schuster.

4

Cultural Competency Model

We are challenged to see that the barriers of yesterday . . . are not replaced by new barriers of apathy, of underdeveloped skills, of lack of training.

—WHITNEY YOUNG, JR. (AS CITED IN JOHNSON, 1995, P. 47)

Key Points

- The Cultural Competency Model is a framework for developing and evaluating one's progress toward becoming a culturally competent health care professional. It emphasizes self-exploration, knowledge, and skills.

- *Self-exploration* is the process of looking inward. It is not always a risk-free or pleasant process, but it is a necessary process to open avenues of learning and growth.

- *Knowledge* promotes understanding. It allows health care providers to modify treatment, adapt the way in which services are delivered, and develop strategies for acquiring additional information.

- *Skill* is the acquiring and mastering of strategies, techniques, and approaches for communicating and interacting with people from different cultures, as well as for enhancing the delivery of care.

CULTURE IS A PART OF EVERYONE'S LIFE. It is a part of every personal encounter, every casual or chance meeting, and every lifelong interaction. Every individual is influenced by a unique combination of different cultural orientations and influences. Every person belongs to many cultural groups that direct and shape his or her multicultural identity. People are the products of multiple cultural memberships. We are multicultural individuals. Whenever people interact and communicate, there are multiple cultural influences on their interactions (Fitzgerald, 1992; Kreps & Kunimoto, 1994).

With culture a part of every clinical encounter, the modern health care system is a cultural smorgasbord composed of individuals from different combinations of national, regional, ethnic, racial, occupational, and generational characteristics, as well as socioeconomic levels, health status, and cultural orientations. As the American population becomes multiracial, multicultural, and multilingual, those seeking and providing health care are increasingly diverse. The modern health care system also is influenced by differences in sexual identity, age, educational background, and occupation of both health care providers and consumers. All these cultural influences affect the provision of effective and quality health care, thereby making every clinical encounter a cross-cultural interaction (Kreps & Kunimoto, 1994; Mead, 1956; Pachter, 1994; Wells, 1994). Health care consumers and providers approach health care situations with their own unique communication characteristics, health beliefs, and customs based on their personal backgrounds. These cultural influences challenge health care providers to perform assessments and develop intervention plans with clients who may not share a common language with them; who may have a different understanding of the nature of work, leisure, and self-care; and who may have differing beliefs, values, attitudes, and behaviors. Understanding the cultural relations between culturally unique participants in the modern health care system is a prerequisite to effective health care delivery (Howe-Murphy, Ross, Tseng, & Hartwig, 1989; McNeil, 1990). By understanding and accepting clients' values and beliefs, providers have a better chance of assessing and facilitating more effective outcomes.

Health care providers have a responsibility to develop an awareness of self, knowledge about other cultures, and skills not only to effectively accomplish the health care goals of their clients but also to interact and communicate within multicultural societies. Accompanying the need to have culturally competent providers is the dilemma of not only quantifying competency in multicultural interaction and integrating culture into the health care procedures and teaching approaches but also identifying a model for developing this competency.

This chapter introduces the *Cultural Competency Model* and outlines a process for becoming a culturally competent health care provider. It explores a framework that providers, students, and systems can use to develop and acquire the knowledge, skills, and awareness needed to increase their ability to function effectively and provide quality care in a multicultural environment.

Importance for Health Professionals

Caring for patients and clients from different cultures presents a variety of challenges. The relationship between culture and health-related behavior is inherently complex. The cultural and ethnic backgrounds of clients and patients can shape their views of illness and well-being in the physical, emotional, and spiritual realms and affect their perceptions of health care as well as the outcomes of treatment (Genao, Bussey-Jones, Brady, Branch, & Corbie-Smith, 2003; Kundhal, 2003). *Health-seeking behaviors,* when and to whom we go for care and the length of time we remain in care, are determined in part by cultural beliefs about illness. Cultural beliefs affect how we communicate our health problems, influence the way we present our symptoms, and define reactions to illness, and these may affect health outcomes. Patterns of trust between the health care system and providers may reflect divergent cultural experiences. Also, differences in beliefs, values, and traditional health care practices are relevant to end-of-life care (Boulware, Cooper, Ratner, LaViest, & Powe, 2003; Crawley, Marshall, Lo, & Koening, 2002; Genao et al., 2003; Hyun, 2002).

Participants of the health care system must share relevant information and coordinate many activities to effectively accomplish their health care goals. Occupational therapists and occupational therapy assistants depend on receiving information from their clients about health histories and symptoms, lifestyles, and concerns to make appropriate intervention decisions. Similarly, clients depend on receiving clear and descriptive information about health care treatment and strategies from their providers. Members of the health care team also depend on sharing pertinent information with one another to provide effective care (Crawley et al., 2002; Kreps & Thornton, 1992). Yet, the client, provider, and team members are all likely to have very different cultural orientations and understandings regarding the provision of health care, based on their personal cultural influences and life experiences as well as on their professional training.

These different points of view can generate a broad base of information that encourages a holistic view of the client's condition, needs, and health care. These different cultural perspectives also can complicate health care if there is a lack of respect and understanding for different cultural orientations and influences. Lack of awareness and knowledge about differences can make it difficult for both the providers and clients to achieve the best, most appropriate care (Fitzgerald, 1992; Good, 1996; Pachter, 1994; Wells, 1994). The plethora of different cultures represented in today's health care system can encroach on personal cultural beliefs about health and life held by consumers, providers, and team members, especially if cultural diversity is not valued (Kreps & Thornton, 1992).

According to Diversity Rx (1997), the medical community often is unaware of differences that can result from a combination of factors, which may include

- *Lack of knowledge,* resulting in the inability to recognize differences;
- *Self-protection/denial,* leading to an attitude that these differences are not significant, or that common humanity transcends differences;
- *Fear of the unknown or the new,* because it is challenging and perhaps intimidating to understand something that is new and does not fit one's viewpoint; and
- *Feeling of pressure due to time constraints,* which can lead to feeling rushed and unable to look in depth at an individual client's needs.

The consequences of cultural incompetency can be significant. Miscommunication, distrust, and misunderstanding can result. The provider may not understand why the client does not comply with the intervention plan. The client may reject the health care provider even before one-on-one interaction occurs because of nonverbal cues that do not fit expectations (Diversity Rx, 1997; McGee, 2001; Rivera-Andino & Lopez, 2000). Accepting societal stereotypes and beliefs about others who differ in some way from the dominant culture or who belong to a different subculture can lead to avoidance, lack of respect, and stigmatization, which can influence how these individuals are treated (Erlen, 1998).

The development and expression of genuine interest and respect for different cultural orientations is needed to enhance the effectiveness of health care delivery. We not only must be tolerant of different cultural perspectives, we also must demonstrate active interest, knowledge, admiration, sensitivity, and awareness of the cultural norms of other cultures. We have an obligation to understand and appreciate the differences that exist and to plan for these differences in the delivery of health care.

Given the need for cultural competency in health care practice, a thorough, systemic, and integrated learning process, which incorporates self-exploration, knowledge, and skills, is needed to address the issue of acquiring cultural competence. Using the premise, goals, and principles of multicultural education and several sociological theories, in 1996, Wells formulated a cultural competence–oriented model, the *Cultural Competency Model,* to be used by health care providers and students to develop the skills needed to be effective in health care delivery.

Conceptual Framework of the Model

The conceptual and theoretical framework for the Cultural Competency Model has been developed from two schools of thought: sociology and education. *Sociology* is the study of human relationships and patterns of behavior. *Education* is the act of acquiring knowledge. Each makes a contribution and should be considered and reviewed in its relationship to becoming culturally competent.

Sociological Perspectives

In sociology, three theoretical perspectives have shaped the study of and described the interaction between minority and majority groups in a society: functional theory, conflict theory, and interactionist theory. *Functional theory* examines the theoretical support for maintaining a harmonious society and seeking new and different adjustments to restore equilibrium when dysfunction occurs. Functionalists believe that a stable, cooperative social system is the basis of society. Rapid social changes, such as demographic changes, require compensating adjustments. If these adjustments do not occur, tension and conflicts are created between the groups (Parrillo, 1997): "The key factor in this analysis of social disorganization is whether to restore the equilibrium as it was, or to seek a new and different equilibrium" (p. 18).

Conflict theory emphasizes the tension and conflicts that result when different groups compete for limited resources. Conflict theorists see disequilibrium and change as the norm because of societal inequalities. Group cohesiveness and struggle against oppression are necessary to effect social change (Levine & Campbell, 1972; Parrillo, 1997; Solomos & Back, 1995). *Interactionist theory* focuses on the personal interaction patterns in everyday life. Essential to this perspective is the belief that people operate within a socially constructed perception of reality. Interactionists conclude that shared expectation and understanding, or lack of the same, explain intergroup relations. And through better communication and intercultural awareness, minority–majority interaction patterns can improve (Ballis, 1995; Berger & Luckmann, 1963; Parrillo, 1997).

The type of interaction between minority peoples and those of the dominant culture promoted by the Cultural Competentcy Model is based on the views and values expressed in the ideology and theory of *cultural pluralism*. The accommodation or pluralism theory of minority integration has emerged as a school of thought in recognition of the persistence of ethnic and racial diversity in a society with a commonly shared core culture (Baptiste, 1979; Parrillo, 1997). Cultural pluralism has been defined as "two or more culturally distinct groups living in the same society in relative harmony" (Parrillo, 1997, p. 548). According to pluralist theorists, minorities can maintain their distinctive subcultures and simultaneously interact with relative equality in the larger society.

In 1915, sociologist Horace Kallen published his classic work, *Democracy Versus the Melting Pot*, in which he expounded that each group tends to preserve its own language, institutions, and cultural heritage. He also stated that the very nature of democracy gave each group the right to do so. Kallen believed that cultural pluralism could be the basis for a great democratic commonwealth. According to Gordon (1964), many minority groups lose their visibility because they have acculturated, but many retain identification with and pride in their heritage, maintaining primary relationships mostly with members of their ethnic or cultural group.

Cultural pluralism was and is a fact of American society. Early settlements were small ethnic enclaves. Chain migration patterns resulted in immigrants settling in clusters—Irish in New York, Germans and Scandinavians in the Midwest, French in Louisiana, Asians in California, and Cubans in Florida. "Assimilation and pluralism have always existed simultaneously among different groups, at different levels. Whether as persistent subcultures or as convergent ones that gradually merge into the dominant culture over several generations, cultural distinct groups have always existed" (Parrillo, 1997, p. 61).

Multicultural Education Perspectives

Grounded in the philosophy of cultural pluralism and the principles of equality, mutual respect, acceptance, understanding, and moral commitment to social justice, multicultural education stresses the importance, legitimacy, and vitality of ethnic and cultural diversity in shaping the lives of individuals, groups, and nations (Baptiste, 1979). According to the Association for Supervision and Curriculum Development Multicultural Education Commission,

> [Multicultural education is] a humanistic concept based on the strength of diversity, human rights, social justice, and alternative lifestyles for all people. It views a culturally pluralistic society as a positive force and welcomes differences as vehicles for better understanding the global society. (Grant, 1977, p. 3)

The literature on multicultural education views *multiculturalism* as a cultural concept that recognizes the diversity of cultural differences that exist in a pluralistic society (Banks, 1994; Darder, 1995; Grant, 1994; Sleeter & Grant, 1994). It places emphasis on the universal acceptance of differences and a society in which individuals of all cultures are accepted and accorded respect (Kanpol & Brady, 1998). Multiculturalists encourage positive acceptance of races, religions, and cultures, and they recognize such diversity as healthy (Banks, 1994; Gay, 1994; Parrillo, 1997). Multiculturalists describe the role and goal of education in a multicultural society as one that

- Develops the potential of each person to the fullest extent;
- Offers both the knowledge and critical thinking skills to allow learners to become active agents of change in their lives;
- Engages the learner as an active participant in the construction of knowledge; and

- Presents learners with a language of critique and possibility (Burnett, 1994; Gay, 1994; Gorski, 1997; Kanpol & Brady, 1998).

Asante (1991) proclaims that the goal of multicultural education is to achieve cultural pluralism without hierarchy. The general goals of multicultural education fall into seven general clusters:

1. Ethnic and cultural literacy
2. Personal development
3. Attitude and value clarification
4. Multicultural social competence
5. Basic skills proficiency
6. Educational equality and excellence
7. Empowerment for societal reform (Banks, 1994; Gay, 1994; Gorski, 1997).

Multicultural education offers a variety of opportunities not only to deal directly with cultural diversity but also to infuse the perspectives of others into the learning process. It encourages learners to view different cultures as sources of learning and enrichment. It focuses on how to learn rather than on specific information; it emphasizes the importance of people sharing their stories and learning from stories of others; and it takes into account the learner, his or her learning style, and the extent to which the learner has changed relative to the material. Multicultural education is an ongoing process that requires long-term investments of time and effort as well as clearly planned and monitored actions (Banks & Banks, 1993). It means learning about, preparing for, and celebrating cultural diversity.

Cultural Competency Model

The Cultural Competency Model refers to a structural process designed to foster understanding, acceptance, knowledge, and constructive relations between people of various cultures and differences. The model is built on the assumptions that

- All people have experienced a variety of multicultural influences;
- Everyone is affected and molded by more than one culture and, therefore, is a multicultural being;
- Becoming culturally competent is a lifelong process;
- Cultural competence is a professional and ethical obligation; and
- Cultural competence enhances the quality of health care delivery.

The model is designed as a tool for developing the knowledge and skills that occupational therapy practitioners will need to provide quality care in the 21st century. It provides a foundation for understanding personal interaction patterns within social and cultural contexts. It can help practitioners adjust to a changing society as well as effect social changes.

The Cultural Competency Model groups the seven goals' cluster of multicultural education (above) into three areas or characteristics:

1. Self-exploration
2. Knowledge
3. Skills.

Other personal components necessary to be culturally competent, such as attitudes, behaviors, and perceptions, are not directly addressed but are infused during the learning process. The model aims to

- Increase the sense of one's own cultural identity;
- Heighten the awareness of one's own cultural perspectives and the effects of those perspectives on individuals from other groups as well and interactions;
- Develop knowledge of and practice in using effective strategies for inter-rupting culturally inappropriate and offensive remarks and behaviors that hinder relationships across cultures; and
- Assist individuals to develop a plan with specific ways to improve cultural self-awareness, acquire knowledge, develop skills, and build alliances with people who are culturally different from oneself.

The Cultural Competency Model furnishes a clear framework for developing and assessing one's progress toward becoming culturally competent (see Figure 4.1).

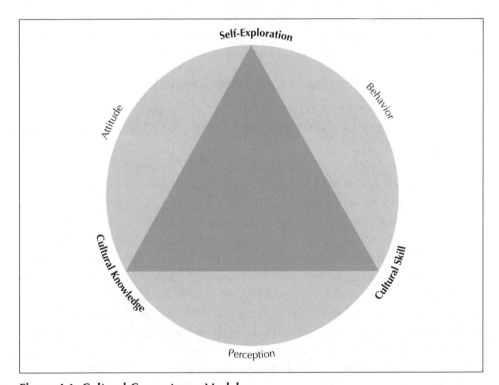

Figure 4.1. Cultural Competency Model.

> To succeed, [health care providers] need an awareness and acceptance of cultural differences, an awareness of their own cultural values, an understanding of the dynamics of differences in the helping process, a basic knowledge about the client's culture, knowledge of the client's environment, and the ability to adapt practice skills to fit the client's context. (Cross, Bazron, Dennis, & Isaacs, 1989, p. 32)

Characteristics

As society becomes increasingly more diverse, it is critical that occupational therapy practitioners and students are prepared for delivering health care as well as living in this multicultural environment. A variety of issues, ranging from ethnocentrism to unity through acceptance and understanding, and from discrimination to equality of experience and opportunity, must be addressed. Practitioners must recognize and understand the dynamics of diversity, explore their own diversity, and acquire knowledge about other groups. It is important for providers to recognize and understand their own biases and prejudices and their effects on others and the clinical interaction. From self-exploration and accumulation of knowledge will come effective and culturally appropriate intervention strategies, as well as improved intercultural communication skills.

There are truly only three areas in which intervention for change can occur—self-exploration and awareness, cultural knowledge, and cultural skills (see Exhibit 4.1).

Self-Exploration and Awareness

The literature has shown that bias, stereotyping, prejudice, and clinical uncertainty by health care providers contribute to racial or ethnic disparities in health care (Betancourt, Alexander, & Carrillo, 2003; Boulware et al., 2003; Taylor, 2005; Tucker et al., 2003). Consequently, self-exploration is an essential requirement to be culturally competent. Knowledge of one's self enables the practitioner to be aware of and take responsibility for his or her own emotions and attitudes as they affect professional behavior. Understanding how differences, oppression, *isms*, discrimination, and stereotyping affect the clinical interaction, as well as the individual personally, also is a must for becoming culturally competent. Self-exploration furnishes the therapist with an understanding of his or her own cultural biases, as well as the medical culture's biases, and the degree to which he or she is conditioned by these (Cross et al., 1989; Devore & Schlesinger, 1981). Self-exploration is an internal, personal experience. It is a process of looking inward, learning to recognize when old information no longer applies, and using this knowledge of self (Pedersen, 1988; Pusch, 1979).

Self-exploration is not always a risk-free and pleasant process. It is looking at and recognizing the *Me*, who is sometimes judgmental and noncaring. It is having

Exhibit 4.1. Areas of Intervention

Self-Exploration and Awareness
Goal: To build an awareness of one's own cultural heritage
Objectives:
1. To expand cultural self-awareness
2. To provide the individual with an understanding of his or her own culture and of the degree to which he or she is conditioned by it
3. To increase tolerance and acceptance of different values, attitudes, behaviors, and perceptions.

Cultural Knowledge
Goals: To understand that no one culture is intrinsically superior to another; to recognize individual and group differences and similarities
Objectives:
1. To foster the affirmation of all cultures, especially those which, because of minority status, have received a disproportionate amount of negative reinforcement from society
2. To prepare for effective personal adjustment to the stress of intercultural experiences
3. To open avenues of learning and growth, which multicultural experiences make accessible.

Cultural Skills
Goal: Mastery of appropriate, relevant, and sensitive strategies and skills in communicating and interacting with people from different cultures
Objectives:
1. To develop intercultural communication skills
2. To integrate cognitive, affective, and experiential learning
3. To develop the ability to seek information about the economic, political, and social stresses and the aspirations of various cultures or ethnic groups within a society.

the ability to recognize when the judgmental, noncaring self interferes with the ability to reach out, to explore, and to help others. Acknowledging vulnerability in self-introspection can encourage direct communication and bolster personal integrity (Devore & Schlesinger, 1981; Kavanagh & Kennedy, 1992). Engaging in introspection will help one determine if he or she has any biases or negative feelings toward particular cultures (Erlen, 1998).

In getting at the *Who* of *Me,* Schulman (1978) posed three questions to answer:

1. Who am I?
2. Who do others think I am?
3. Who would I like to be?

The answers begin to help us recognize, with some accuracy, our perceptions of ourselves, the perceptions of others about us, and our dreams of what we might be. The awareness of one's own race, ethnicity, and cultural diversity, as well as the ability to recognize how these may affect practice, is also crucial to this process. In actuality, more culturally appropriate questions to be answered are

1. Who am I in the racial, ethnic, or cultural diversity sense?
2. What does it mean to me?
3. How does it shape my perceptions of persons who are my clients?

A heightened self-awareness and a greater awareness of diversity lead to a realization that, for many individuals, race, ethnicity, gender, religion, sexual identity, appearance, and disability are forces that shape movement through the life cycle, determining appropriate marriage partners, language, dietary selections, and the various subtleties of daily life. Self-exploration opens avenues of learning and growth.

Outcomes of Self-Exploration and Self-Awareness. Culturally competent health care providers have knowledge

- About their own racial or ethnic cultural heritage and how it personally and professionally affects their definitions of normality and abnormality and the process of providing services;
- Insight about how oppression, *isms,* discrimination, and stereotyping affect them personally and professionally; and
- About their social impact on others, including an awareness of their communication style differences.

Cultural Knowledge

Cultural knowledge about other groups promotes understanding and allows occupational therapy practitioners and students to adapt the way in which services are delivered. The greater the shared knowledge, the less likely misunderstandings will occur. Many of us often have experienced situations in which we are aware of and sensitive to differences but lacked the specific knowledge of the other cultures or systems involved to avert problems, develop solutions, or acknowledge interplay of cultures. Cultural knowledge provides the framework that can help practitioners understand the experiences of the client and to intervene at an appropriate cultural and individual level (Cross et al., 1989; Fitzgerald, 1992; Good, 1996; Kavanagh & Kennedy, 1992). It also allows the therapist to look at interaction from multiple perspectives, including the culture in which the interaction occurs, cultures of the individuals involved, and the culture of the society or system.

According to Kavanagh and Kennedy (1992) "patterns of social interaction, social organization, distribution of resources, and social changes are directly relevant to social experiences" (p. 4) and behaviors. Individual behaviors often reflect the influences of these social factors. Communication styles, for example, such as eye contact, tone of voice, or greetings, may vary with social characteristics such as age, gender, or ethnic or racial background. A basic understanding and knowledge of the effects of the following are necessary:

- Social organization, interaction, and processes in the United States
- Sociopolitical systems operating within the United States with respect to treatment of minorities

- Cultural characteristics and life experiences of racial and ethnic populations
- Similarities and differences among racial, ethnic, and culturally diverse groups
- Human development and the life cycle as they relate to ethnicity, race, gender, religion, sexual orientation, disability, and appearance
- Professional behaviors and values with respect to dealing with consumers, clients, and families (Dillard et al., 1992; London & Devore, 1988; Sayles-Folks & People, 1990; Wells, 1994).

Gaining enough knowledge to know *what, who,* and *how* to ask for information should be a desirable goal for a culturally competent practitioner (Green, 1982). Information that will add to the occupational therapist's knowledge is a must because of the diversity within groups. Cultural knowledge also includes knowledge of health-related beliefs, values, disease incidence and prevalence, and treatment efficacy among diverse groups.

The average practitioner cannot achieve comprehensive knowledge about any group, population, or culture. More important is knowing *where* and *how* to obtain the necessary detailed information for use in specific cases (Cross et al., 1989). Specific knowledge about a client's culture adds a critical dimension to the helping process. It is necessary to know what symbols are meaningful, how health is defined, and how primary support networks are configured. Building a knowledge base is not an end in and of itself (Cross et al., 1989; Fitzgerald, 1992). The therapist must be able to acquire knowledge to use in modifying intervention approaches, adapting the way in which services are delivered, or developing strategies for acquiring additional information.

Outcomes for Cultural Knowledge. A culturally competent health care provider has

- Specific and extensive knowledge of the language, values, customs, and beliefs of another culture;
- An understanding about the effects of gender, race, ethnicity, religion, disability, sexual identity, appearance, nationality, geographic location, and lifestyle on human development;
- A basic knowledge about the effects, real or perceived, of institutional and individual discrimination on interaction and utilization of services; and
- Knowledge about the influence of culture on behaviors and needs.

Cultural Skills

Cultural skills refers to acquiring and mastering strategies, techniques, and approaches for communicating and interacting with people from different cultures. It includes the ability to collect culturally relevant data during assessments. It is stepping out of one's value orientation to identify and interpret what is important in understanding another cultural group (Taylor, 2005). It is making the shift from authority figure to learner in cross-cultural interactions. Cultural skills also include having the cultural desire to become culturally competent (Campinha-Bacote, 2002). Cultural skills are manifested in a therapist's ability to accurately interpret and respond to nonverbal or other cultural cues (Agency for Healthcare Research and Quality [AHRQ], 2004). This can lead to the behavioral adaptations needed for culturally competent care.

Cultural skills are based on awareness of attitude, knowledge, and dedication to effective communication. *Skill* is the translation of knowledge into "telephone behaviors, receptionist practices, client interactions which build trust, establish credibility, and help create a culture-friendly environment" (Arkansas Research and Training Center in Vocational Rehabilitation, 1992, p. 48) when working with people from diverse ethnic backgrounds. Communication encompasses a wide range of activities, including oral, nonverbal, and written, that describe the flow and exchange of information among those involved in the provision and receipt of care,

Cultural factors affect consumer–provider communication.

including interpersonal exchanges and exchanges between individuals and organizations. Cultural factors affect consumer–provider communication.

Proficiency in cultural communication has been described as skills in communicating with members of diverse cultural groups to achieve desired objectives (Kreps & Kunimoto, 1994). Kavanagh and Kennedy (1992) state that "effective cross-cultural communication requires awareness that communication is possible and that mistakes will occur, sensitivity to the communication process, knowledge of expectable patterns of communication styles that are appropriate to the client, and a set of practice skills" (p. 42). The development of specific skill areas, such as articulating the problem, managing resistance and defensiveness, and recovering when mistakes are made, is needed to examine communication patterns and their potential for creating barriers or mutual respect. Such skills empower or enable the communicator professionally and personally (Ivey, 1980; Pedersen, 1988). "Intercultural communication proficiency empowers one in the decision-making process of personal health" (Kreps & Kunimoto, 1994, p. 26).

Mutual communication conveys a commitment to involvement in an interactive process that affords respect, recognition and value of human dignity, and a willingness to alter personal behaviors in response to the communication process. Developing the skills to empathize and understand others' beliefs, assumptions, perspectives, and feelings are important communication strategies (Pedersen, 1988). Possessing the willingness to risk and expose oneself as limited and still developing sensitivity, knowledge, and skills, also is crucial to the mutual communication process. Mutual and shared communication and understanding—an effective goal of health care professionals—promotes the ability to help clients and others find and accept appropriate intervention (Kavanagh & Kennedy, 1992). Cultural competence leads to actions creating concordance in communication styles and increases the availability and accessibility of language services (e.g., interpretation and translation) to improve communication. Improved communication can lead to increased consumer satisfaction and an improved understanding of and compliance with diagnoses and treatment regimens (AHRQ, 2004).

Through training and experience, the therapist can gain skills to adapt and adjust the helping process to compensate for cultural differences. Interviewing styles, knowing who is included in family intervention, and developing intervention goals are a few of the things that can be changed to meet cultural needs (Cross et al., 1989). Beyond multicultural communication skills, providers can be taught interviewing skills that are reflective of the individual's understanding of culture and diversity; techniques for learning the culture of their client groups; and strategies for managing feelings and attitudes, both personally and for others. Proficiency in the area of cultural skill enables the occupational therapist to communicate effectively with people of different backgrounds, to learn about others, and to adapt to the constraints of their lives. It enables one to obtain information from other health care therapists and professionals in diverse cultural settings, enables therapists to build supportive environments and to begin institutionalizing cultural interventions as legitimate helping approaches, and allows therapists to continue to acquire skills and behaviors that would enhance the delivery of health care services to all people (AHRQ, 2004; Arkansas Research and Training Center in Vocational Rehabilitation, 1992; Cross et al., 1989; Kavanagh & Kennedy, 1992; Kreps & Kunimoto, 1994).

Outcomes for Cultural Skill. Culturally competent health care providers have the
- Ability to generate, modify, and adapt a variety of intervention strategies to accommodate the particular need of the client and his or her family;
- Knowledge to be creative and resourceful in identifying and using cultural value systems on behalf of clients;
- Ability to use, send, and interpret a variety of verbal and nonverbal communication skills to bridge the gap between cultures;
- Skills and knowledge to learn about cultures; and
- Capability to assess discriminatory intent and discriminatory effect in their interactions and services.

Summary

The Cultural Competency Model focuses on the process of developing cultural competency in health care practice. MacDonald (1998) states that this model can be used to structure teaching and learning strategies:

It provides a clear framework for curriculum development and assessment. It is suggested that educational establishments are the best equipped to assess the knowledge and self-exploration components of the model and that the skills component is best assessed while on fieldwork. (p. 325)

In occupational therapy academic and fieldwork settings, it is critical that educators are prepared to teach, facilitate, promote, and develop cultural competence among students. Educators must take students beyond their own individual experiences and encourage active and lifelong learning and positive attitudes about groups of people who are different from them. They must model and facilitate ways of evaluating knowledge from different perspectives. More importantly, educators must help students understand their personal values and beliefs and how they affect the therapeutic relationship and interactions. Finally, educators must give students the skills and strategies to interact effectively in multicultural environments.

In many practice settings, occupational therapy practitioners still wonder if it is possible to provide culturally competent care. The Cultural Competency Model can be used to help practitioners answer that question in the affirmative. It can be used to develop plans for individuals as well as systems to practice in a multicultural environment, celebrating and respecting cultural differences. As occupational therapy practitioners examine their practice and articulate effective, culturally appropriate intervention strategies, health care delivery will improve. Each person will add to his or her knowledge base, through both positive and negative experiences, developing his or her expertise over time (Cross et al., 1989). This requires staying abreast of contemporary theories, practice, and research in this area.

Reflection

1. Discuss how you can use the Cultural Competency Model to become culturally competent.

2. Answer the following questions (be honest with yourself):

   a. Who am I in the racial, ethnic, or cultural diversity sense?

   b. What does it mean to me?

   c. How does it shape my perceptions of persons who are my clients?

   d. Am I a culturally competent person/professional? If not, what must I do to move toward cultural competence?

References

Agency for Healthcare Research and Quality. (2004). *Setting the agenda for research on cultural competence in health care.* Retrieved January 6, 2006, from http://ahrq.gov/research/cultural.htm

Arkansas Research and Training Center in Vocational Rehabilitation. (1992). *Cultural diversity in rehabilitation: Nineteenth institute on rehabilitation issues.* Hot Springs: Author.

Asante, M. (1991). Afrocentric curriculum. *Educational Leadership, 49,* 28–39.

Ballis, L. B. (1995). Symbolic interaction theories. *American Behavioral Scientist, 38,* 421–441.

Banks, J. A. (1994). *An introduction to multicultural education.* Boston: Allyn & Bacon.

Banks, J. A., & Banks, C. A. (1993). *Multicultural education: Theory and practice* (2nd ed.). Boston: Allyn & Bacon.

Baptiste, H. P. (1979). *Multicultural education: A synopsis.* Washington, DC: University Press of America.

Betancourt, J. R., Alexander, R. G., & Carrillo, J. E. (2003). Defining cultural competence: A practical framework for addressing racial/ethnic disparities in health and health care. *Public Health Reports, 118,* 293–302.

Berger, P. L., & Luckmann, T. (1963). *The social construction of reality.* Garden City, NJ: Doubleday.

Boulware, L. E., Cooper, L. A., Ratner, L. E., LaViest, T. A., & Powe, N. R. (2003). Race and trust in the health care system. *Public Health Reports, 118,* 358–365.

Burnett, G. (1994). *Varieties of multicultural education: An introduction.* [ERIC Digest Online]. Retrieved July 2007 from http://eric-web.tc.columbia.edu/digests/dig98.html

Campinha-Bacote, J. (2002). The process of cultural competence in the delivery of health-care services: A model of care. *Journal of Transcultural Nursing, 13,* 181–184.

Crawley, L. M., Marshall, P.A., Lo, B., & Koening, B.A. (2002). Strategies for culturally effective end-of-life care. *Annals of Internal Medicine, 136,* 673–679.

Cross, T. L., Bazron, B. J., Dennis, K. W., & Isaacs, M. R. (1989). *Towards a culturally competent system of care* (Vol. I). Washington, DC: CASSP, Georgetown University Child Development Center, Technical Assistance Center.

Darder, A. (Ed.). (1995). *Culture and difference.* Westport, CT: Bergin & Garvey.

Devore, W., & Schlesinger, E. G. (1981). *Ethnic-sensitive social work practice.* St. Louis, MO: Mosby.

Dillard, M., Andonian, L., Flores, O., Lai, L., MacRae, A., & Shakir, M. (1992). Culturally competent occupational therapy in a diversely populated mental health setting. *American Journal of Occupational Therapy, 46,* 21–26.

Diversity Rx. (1997). *Why is cultural competence important for health professionals?* Retrieved July 27, 2007, from www.diversityrx.org

Erlen, A. (1998). Culture, ethics, and respect: The bottom line is understanding. *Orthopaedic Nursing, 17*(6), 79.

Fitzgerald, M. H. (1992). Multicultural clinical interactions. *Journal of Rehabilitation, 58,* 38–42.

Gay, G. (1994). *A synthesis of scholarship in multicultural education* [NCREL's Urban Education Monograph Series]. Oak Brook, IL: North Central Regional Educational Laboratory.

Genao, I., Bussey-Jones, J., Brady, D., Branch, W. T., & Corbie-Smith, G. (2003). Building the case for cultural competence. *American Journal of Medical Sciences, 326,* 136–140.

Good, D. (1996). Cultural sensitivity: Integrating cultural concepts into clinical practice. *WORK, 6,* 61–65.

Gordon, M. (1964). *Assimilation in American life.* New York: Oxford University Press.

Gorski, P. (1997). *A working definition: Initial thoughts on multicultural education.* Retrieved July 2007 from http://curry.edschool.virginia.edu/go/multicultural/activityarch.html

Grant, C. (1977). *Multicultural education: Commitments, issues, and applications.* Washington, DC: Association for Supervision and Curriculum Development.

Grant, C. (1994). Best practice in teacher preparation for urban schools: Lessons from the multicultural teacher education literature. *Action in Teacher Education, 16*(3), 1–18.

Green, J. W. (1982). *Cultural awareness in the human services.* Englewood Cliffs, NJ: Prentice Hall.

Howe-Murphy, R., Ross, H., Tseng, R., & Hartwig, R. (1989). Effecting change in multicultural health promotion: A systems approach. *Journal of Allied Health, 18,* 291–305.

Hyun, I. (2002). Waiver of informed consent, cultural sensitivity, and the problem of unjust families and traditions. *Hasting Center Report, 32*(5), 14–22.

Ivey, A. (1980). *Counseling and psychotherapy: Skills, theories, and practice.* Englewood Cliffs, NJ: Prentice Hall.

Johnson, V. (1995). *Heart full of grace: A thousand years of Black wisdom.* New York: Simon & Schuster.

Kallen, H. (1915, February 18). Democracy versus the melting pot. *Nations,* pp. 190–194.

Kanpol, B., & Brady, J. (1998). Teacher education and the multicultural dilemma: A "critical" thinking response. *Journal of Critical Pedagogy, 1*(2), 62–66

Kavanagh, K. H., & Kennedy, P. H. (1992). *Promoting cultural diversity: Strategies for healthcare professionals.* Newbury Park, CA: Sage.

Kreps, G. L., & Kunimoto, E. N. (1994). *Effective communication in multicultural health care settings.* Thousand Oaks, CA: Sage.

Kreps, G. L., & Thornton, B. C. (1992). *Health communication: Theory and practice* (2nd ed.). Prospect Heights, IL: Waveland.

Kundhal, K. K. (2003). Cultural diversity: An evolving challenge to physician–patient communication. *Journal of the American Medical Association, 289*(1), 94–96.

Levine, R. A., & Campbell, D. T. (1972). *Ethnocentrism theories of conflict, ethnic attitudes, and group behavior.* New York: Wiley.

London, H., & Devore, W. (1988). Layers of understanding. *Family Relations, 37,* 310–314.

MacDonald, R. (1998). What is cultural competency? *British Journal of Occupational Therapy, 61,* 325–328.

McGee, C. (2001). When the golden rule does not apply: Starting nurses on the journey toward cultural competence. *Journal for Nurses in Staff Development, 17,* 105–112.

McNeil, C. (1990). Culture: The impact on healthcare. *Journal of Cancer Education, 5,* 13–16.

Mead, M. (1956). Understanding cultural patterns. *Nursing Outlook, 4,* 260–262.

Pachter, L. M. (1994). Culture and clinical care: Folk illness beliefs and behaviors and their implications for health care delivery. *Journal of the American Medical Association, 271,* 690–694.

Parrillo, V. N. (1997). *Strangers to these shores: Race and ethnic relations in the United States* (5th ed.). Boston: Allyn & Bacon.

Pedersen, P. (1988). The three stages of multicultural development: Awareness, knowledge, and skill. In P. Pedersen (Ed.), *A handbook for developing multicultural awareness* (pp. 3–18). Alexandria, VA: American Association for Counseling and Development.

Pusch, M. D. (1979). *Multicultural education: A cross-cultural approach.* Yarmouth, ME: Intercultural.

Rivera-Andino, J., & Lopez, L. (2000). When culture complicates care. *RN, 63*(7), 47–49.

Sayles-Folks, S., & People, L. (1990). Cultural sensitivity training for occupational therapists. *Physical Disabilities Special Interest Section Newsletter, 13*(3), 4–5.

Schulman, E. D. (1978). *Intervention in human services* (2nd ed.). St. Louis, MO: Mosby.

Sleeter, C. E., & Grant, C. A. (1994). Multicultural education. In C. E. Sleeter & C. A. Grant (Eds.), *Making choices for multicultural education: Five approaches to race, class, and gender* (2nd ed., pp. 136–173). Columbus, OH: Merrill.

Solomos, J., & Back, L. (1995). Marxism, racism, and ethnicity. *American Behavioral Scientist, 38,* 407–420.

Taylor, R. (2005). Addressing barriers to cultural competence. *Journal for Nurses in Staff Development, 21*(4), 135–142.

Tucker, C., Herman, K., Pedersen, T. R., Higley, B., Montrichard, M., & Ivery, P. (2003). Cultural sensitivity in physician–patient relationships: Perspectives of an ethnically diverse sample of low-income primary care patients. *Medical Care, 41,* 859–870.

Wells, S. A. (1994). *A multicultural education and resource guide for occupational therapy educators and practitioners.* Bethesda, MD: American Occupational Therapy Association.

II

Understanding the Components of Cultural Competence

If any of the three stages of awareness, knowledge, or skill is missing from [one's] training, difficulties are likely to arise. If they neglect awareness, they are more likely to build on wrong or inappropriate assumptions. If they neglect knowledge, they may be inaccurate in their description of a situation. If they neglect skill, they may be changing the situation in counterproductive directions.

—PEDERSEN & IVEY, (1993, P. 19)

Objectives

The information in Part II will help readers

- Recognize the three characteristics of cultural competence, self-awareness, knowledge, and skill;

- Understand the inherent complexity of developing and integrating these three characteristics;

- Understand the concept of power in client–practitioner relationships and apply this information to current or future practice; and

- Develop a personal plan for the development of cultural competence.

Section A

*Cultural Self-Awareness
and the Concept of Power*

5

Cultural Self-Awareness

*The starting point of any education programme [in cultural competence]
should therefore be an exploration of the students' own cultural values,
beliefs, and practices, including their own prejudices.*

—GERRISH & PAPADOPOULOS (1999, P. 1454)

Key Points

- Cultural self-awareness may be the most important characteristic necessary for cultural competence.

- Cultural self-awareness is more complex than understanding one's strengths and weaknesses.

- Cultural self-awareness means engaging in a critical self-examination that involves careful study of our culture and subcultures and our beliefs and values, as well as understanding where we are in the sociocultural hierarchy of our society.

- Cultural self-awareness is the bridge to understanding other cultures.

ONE OF THE MAIN CHARACTERISTICS identified in the Cultural Competency Model for someone moving toward cultural competence is that of cultural self-awareness or self-exploration. Many, including the authors of this book, believe self-awareness is not only the most important of the three characteristics, but also the necessary first step in the development of cultural competence (Chan, 1990; Harry, 1992; Lynch & Hanson, 1998; Weaver, 1999; Wells & Black, 2000). Leonard and Plotnikoff (2000) refer to self-awareness as the "heart of cultural compe-tence"(p. 51).

Occupational therapists and occupational therapy assistants often are quite skilled in identifying their own strengths and weaknesses, which is one aspect of self-awareness. Cultural self-awareness, however, is more complex and goes beyond those skills. Individuals with cultural self-awareness know and understand them-selves at a deeper level. Developing this kind of self-awareness involves engaging in a critical self-examination, which allows people to carefully study their culture and subcultures and the beliefs and values that emerge to help form their identity and worldview, including recognition of the role they each play in an imperfect world. They reflect on how they value and respond to people who differ from themselves in age, gender, class, race, ethnicity, sexual orientation, religion, and ability. This self-discovery process gives students and practitioners not only a sense of self in a diverse world but also an openness that enhances their empathy with those from different cultural backgrounds (Black, 2002).

Culturally aware individuals recognize the characteristics of their own cul-ture and social location and know how these influence their values, beliefs, behav-iors, and choices; they are mostly comfortable with cultural differences between themselves and others and are sensitive to issues of culture in all interactions (Wells & Black, 2000). McPhatter (1997) refers to this increased self-awareness as *enlightened consciousness.* She believes it is a fundamental transformational process that results in the

> Reorienting [of] one's primary worldview. . . . It often requires a radical
> restructuring of a well-entrenched belief system that perceives oneself
> and one's culture, including values and ways of behavior, as not only
> preferred, but clearly superior to another's. The ultimate goal of this shift
> in mind-set is to create a belief in, and acceptance of others on the basis
> of equality solely because of a sense of shared humanity. (pp. 262–263)

McPhatter (1997) is not talking about simply completing a few self-awareness exercises. Rather, she emphasizes the gravity of this work and the need for ongoing and sustained practice. Analyzing oneself is not always easy, especially for students and practitioners with characteristics of the dominant societal group. In the United States, that group consists of those who are White, middle or upper class, financial-ly secure, able-bodied, heterosexual, and male. This self-analysis necessitates recognizing and grappling with one's unearned privilege (McIntosh, 1988) and reflecting on how it may affect client–practitioner interactions:

> It should be apparent that this dynamic process cannot even begin in short-term or brief overtures into another's world. It must be a sustained effort motivated by true desire to become accepting and comfortable in personal cross-cultural interactions and effective in providing services to clients whose cultural realities differ markedly from one's own. (McPhatter, 1997, p. 264)

In occupational therapy practice, as in other health care arenas, "students must be able to acknowledge their own cultural backgrounds and not feel threatened by their own cultural identifications, especially when they differ with that of the client" (Chau, 1990, as cited in Sowers-Hoag & Sandau-Beckler, 1996, p. 43). Cultural self-awareness "is the bridge to learning about other cultures" (Lynch & Hanson, 1998, p. 55), and every occupational therapy education program should include an opportunity for "an exploration of the students' own cultural values, beliefs, and practices, including their own prejudices" (Gerrish & Papadopoulos, 1999, p. 1454).

An aspect of understanding oneself is the awareness of cultural power and its affect on occupational therapy practice. The following chapters deepen the process of self-examination by exploring the relationship of power to privilege and prejudice, the power of being White, and the power inherent within the professional role.

Reflection

1. Choose a favorite activity.

   a. Why is this a favorite of yours?

   b. From whom did you learn this activity?

   c. How does the activity reflect your culture?

   d. What personal values are reflected in this activity?

   e. How would it feel if you were told you could never engage in this activity again?

2. Consider your social location.

   a. How does your age, nationality, gender, sexual identity, religion, race or ethnicity, class, or ability affect your social status?

   b. What aspects above can you change?

   c. What aspects above would you want to change? Why?

   d. How do your unique characteristics benefit you in your society?

   e. Do any of your unique characteristics limit you in some way?

References

Black, R. M. (2002). *The essence of cultural competence: Listening to the voices of occupational therapy students.* Unpublished doctoral dissertation, Lesley University, Cambridge, MA.

Chan, S. Q. (1990). Early intervention with culturally diverse families of infants and toddlers with disabilities. *Infants and Young Children, 3*(2), 78–87.

Gerrish, K., & Papadopoulos, I. (1999). Transcultural competence: The challenge for nurse education. *British Journal of Nursing, 8,* 1453–1457.

Harry, B. (1992). Developing cultural self-awareness: The first step in values clarification for early interventionists. *Topics in Early Childhood Special Education, 12,* 333–350.

Leonard, B. J., & Plotnikoff, G. A. (2000). Awareness: The heart of cultural competence. *AACN Clinical Issues, 11*(1), 51–59.

Lynch, E. W., & Hanson, M. J. (1998). *Developing cross-cultural competencies: A guide for working with children and their families* (2nd ed.). Baltimore: Paul H. Brookes.

McIntosh, P. (1988). *White privilege and male privilege: A personal account of coming to see correspondences through work in women's studies* (Working Paper No. 189). Wellesley, MA: Wellesley College, Center for Research on Women.

McPhatter, A. R. (1997). Cultural competence and child welfare: What is it? How do we achieve it? What happens without it? *Child Welfare, 76*(1), 255–278.

Pedersen, P. B., & Ivey, A. (1993). *Culture-centered counseling and interviewing skills.* Westport, CT: Praeger.

Sowers-Hoag, K. M., & Sandau-Beckler, P. (1996). Educating for cultural competence in the generalist curriculum. *Journal of Multicultural Social Work, 4*(3), 37–56.

Weaver, H. N. (1999). Indigenous people and the social work profession: Defining culturally competent services. *Social Work, 44,* 217–225.

Wells, S. A., & Black, R. M. (2000). *Cultural competency for health professionals.* Bethesda, MD: American Occupational Therapy Association.

6

Prejudice, Privilege, and Power

We do not really see through our eyes or hear through our ears, but through our beliefs. To put our beliefs on hold is to cease to exist as ourselves for a moment, and it is not easy. It is painful as well, because it means turning yourself inside out, giving up your own sense of who you are and being willing to see yourself in the unflattering light of another's angry gaze. We must learn to be vulnerable enough to allow our world to turn upside down in order to allow the realities of others to edge themselves into our consciousness.

—DELPIT (1988, PP. 46–47)

Key Points

- Sociocultural power always is part of the client–practitioner relationship.
- White Americans experience unearned privilege simply because of the color of their skin.
- People who are not part of the dominant social group suffer varying levels of prejudice, stereotyping, and discrimination.
- Discrimination can occur at multiple levels: personal, institutional, and structural.
- Occupational therapists and occupational therapy assistants must be aware of their sociocultural power and how it may affect clients and colleagues.
- Each practitioner must evaluate her or his own values, beliefs, biases, and prejudices to prevent engaging in discriminatory practices.

POWER, OR THE LACK OF IT, is an issue dealt with daily, whether consciously or unconsciously. As part of self-reflection, we must recognize this issue. In occupational therapy, researchers have written about the empowerment of clients (Crepeau, 1994; Kronenberg & Pollard, 2005; MacKinnon & Froehlich, 1994; Townsend & Whiteford, 2005), but the reality is that as long as one is in a position of authority in the client–practitioner interaction, a power differential exists between practitioners and clients.

Power issues also are apparent in classrooms, both among students and between students and faculty. In addition, power issues occur among various cultural groups that influence the way people interact with one another. It seems obvious that we must explore the issue of power in occupational therapy practice and education, especially when discussing issues of diversity in practice and multicultural content within a curriculum.

To help students and practitioners put their thinking and self-reflection around issues of culture into context, this chapter introduces the sociocultural power and privilege concept, especially in examining the dominant culture in the United States. It differentiates the concepts of prejudice, stereotyping, and discrimination, explores how these affect behaviors, and ends with a brief discussion of strategies for prejudice reduction.

Sociocultural Power and Privilege

History

U.S. history is a story about power and control—success and growth for some, loss and despair for others. It is a story that has been revisited, reimagined, and revised during the past four decades to now include the perspectives of all participants rather than those of just a privileged few. The following short summary is woefully inadequate, but it provides a point of view prevalent in many of today's history books. This is not a story about blame but a narrative perceived as true by many.

Before being colonized by the Spanish, British, and other Europeans, native people, now referred to as Native Americans, inhabited what is today the United States. White immigrants brought with them a sense of entitlement and ownership that devalued the native inhabitants' lives. White men of power arrived in this country laden not only with their families and material goods but also with their own ideas, beliefs, and values—their culture, which quickly became the dominant manner of thinking and acting. They believed in independence, self-control, and mastery. This belief system ultimately resulted in control of the land, goods and products, education, commerce, religion, and even others (Tai & Kenyatta, 1999). This need for ownership, control, and power resulted in the seizure of lands previously inhabited by native tribes and the large-scale possession of other human beings as slaves to work on those lands. Thus, a hierarchy developed that placed prominent White men at the top of the social ladder with others in inferior positions depending on culture, race, ethnicity, gender, and economic status (Ignatiev, 1995).

Although slavery was legally eradicated in this country, a legacy of oppression, including racism, sexism, classism, heterosexism, ageism, and ableism remains. Despite the work of many to eradicate oppression and support social justice, these sociocultural issues are sustained by power and politics and supported by the economics of capitalism (Omi, Winant, & Winant, 1994). Sociocultural power gives status and control to the dominant social group, which continues to be White, middle- and upper-class heterosexual men. Although today's White men did not cause the sociopolitical power structure within which all participate and many work to lessen its effects, they do benefit the most from it. Power and privilege also are meted out at varying levels to those with any of the characteristics of the dominant group. White Americans in this country, for example, both men and women, are awarded unearned privilege because of their skin color (McIntosh, 1988). Maleness, another privileged characteristic, gives Hispanic American men more power than Hispanic American women. Heterosexual women and men of any race and ethnicity have more freedom and opportunities than homosexual or transgendered women and men.

These characteristics, however, become blended and multilayered, and the complexity of the issue of power and access to goods and services becomes dependent on the context of the social situation. To use an example, a former occupational therapy student is a White, Franco-American male. During a discussion of the history of White male privilege, he disclosed that he never felt privileged because he came from a poor ethnic background and had to work very hard to achieve the status of a master's-degree student. His social location or context certainly affected his perception and reality of privilege. It is important, therefore, to recognize each person's individuality and the complex intersection of issues of race, ethnicity, class, and culture that affects lives.

Sociocultural Location and Standpoint Theory

Each person comes into this world within a particular *social location*. The term refers not just to geography but rather to the context of people's lives. It refers to race, ethnicity, gender, sexual identity, family position, religion, town or city and country of birth, and socioeconomic class; in other words, all of the identifying characteristics that make each person unique. These identifiers fundamentally shape a person's self-perception and worldview, as well as participation in class, gender, racial, age, geographical, and national groups. They also shape the perceptions of those who know that person. Each person's social location "differs on the basis of what is valued by the culture, resulting in variation[s] of social privilege" (Kubiak,

2005, p. 453). People are "fundamentally shaped by the power and authority (or lack thereof) of roles given to us and expectations on us as members of those groups" (Haney, 1994, p. 2). Because I am a White, single, middle-class, heterosexual, educated woman from the rural northeastern United States, born at the end of World War II to working-class parents, others view me in a particular way, while my own worldview is different from that of any other person. My skin color and current socioeconomic status privilege me in ways unavailable to my sisters of color or to those viewed as coming from a lower socioeconomic class.

A recent study by McMillan (2004) examined the academic behaviors of a group of "coloured" working-class women. She found that their identities, which were based on their social location, influenced their beliefs about their academic abilities and which they then allowed to limit their options. As these women conflated their race and class identities, "they associated this conflated social location with a lack of necessary resources, skills, and deportments to perform well" at their colleges (p. 118).

Social location produces subjectivity and influences construction of knowledge (Banks, 1996). People's understanding of the world is influenced by their intersections with race, class, gender, age, and sexual identity, as well as the sociocultural value placed on those characteristics. An example is feminist standpoint theory, which developed from the understanding that women, because of their social location within U.S. culture, understand and interpret their world in a particular way (Harding, 1991; Hekman, 1997). Harding (1991) points out, however, that instead of one "woman's way" of thinking and responding, contradictory

People's understanding of the world is influenced by their intersections with race, class, gender, age, and sexual identity.

social locations exist, for feminists in particular. Where women stand socioculturally determines the expectations for certain behaviors. Women traditionally have been relegated to an inferior place where excellence in thinking not only is not expected but also is often negated and punished in subtle ways. Harding notes that "a woman thinker is a contradiction in terms . . . bearing an identity or speaking from a social location that is perceived as a contradiction in terms can be a serious disadvantage within political, economic, and social structures" (p. 275). One would hope the notion that women do not engage in excellent thinking has been somewhat disabused during the past 15 years, but many occupational therapists have experienced this in their lives; as a female-dominated profession, occupational therapy has felt its effects as well.

Feminist standpoint theory may be a somewhat simplified way to examine the worldview of women because it seems to look at only the gender issue. In reality, everyone has multiple contextual cultural layers that influence the way one perceives the world. Collins (1991), for instance, does an excellent job explaining how African American feminist women think and experience their world, not only from a female standpoint but also from the experience of being African American in a racist society.

People's specific cultural characteristics elicit varying responses *from* and *of* the society in which they live. Although people can, and often do, change some aspects of their social location—such as geography, educational status, language, marital status, and sometimes class—other aspects, such as race, gender, sexual orientation or identity, age, and ability, are not so easily altered. These characteristics determine insider or outsider status within a society and culture.

Insider Status and Privilege as a Member of the Dominant Group

Being a member of the dominant sociocultural group also affords sociopolitical power and privilege. Power in this context is "the capacity to produce desired effects on others; it can be perceived in terms of mastery over self as well as over nature and other people" (Pinderhughes, 1989, p. 109). Sociopolitical power gives dominant group members not only mastery over self and others but also access to better jobs, education, housing, health care, and material goods. People can become decision-makers, participants, and policymakers in the dominant discourse of a society more easily.

Unearned Privilege

The dominant group affords members certain *unearned* privileges (Frankenberg, 1993; Haney, 1994; McIntosh, 1988). Unearned privilege, says Haney, includes "freedoms or other benefits given to us simply because we are White, heterosexual, or born into middle-strata economic and social location. Such unearned privilege allows us to generalize from our own experience, to assume that everyone else's is like ours" (p. 5). McIntosh (1988) compellingly writes about the privilege of being White:

> I have come to see White privilege as an invisible package of unearned assets which I can count on cashing in each day, but about which I was meant to remain oblivious. White privilege is like an invisible weightless knapsack of special provisions, assurances, tools, maps, guides, codebooks, passports, visa, clothes, compass, emergency gear, and blank checks. (pp. 1–2)

One amazing thing about being White or male, or possessing other characteristics of power or privilege, is that these characteristics often are invisible to those who have them. People who are White are taught not to see the mantle of privilege within which they are wrapped, reminiscent of the emperor and his new clothes. By not acknowledging these unearned privileges, White individuals and males can evade recognizing the power they represent and the responsibility that comes from that awareness (Frankenberg, 1993).

Those who do not share the privileges of the dominant group often are very aware of the differences in power and in access to goods and services. Sometimes these oppressive differences are readily apparent, as in the blatant racism that denies people of color access to good education and employment. More often, oppression or discrimination is subtle, affecting each person in ways apparent only to those slighted or misused. Shirley and I, for example, were walking in a well-known department store during one of my visits with her in Maryland, when we passed a cosmetic counter where foundation creams were displayed in various shades of beige and cream. When I recognized none of these creams matched the color of Shirley's skin, I commented on this and asked how she could stand it. She responded that it is frustrating and typical, and that she retaliates by never shopping in that particular store. This interaction clearly exemplifies the subtle yet clear discrimination Shirley faces as an African American woman and the privilege I enjoy as a White woman.

McIntosh (1988) identifies 46 ways in which she, as a White woman, benefits from skin color privilege that most people of color cannot count on, including the following:

- If I should need to move, I can be pretty sure of renting or purchasing housing in an area I can afford and in which I would want to live.
- I can go shopping alone most of the time, fairly well assured that I will not be followed or harassed.
- I can turn on the television or open to the front page of the paper and see people of my race widely represented.
- I can be sure that my children will be given curricular materials that testify to the existence of their race.
- I can do well in a challenging situation without being called a "credit to my race."
- I am never asked to speak for all people of my racial group.
- I can be pretty sure that if I ask to talk to the person in charge, I will be facing a person of my race.

Those who are White may consider few of these items relevant to their lives. Because White people have privileged status, they expect to be responded to in a particular way without even being aware of these expectations or the status associated with them. Most White Americans unconsciously expect that all people are treated as they are, but the previous list is a reminder that this is not the case.

Insider and Outsider Status

People assume they know things about groups different from their own based on what they may have learned from family, friends, the media, books, and formal education. But what they know, or what they think they know, may be only partial truths. Those in privileged groups often are seen as the *insiders,* whereas others are seen as *outsiders.* Merton (1972) used these terms while discussing the validity of group knowledge. He wrote that insiders claim their knowledge of the group is more valid because they understand the group's values, perspectives, and culture. Those who function outside the group, however, claim they have a more objective, and thus more valid, understanding. Both viewpoints are important when trying to understand a particular group: "The perspectives of both outsiders and insiders provide important insights into social reality. Our understanding of a group remains incomplete when the perspective of either the insider or the outsider is overlooked" (Banks, 1996, p. 8). Just as McIntosh (1988) had to consult with many of her friends of color to develop the list of privileges enjoyed by Whites, everyone must listen to both insider and outsider voices to understand the truth about any group of people.

The multilayered nature of people's lives ensures that many maintain both insider and outsider status concurrently because of their social location and the groups to which they belong. Despite the recognition and reality of male privilege in the United States, a study by Blank and Slipp (1994) found that many White men often believe they are powerless and vulnerable, just as the former occupational therapy student stated earlier in this chapter. Other examples of insider and outsider status include the young female engineer who may be considered a social insider because she is White but may experience outsider aspects in her field because of her gender and the Hispanic health care provider who might be considered an insider because of her position's authority but is once again reminded of her outsider status when a White client refuses her treatment. The constant fluctuation and negotiation between and within levels of sociocultural power complicates the concepts of privilege as well as insider and outsider status. Bias and discrimination hold these various levels in place.

Prejudice, Stereotyping, and Discrimination

One element that helps determine and maintain positions of power and status is prejudice. Prejudice is an erroneous judgment, usually negative, held against people based on incomplete or faulty information (Bennett, 1995). When used to label most or all members of a particular group, prejudice becomes a stereotype. Age prejudice, for example, leads one to stereotype all older people as frail and cranky, with nothing left to contribute to society.

No one is born with prejudicial thoughts, and most would choose not to be prejudiced. Prejudice is learned, however, and each of us is well taught. Although some people and groups are very clear about their negative beliefs about others, many others are unaware of their prejudices; they may not realize they hold members of a particular group in low esteem. They may not even be aware that prejudice is what disallows them to accept someone to their own insider status. Rothenberg (1998) defines *prejudice* as a

> General feeling of dislike for people, perhaps even hatred of them, on the basis of some characteristic they have or are believed to possess. Prejudice may be based on race, gender, or ethnicity; or on hair color, religion, or style of dress; or just about any imaginable characteristic. (p. 132).

Considering Rothenberg's (1998) definition, someone may be prejudiced about young men with long hair, men and women with tattoos, or people in wheelchairs. She differentiates between these kinds of prejudicial thoughts and those encompassed in racism or sexism, which require not prejudice alone but "prejudice plus power":

> When we use these terms rather than *prejudice* or *discrimination,* we highlight the unequal distribution of power in U.S. society and draw attention to the elaborate, interlocking system of rituals, stereotypes, institutions, punishments, and rewards that have functioned historically to reinforce *male privilege* and *White skin privilege.* (Rothenberg, p. 132, italics added)

I would suggest that prejudice, plus power, is seen not only with racism and sexism but also with heterosexism, classism, ageism, and ableism. The unequal distribution of power in the United States is apparent when one examines laws that do not support the safety of homosexuals or those who live in poverty and the lack of access to health care and productive work for older Americans and people with disabilities.

Young-Bruehl (1996, cited in Marsiglia & Hecht, 1998) recognizes not all prejudices are the same. She argues that "racism, anti-Semitism, sexism, and homophobia differ in their internal (il)logic; that is, although all expressions of prejudice are oppressive, they may differ in intensity and scope" (p. 290). That difference becomes clear when one hears and reads daily media reports about hate crimes perpetuated by White supremacist groups against African Americans, Jews, homosexuals, and immigrants.

Definition of Terms

Within multicultural literature, the terms *stereotype, prejudice,* and *discrimination* are used somewhat interchangeably when discussing sociocultural power. The simplest way to differentiate these terms is to recognize *prejudice* as preconceived ideas and attitudes—usually negative—about a particular group of people, often without full examination of the facts; *stereotype* is a particular belief about a person or members of a group that may or may not have some basis in fact; and *discrimination* is the overt action people take to exclude, avoid, or distance themselves from others (Hecht, 1998).

Stereotype

Stereotyping occurs when one sees a characteristic in one or a few members of a particular group and generalizes it to the entire group. Some common stereotypical statements include the following:

- All African Americans can dance.
- All Native Americans are alcoholics.
- Obese people are morally weak.
- All Jewish Americans are good with money management.
- All single mothers are on welfare.
- All White Americans are racist.
- Poor people do not want to improve their lot in life.
- All women are emotional.
- People in wheelchairs are powerless.
- All Asian Americans are smart and work hard.

These statements may be true for a few members in the identified groups, but by assuming all members of the groups carry these characteristics, one negates the individuality of each member, rendering them invisible.

Allport (1974, cited in Hecht, 1998) believes categorization is necessary to daily functioning because it enables people to react quickly to new, incoming stimuli. Knowing that White Americans are taught to shake hands when greeting one another, for example, enables a stranger to respond appropriately when first introduced. Allport suggests, however, that categorization done with stereotyping moves to overgeneralization, which actually can impede the process of encoding, storing, and retrieving information. If people expect an Asian woman to be shy and self-effacing, that is what they will see, even if the evidence is contrary. They then interact with this person based on what they expect to be true rather than on what the reality actually is, often resulting in what Neuberg (1991) and others refer to as a *self-fulfilling prophecy*. If someone is working with an Asian or Asian American woman in a therapeutic encounter, he or she may overlook a vital factor of her condition or belief system during assessment if he or she unwittingly stereotypes her and does not probe for important and necessary information.

Goldstein (1997) warns of the "powerful cognitive, affective, and behavioral impact of stereotypes on the perceiver as well as the target." (p. 256). Targets of stereotyping may alter their behavior in anticipation of being stereotyped, whereas those who stereotype will respond to people in a particular way because of their belief in the stereotype. If the stereotype is positive—all Asian Americans are good students, for example—positive behaviors may result. On the other hand, if the stereotype is negative—young Hispanic men are lazy—the stated "poor" behavior may strengthen.

Prejudice and Discrimination

Prejudice (one's attitude) and stereotyping (one's beliefs about a group) may lead to discrimination (overt action). Lott (1995, cited in Hecht, 1998) argues that, although prejudice and stereotyping are deplorable, discrimination is the social problem. Although people may have prejudicial thoughts, attitudes, and stereotypical beliefs (most raised in the United States do), it is only when they act on these that they see the evidence of sociopolitical power.

Discrimination occurs in many forms and at multiple levels. Although maintained through individual actions, discrimination is evident in national patterns of inequality and underrepresentation as well. Rothenberg (1998) identifies three levels of discrimination: individual, organizational, and structural.

At an individual or interindividual level (i.e., face to face), discrimination may be either *intentional* or *unintentional* and may not be motivated by conscious prejudice (Lott, 1995). Although some people are clearly aware of their prejudicial thoughts, others are not, nor would they wish to act in a discriminatory manner. They may perform acts of discrimination, however, because many people have not done much or any self-reflection about their attitudes and behaviors about intercultural interactions. These discriminatory acts "build on and support prejudicial stereotypes, deny their victim's opportunities provided to others, and perpetuate discrimination, regardless of intent" (Rothenberg, 1998, p. 137). The following are a few examples of *individual discrimination:*

- Personnel officers with stereotyped beliefs about women, minorities, and people with disabilities who justify hiring them for low-level and low-paying jobs exclusively, regardless of their potential, experience, or qualifications for high-level jobs.
- Teachers who interpret linguistic and cultural differences as indications of low potential or lack of academic interest on the part of minority students.
- Medical office receptionists who make lower income clients wait longer than paying clients, even when the lower income clients made appointments (Rothenberg, 1998).

Banks and Banks (1997) point out that individual prejudice and discrimination do not occur in only one direction, such as from Whites to African Americans, but often in all directions and even within groups. They believe, however, that as hurtful as individual discrimination can be, "it does not have the long-range and life-limiting effects of institutional [discrimination] and bias" (p. 392).

Institutional or *organizational discrimination* (Rothenberg, 1998) reinforces individual discrimination by instituting rules, policies, and practices that have an adverse effect on nondominant groups such as minorities, women, older people,

people with disabilities, and people with varying sexual identities. This type of discrimination includes

- Height and weight requirements that are unnecessarily geared to the physical proportions of White men, excluding women and some minorities from certain jobs;
- The use of standardized academic tests or criteria geared to the cultural and educational norms of middle-class Whites and that are not relevant indicators of successful academic or job performance;
- Preferences of many law and medical schools in admitting students who are children of wealthy and influential alumni, nearly all of whom are White Americans; and
- Questions about mental illness on a job application, which then affects the applicant's chance of being hired (Rothenberg, 1998).

Organizational discrimination often is not an act of conscious prejudice but is just considered the "normal way" things are done. It becomes part of the organizational climate. People, therefore, are unaware that the practices must be changed despite their discriminatory results, making organizational discrimination harder to change than individual discrimination.

Rothenberg (1998) calls the last level of discrimination *structural discrimination,* which occurs among the fields of employment, education, housing, and government. She describes a classic style of structural discrimination that reproduces itself in the following way:

Discrimination in education denies the credentials to get good jobs. Discrimination in employment denies the economic resources to buy good housing. Discrimination in housing confines minorities to school districts providing inferior education, closing the cycle in the classic form. (p. 140)

Structural discrimination is systemic, and the integration of all aspects of the system (employment, education, housing, and government) results in a lack of access to all for those discriminated against. The complexity of structural discrimination makes change very difficult.

Having an awareness of the prejudice that leads to the varying levels of discrimination is important, but this awareness must be coupled with the means to reduce or eradicate the prejudice altogether. Many people and groups are moved to action by using particular prejudice reduction strategies.

Prejudice Reduction Strategies

Vorauer and Turpie (2004) cited research that indicates engaging in unprejudiced behaviors is a skill individuals can improve on over time. The literature identifies many approaches to help reduce prejudicial attitudes as they relate to sociocultural issues, resulting in changes in behavior (Hill & Augoustinos, 2001; Kiselica & Maben, 1999; Levy, 1999; Zarate & Garza, 2002). Hecht (1998) identifies four locations where intervention to change behaviors can occur: (1) at the personal and interpersonal level, (2) within organizational structures, (3) through educational interventions, and (4) through changes in public policy. This chapter discusses interventions at the personal level and through educational methods.

At the personal level, some believe that if people have an opportunity to meet and work with others from different groups, their attitude toward those group members will shift. One of the earliest and most well-known theories that supports this idea is the *contact hypothesis,* developed by Allport (1954). This theory, now further developed and recognized as *social contact theory,* provides useful guidelines for developing more positive interracial attitudes and actions. It emphasizes the social situation and targets individual prejudicial attitude change. Allport believed that while contact between groups improves intergroup relations, the contact must be characterized by the following conditions:

1. Members of various groups must share equal status.
2. The contact situation should lead people to work cooperatively rather than in competition with one another.
3. Institutional sanction and support should come from authorities, such as teachers and administrators, or a social climate that encourages intergroup contact should exist.
4. Contact must be characterized by interpersonal interactions in which various group members become acquainted as individuals in such a way to produce reciprocal knowledge and understanding between groups (Banks & Banks, 1997; Bennett, 1995).

In addition to these four conditions, Cook (1978, cited in Wittig & Grant-Thompson, 1998) emphasized another condition: (5) The interaction must encourage behavior that disconfirms the stereotypes groups hold of each other.

One of Allport's most difficult conditions to establish is an equal-status environment for different racial groups. Within schools, where this theory mostly has been applied, major socioeconomic differences and differences in the initial achievement levels between Whites and other students of color often exist (Bennett, 1995). These discrepancies often are seen in higher education as well, even though socioeconomic differences are less pronounced.

Social contact theory has been extensively researched (McKown, 2005; Wittig & Grant-Thompson, 1998) and found to reduce prejudicial attitudes, but not without serious planning and commitment. Sutliff (1996) states

> Simply creating a group initiative or trust-building activity will not be
> enough to encourage prejudice reduction. The teacher must create an

environment conducive to social awareness and sensitivity. Without a climate of respect and openness that supports equal status, having contact with someone from a different cultural group may not reduce prejudice at all. (p. 158)

In the United States, prejudice reduction programs such as Teaching Tolerance, Days of Dialogue, Study Circles, and the National Coalition Building Institute have been used with promising results, as reported by the 1997–1998 Presidential Advisory Commission Race (Wittig & Grant-Thompson, 1998), but "most researchers acknowledge the need to employ multifaceted approaches in such efforts"(p. 796). McKown (2005) believes many of these programs are "narrowly focused short-term efforts . . . that have not had a lasting and pervasive impact" (p. 178). He proposes using ecological theory as a model for integrating three approaches toward prejudice reduction into a "coordinated theoretical system" (p. 178), which would have a greater effect than one approach. By targeting several levels of social prejudice at once, an approach to reduce prejudice can be developed to "fit a particular setting" (p. 186). He summarizes, "Ecological theory serves as a framework within which educators may select and implement multiple compatible prejudice-reduction intervention approaches, as fits the local context" (p. 188).

Summary

Bias, prejudicial attitudes, and discriminatory behaviors are part of the social structure of the United States. Power and privilege are awarded to members of the dominant sociocultural group by virtue of their race, ethnicity, class status, gender, sexual identity, and religion. Those who do not possess the valued characteristics of the dominant group often are not treated with equal respect, are stereotyped, and endure prejudice and discrimination. It is vital for health care practitioners to be aware of the differences in sociocultural power and that they interact with each person in their care in a fair and equal manner.

Equal-status environments are difficult to achieve in the health care setting. When the occupational therapy practitioner and his or her client come from different racial and ethnic groups and one is a White American, not only does inequality in the level of authority occur but also an unequal racial relationship. It is doubly challenging for practitioners to establish a more equitable climate when they must deal with multiple levels of hierarchy.

It is imperative that occupational therapy practitioners who strive to be culturally competent be aware of power issues within American society and know how those issues are reflected within each health care setting. White American practitioners must be sensitive to their own privileges and how they may influence client-centered interaction and rapport, especially if the client is not White. As part of cultural self-awareness development, everyone must evaluate his or her own values, beliefs, biases, and prejudices so that he or she never engages in discriminatory workplace practices. All people are responsible for working toward sociopolitical equality and justice within their professional and personal lives.

Reflection

1. Consider a time when you were discriminated against. What was this like for you?

    a. Share this experience with another student or colleague.

    b. Determine what societal values supported this discrimination.

    c. Share whether either of you have seen this kind of discrimination in school or in the workplace.

    d. Discuss how this behavior may affect clients in a health care institution.

2. Reflect on your own personal biases or stereotypes toward certain groups of people.

    a. Try to recall where you learned these.

    b. Have you ever discriminated against members of these groups based on your biases?

    c. Think about how these biases might affect your occupational therapy practice.

3. Consider your in-group or out-group status.

    a. Make a list of the groups and subgroups in which you have insider status.

    b. What are the privileges of that status?

    c. Identify any groups where you are an outsider but would like to be an insider.

    d. Why would you like to be a member of that group?

    e. Identify any benefits of being a group outsider.

References

Allport, G. W. (1954). *The nature of prejudice.* Reading, MA: Addison-Wesley.

Banks, J. A. (1996). *Multicultural education, transformative knowledge, and action.* New York: Teachers College.

Banks, J. A., & Banks, C. A. M. (1997). *Multicultural education: Issues and perspectives* (3rd ed.). Newton, MA: Allyn & Bacon.

Bennett, C. I. (1995). *Comprehensive multicultural education: Theory and practice* (3rd ed.). Newton, MA: Allyn & Bacon.

Blank, R., & Slipp, S. (1994). *Voices of diversity: Real people talk about problems and solutions in a workplace where everyone is not alike.* New York: American Management Association.

Collins, P. H. (1991). *Black feminist thought: Knowledge, consciousness, and the politics of empowerment.* Boston: Routledge & Kegan Paul.

Crepeau, E. B. (1994). *Uneasy alliances: Belief and action on a geropsychiatric team.* Unpublished doctoral dissertation, University of New Hampshire, Durham.

Delpit, L. (1988). The silenced dialogue: Power and pedagogy in educating other people's children. *Harvard Educational Review, 58,* 280–298.

Frankenberg, R. (1993). *White women, race matters: The social construction of Whiteness.* Minneapolis: University of Minnesota.

Goldstein, S. B. (1997). Methods and techniques. The power of stereotypes: A labeling exercise. *Teaching of Psychology, 24,* 256–258.

Haney, E. (1994). *Social location and alliance building.* Unpublished manuscript.

Harding, S. (1991). *Whose science? Whose knowledge? Thinking from women's lives.* Ithaca, NY: Cornell University.

Hecht, M. L. (1998). *Communicating prejudice.* Thousand Oaks, CA: Sage.

Hekman, S. (1997). Truth and method: Feminist standpoint theory revisited. *Signs: Journal of Women in Culture and Society, 22,* 341–365.

Hill, M. E., & Augoustinos, M. (2001). Stereotype change and prejudice reduction: Short- and long-term evaluation of a cross-cultural awareness programme. *Journal of Community and Applied Social Psychology, 11,* 243–262.

Ignatiev, N. (1995). *How the Irish became White.* New York: Routledge.

Kiselica, M. S. & Maben, P. (1999). Do multicultural education and diversity appreciation training reduce *prejudice* among counseling trainees? *Journal of Mental Health Counseling, 21,* 240–254.

Kronenberg, F., & Pollard, N. (2005). Overcoming occupational apartheid: A preliminary exploration of the political nature of occupational therapy. In F. Kronenberg, S. S. Algado, & N. Pollard (Eds.), *Occupational therapy without borders: Learning from the spirit of survivors* (pp. 58–86). Edinburgh, Scotland: Elsevier/Churchill Livingstone.

Kubiak, S. P. (2005). Trauma and cumulative adversity in women of a disadvantaged social location. *American Journal of Orthopsychiatry, 75,* 451–465.

Levy, S. R. (1999). Reducing prejudice: Lessons from social–cognitive factors underlying perceiver differences in prejudice. *Journal of Social Issues, 55,* 745–765.

Lott, B. (1995). Distance from women: Interpersonal sexist discrimination. In B. Lott & D. Maluso (Eds.), *The social psychology of interpersonal discrimination* (pp. 12–49). New York: Guilford.

MacKinnon, S., & Froehlich, J. (1994, January 6). Cultural diversity: Empowerment. Empowering others by empowering yourself. *OT Week,* pp. 18–19.

Marsiglia, F. F., & Hecht, M. (1998). Personal and interpersonal interventions. In M. L. Hecht (Ed.), *Communicating prejudice* (pp 287–301). Thousand Oaks, CA: Sage.

McIntosh, P. (1988). *White privilege and male privilege: A personal account of coming to see correspondences through work in women's studies* (Working Paper 189). Wellesley, MA: Wellesley College, Center for Research on Women.

McKown, C. (2005). Applying ecological theory to advance the science and practice of school-based prejudice reduction interventions. *Educational Psychologist, 40,* 177–189.

McMillan, W. (2004). "I could go work in a factory, but this is something I want to achieve:" Narratives into social action. *Race, Ethnicity, and Education, 7,* 115–134.

Merton, R. K. (1972). Insiders and outsiders: A chapter in the sociology of knowledge. *American Journal of Sociology, 78*(1), 9–47.

Neuberg, S. L. (1991). Expectancy-confirmation processes in stereotype-tinged social encounters: The moderating role of social goals. In M. P. Zanna & J. Olson (Eds.), *Ontario Symposium on Personality and Social Psychology, Volume 7: The psychology of prejudice* (pp. 103–130). Hillsdale, NJ: Lawrence Erlbaum.

Omi, M., Winant, H. A., & Winant, H. (1994). *Racial formation in the United States: From the 1960s to the 1990s.* London: Routledge.

Pinderhughes, E. (1989). *Understanding race, ethnicity, and power: The key to efficacy in clinical practice.* New York: Free Press.

Rothenberg, P. S. (1998). *Race, class, and gender in the United States: An integrated study* (4th ed.). New York: St. Martin's Press.

Sutliff, M. (1996). Multicultural education for Native American students in physical education. *Physical Educator, 53,* 157–163.

Tai, R. H., & Kenyatta, M. (1999). *Critical ethnicity: Countering the waves of identity politics.* Lanham, MD: Rowman & Littlefield.

Townsend, E., & Whiteford, G. (2005). A participatory occupational justice framework. In F. Kronenberg, S. S. Algado, & N. Pollard (Eds.), *Occupational therapy without borders: Learning from the spirit of survivors* (pp. 110–126). Edinburgh, Scotland: Elsevier/ Churchill Livingstone.

Vorauer, J. D., & Turpie, C. A. (2004). Disruptive effects of vigilance on dominant group members' treatment of outgroup members: Choking versus shining under pressure. *Journal of Personality and Social Psychology, 87,* 384–399.

Wittig, M. A., & Grant-Thompson, S. (1998). The utility of Allport's intergroup contact for predicting perceptions of improved racial attitudes and beliefs [Electronic version]. *Journal of Social Issues, 54,* 795–812.

Zarate, M. A., & Garza, A. A. (2002). In-group distinctiveness and self-affirmation as dual components of prejudice reduction. *Self and Identity, 1,* 235–242.

7

The Challenge of Being White

Whiteness is a problem to be investigated and confronted.

—ROEDIGER (2006, P. B8)

Key Points

- Whiteness is socially constructed and must be examined.
- Being White often results in a kind of cultural blindness, which becomes a barrier to cultural self-awareness.
- Unexamined Whiteness becomes a barrier for effective cross-cultural interactions, often resulting in denial, hostility, fear of diversity, and the choice to remain unaware.
- White practitioners must engage in cultural self-exploration and the development of cultural skills to provide culturally competent care.
- Effective White occupational therapy educators of diversity share several positive characteristics.

LIKE THE MAJORITY OF OCCUPATIONAL THERAPY PRACTITIONERS in the United States, I am a White (Caucasian) woman, although I do have Native American ancestry. It is vital to consider the effect Whiteness has on cross-cultural interactions because the occupational therapy profession historically has been, and currently still is, composed predominantly of White women. If practitioners are truly to become culturally self-aware, then they must recognize the power and privilege inherent within the color of their skin and how it may affect others not so privileged. Most people never have had to examine the concept of Whiteness or think about their skin color because they live in a society where they are part of the dominant group. This lack of awareness becomes challenging in cross-cultural interactions.

White Social Identity

In today's literature, an interdisciplinary interest in examining Whiteness as a social construct is increasing (Nakayama & Martin, 1999; Roediger, 2006). As a result, the invisibility of Whiteness is shifting, and White racial identity is becoming more apparent and recognized. Nakayama and Martin (1999) argue that Whiteness is best understood "as a communication phenomenon" (p. viii). In this chapter, the connection between Whiteness and communication is examined.

Although the preceding chapter discusses the privileges and benefits White Americans are given solely because of their skin color, challenges and problems are inherent within these benefits, especially when one considers becoming culturally competent. Much of the earlier work on race relations and multicultural theory has focused on understanding the lives and cultural experiences of nondominant groups, including African Americans, Hispanics, Asians, and Native Americans (Howard, 1993). "Studies of racial and cultural identities have tended to view the range of potential subjects of research as limited to those who differ from the (unnamed) norm" (Frankenberg, 1993, p. 17). For decades, White Americans have been allies with oppressed groups and have worked for, written about, and spoken up for social justice. Yet little of the rhetoric actually had examined what it meant to be White.

Only recently (within the past 15 years) have White American authors focused on Whiteness as a racial category or written about White racial identity. McLaren (1997), in an extensive and in-depth sociopolitical analysis, states that *Whiteness* became racialized from the mid-1700s to early 1800s, after racism was established in the United States. By the early 1860s, "Whiteness had become a marker for measuring inferior and superior races" (p. 259). Today, the broadened concept of Whiteness as a cultural construct "constitutes and demarcates ideas, feelings, knowledge, social practices, cultural formations, and systems of intelligibility that are identified with or attributed to White people and that are invested in by White people as White" (p. 267). In simpler terms, the social construct of Whiteness connotes superiority. It is an elitist category. As such, the concept of Whiteness "not only allows millions of non-whites to fall through the cracks, but also millions of whites—men, women, and children [who may be poor, disabled, or otherwise disadvantaged] as well" (Wander, Martin, & Nakayama, 1999, p. 21). Because of this well-established and accepted, albeit invisible, societal worldview in the United States, most people who are not White are disempowered and disadvantaged, as are Whites who do not fit the elitist social construct.

Inherent Challenges in Whiteness

One might ask, if Whiteness is identified as privileged, where then is the challenge? McIntosh (1988) characterizes Whiteness within American culture as coming with an "invisible knapsack of unearned privilege" (p. 11). What she means is that as a privileged, dominant group, White Americans have not had to examine or think about what it means to be White. White just is! It is the standard by which others are measured. The privileges are generally invisible to White Americans, who have numerous expectations, some of which McIntosh delineates (see Chapter 6).

The invisibility of Whiteness is so complete that people rarely use it as an adjective to describe a specific person or group. One rarely hears: *the White teacher* or *White doctor* or *White lawyer,* because White people are the expected standard—the dominant group in society. On the other hand, roles held by other group members described by their race or ethnicity are common: the *Black professor, the Mexican banker,* or *the Chinese lawyer,* indicating that person is not White.

To become culturally competent and have a better understanding of themselves and their values and beliefs, White American occupational therapists also must examine what it means to be White. It is imperative for those who are White to be aware not only of the power and authority they are given by virtue of their positions as health care professionals but also the inherent power and privilege they have simply because of the color of their skin. Herein lies the challenge.

Unexamined Whiteness is maintained partly by the emotion elicited when White Americans begin to evaluate what being White means in the sociopolitical reality of the United States. When discussing racism or multiculturalism, an examination of the privilege and power often brings feelings of guilt, shame, embarrassment, and hopelessness, which often lead to fear, anger, defensiveness, or confusion (Kivel, 1996). *White guilt* often is a byproduct of this examination (Holzman, 1995).

White Guilt

Essayist and culture critic Shelby Steele has written quite extensively about White guilt (1990, 1998/1999, 2002, 2003). He (1990) believes "white guilt, in its broad sense, springs from a knowledge of ill gotten advantage. More precisely, it comes from the juxtaposition of this knowledge with the inevitable gratitude one feels for being white rather than black in America" (p. 499). From his African American per-spective, Steele's contention is that awareness of White people's subjugation of an entire race leads to a sense of guilt and fear, "the fear of what the guilty knowledge says about us" (p. 501).

Steele (2003) insists White guilt has given Blacks an advantage, allowing them to develop a different kind of identity than that of the 1960s and earlier, when racism was more prevalent. Steele (1990) believes White guilt also has changed social policy. His writing gives African Americans a fascinating point of view on the consequences of White guilt.

Within my experience and perspective, I have witnessed White Americans become somewhat paralyzed by feelings of White guilt. As people begin the work of cultural self-analysis and recognize that Whites have oppressed people in other groups, they often experience shame and embarrassment. This phenomenon seems to be natural in this work. Instead of moving on to positively resolve these feelings, however, some people seem to get stuck. They remain apologetic and may feel remorse for oppressed groups but never become agents of social change themselves.

In a culture that extols the virtues of strength, confidence, and rational think-ing, a sense of vulnerability and discomfiture results from these feelings. These reac-tions are expected of those seen as the dominant and most powerful individuals in a society. It is important, at this point, to remember Kivel's words (1996):

> There's absolutely nothing wrong with being White or with noticing the difference that color makes. We were born without choice into our families. We did not choose our skin color, native language or culture. We are not responsible for being White or being raised in a White-dominated, racist society in which we have been trained to have particular responses to persons of color. We are responsible to how we respond to racism . . . and we can only do that consciously and effectively if we start by realizing that it makes a crucial difference that we are White. (p. 14)

As Kivel reminds readers, they are responsible for their actions, not their thoughts or what they've been taught. Occupational therapists know the importance of action, of doing. So, how do they tend to respond in cross-cultural situations? This is another challenge of Whiteness.

Typical Responses of Whites in Cross-Cultural Interactions

Unfortunately, White Americans do not always respond to racism or oppression in responsible ways. As people learn about the sociopolitical power of Whiteness, new information challenges feelings of security, pride, and satisfaction and shifts the real-ity of who they think they are. This shift results in what Howard (1993) describes as a classic state of *cognitive dissonance* (p. 38). Combined with the emotions listed above, cognitive dissonance often is hard to bear. One way many White Americans deal with it is by choosing to remain unaware. Howard (1993) reports this luxury of ignorance is available only to members of the dominant group. He states, "throughout most of history, there has been no reason why White Americans, for their own survival or success, have needed to be sensitive to the cultural perspectives of other groups" (p. 41). If someone is African American, Hispanic, Native American, Asian, or from any other non-White ethnicity, his or her success and daily survival depends on knowing the expectations and behaviors of the White American community.

Another strategy many White Americans adopt in dealing with the realities of the country's oppressive history is *denial.* By denying the reality of White privilege, discrimination, or inequitable resources or access for minority groups, people can abdicate any responsibility for changing the social injustices that occur. While maintaining this blindness, White Americans can avoid eye contact with the panhandler on the street, refuse to acknowledge racial discrimination in public school classrooms (Kozol, 1991), and choose not to see the poverty and lack of access to health care and other health disparities for many nondominant people.

Along with denial, Howard (1993) identifies two "emotions that kill": *hostility* and *fear of diversity* (p. 37). The move from blatant hostility to violent action is apparent every day in the media and on the streets in reports about the murder of Matthew Shepard, a gay man in Wyoming (Loffreda, 2001); the beating of Rodney King, an African American man in Los Angeles (Jacobs, 1996); the murder of Alan Berg, a Jewish talk show host by a neo-Nazi group in Denver (Singular, 1989); and increased racial incidents and hate crimes on college campuses.

Howard (1993) believes fear of diversity underlies the denial and hostility of many White Americans. Historically, people often have feared those who are different from them. Fear often turns to hatred—the kind of hatred apparent in White supremacist groups, like the one that went to Lewiston, Maine, to terrorize a Somali community (Hamzeh, 2003). Fear also comes from ignorance—an ignorance supported by lack of information and education

> *Historically, people often have feared those who are different from them.*

about diverse groups in society and ignorance kept in place by dominant groups that fear a loss of sociopolitical power and control.

For White occupational therapists working with diverse groups of people, denial, hostility, and fear of diversity have no place. Rather, a knowledge of self, including an awareness and understanding of the power and reality of Whiteness, an openness to and respect for difference that leads to knowledge about groups different from one's own, and a commitment to providing equitable and just care to all people is what all occupational therapists must strive for.

Considerations for a White Practitioner

What must White American occupational therapists and occupational therapy assistants know in their practice? There are many things to consider. First, although the demographics of the United States are changing rapidly, the majority of the workforce in the major health professions remains White. Because Whites will undoubtedly continue to dominate medicine and allied health for the near future, policies and practices will continue to reflect this group's attitudes, language, expectations, and other values and beliefs. This trend, in turn, will decrease representation for the growing numbers of non-White clients, automatically placing non-majority groups and people in vulnerable and unequal power positions, simply because of their race or ethnicity.

Additionally, occupational therapy practitioners are in an authoritative position because of their role in the client–practitioner dyad. Clients are in a vulnerable state—physically, emotionally, and socially—and they depend on their health care provider to treat them effectively and fairly. Most do. The experience of being a non-White client, however, places that person in a double-jeopardy situation that often disempowers him or her much more than a White client. It then becomes the responsibility of the practitioner to try to lessen this power inequity as much as possible within the context of the health care system. Practitioners can do this by striving for and achieving an attitude of acceptance and developing skills that demonstrate it.

An accepting attitude is based on honesty, humility, and respect. Howard (1993) believes that White Americans must face the fact that they have benefited from racism and that they are given sociocultural privileges as a result. Within a client–practitioner relationship, honesty is enhanced when the White practitioner examines his or her beliefs and values and determines whether he or she harbors biases or prejudices that would affect the care offered the client:

> Awareness of one's attitudes and behavior becomes a critical component of preparation to remove barriers for effective cross-cultural interaction. Such awareness means identifying distortions born of cultural indoctrination as well as psychological need, and it requires an in-depth understanding of one's own cultural background and its meaning. (Pinderhughes, 1989, p. 20)

If cultural differences exist between client and practitioner, an honest attempt to learn more about the client's culture and beliefs will help develop trust and rapport, facilitate client-centered care, and reduce potential cultural misunderstandings and mistakes.

Humility, or giving up one's power and humbly admitting the need for additional knowledge about a client's cultural background, also is necessary for White practitioners. In a client-centered approach to intervention, the occupational therapist must recognize the client's uniqueness and work collaboratively with that person and family to develop goals and an intervention plan. To do this process effectively, knowledge must be shared about the client's desires, as well as beliefs about illness, wellness, therapeutic care, and independence. These beliefs are grounded in one's culture.

Respect for each individual client provides the foundation for honest and humble interactions. "One of the greatest contributions White Americans can make to cultural understanding is simply to learn the power of respect" (Howard, 1993, pp. 39–40). Respecting each client's dignity and uniqueness is a necessary attitude for the culturally competent practitioner. Without respect, no mutuality or social equality can occur within the client–practitioner relationship. White practitioners must practice additional skills to be effective within a diverse environment. Although not exhaustive, the list in Exhibit 7.1 is a place to begin.

In conclusion, being a White American occupational therapist or occupational therapy assistant is a privilege and a challenge. To be an effective and culturally competent practitioner, one must have an awareness of self, of one's beliefs and attitudes, and an understanding of the inherent power within the whiteness of one's skin. Additionally, the White practitioner has a responsibility to develop the attitudes and skills necessary to competently and effectively establish rapport and trust within a cross-cultural client–practitioner relationship. It is vital to "know how to manage the dynamics of race, ethnicity, and power in ways that celebrate the differences among people, while also promoting mutual understanding, empathy, and respect" (Pinderhughes, 1989, p. 210).

White Teachers Teaching About Diversity

Considerations of Whiteness also must take place in occupational therapy academic programs. Can a White teacher teach about diversity? The answer often is an enthusiastic "Of course! Good teachers can teach about anything." But any White teacher sensitive to diversity issues and aware of the power of Whiteness often questions his or her ability to present these concepts effectively and with an awareness

---

Exhibit 7.1. Skills for the White American Practitioner

- Use inclusive language
- Make no assumptions about a person
- Ask culturally inquisitive questions
- Listen well
- If there is a language barrier, seek a translator
- Learn about the client's culture
- Explain what you are doing and why
- Engage the client's family if appropriate for the culture
- Approach each client with openness and willingness to learn

and appropriate use of power supporting the empowerment of all students (Kivel, 1996; McLaren, 1998; Paley, 1989; Sleeter, 1995). Many White teachers of diversity issues question their ability to teach students how to critically analyze the power structure of White America; they not only are a part of that structure and benefit from it but also benefit from the authoritative and powerful position of teacher. They face a conundrum, and their concerns echo those of Kivel (1996):

> People of color have addressed all the issues much more powerfully than I could. I would make mistakes. I would leave important pieces out. People of color would be angry with me. Other White people would call me racist. People would expect me to have all the answers. The entire task felt formidable, scary, fraught with problems, and I felt ill-equipped to carry it out successfully. (pp. xi–xii)

So, what can a teacher do? First, White American occupational therapy faculty members must continue to teach about diversity simply because there are more of them than non-White colleagues to do so. With far greater numbers of White teachers in occupational therapy educational programs and the Accreditation Council in Occupational Therapy Education's (2007) mandate that culture and diversity issues be included in curricula, more White teachers will be teaching about diversity than will non-Whites.

Additionally, many White teachers are sincerely interested in becoming culturally competent and facilitating students toward cultural competence. Sensitive, knowledgeable, and skilled White teachers make excellent allies for those who are non-White. If there is interest and knowledge, there also is a responsibility to make a difference. A quote by Rabbi Tarfon (cited in Kivel, 1996) supports this: "It is not upon you to finish the work. Neither are you free to desist from it" (p. xii). Educators cannot ignore this issue because they feel unprepared or uncomfortable with it.

White American teachers are responsible for presenting an inclusive and multicultural curriculum to all students. If they are concerned that they do not have enough knowledge, then it is imperative they obtain it. Many references and resources in this book provide a place to begin. Another approach to meeting the need for more knowledgeable professors to teach diversity issues is to identify one faculty member from each occupational therapy program who has an interest in this area. The program must then support that person through allocation of funding and time to increase his or her knowledge and share that knowledge with colleagues and students.

There are multiple ways to present this kind of information in an academic setting, many of which are described in Chapter 18. The attitude of the White teacher, however, will determine the success of any of the approaches used. The following section is a list of important characteristics for teachers to effectively do this work (also see Exhibit 7.2).

Exhibit 7.2. Characteristics of a Teacher of Diversity

- Courage
- Humility
- Open-mindedness
- Capacity to deal with emotions
- Introspection
- Hunger for knowledge

1. *Courage.* As mentioned earlier, White American teachers of diversity issues often are concerned about whether they can be effective. It takes courage to put one's self in a situation where one feels vulnerable. Yet, teachers must take a bold stance to be successful. They must be willing to make mistakes, offer unpopular theories and ideas, sometimes say the wrong thing, and become co-learners in the classroom. This stance means giving up some of their authority, which may be difficult for some faculty members, particularly those who are not confident in their role as educator.

2. *Humility.* Giving up one's power results in humility (Howard, 1993). White American teachers must be aware of the unearned power of Whiteness and its effect on non-Whites. They must be willing to share authority with their students. Shor (1992) discusses a student-centered approach he calls *democratic authority,* where students collaborate with teachers in the teaching and learning process. To listen well and be willing to learn from students, a teacher must approach the classroom with humility.

3. *Open-mindedness.* Although giving up the ethnocentric beliefs and ideas of being White is difficult, White American teachers of diversity issues must be willing to hear comments and ideas from people different from them, to honestly believe they can learn from others, and to know that different perspectives have value. Being open-minded may result in students and faculty questioning many of the assumptions, beliefs, attitudes, and behaviors of American society previously accepted without critique. That, in turn, may result in cognitive dissonance, as described by Howard (1993).

4. *Capacity to deal with emotions.* Teaching about issues of diversity rarely is objective. Students often have strong and sometimes unexamined feelings about the issues raised. Excitement, passion, fear, and sadness are not uncommon in these classrooms. I agree with bell hooks (1994), who states, "If we focus not just on whether the emotions produce pleasure or pain, but on how they keep us aware or alert, we are reminded that they enhance classrooms" (p. 155). Diversity classrooms are engaging and alive. A faculty member must be comfortable with and skilled in handling the energy often elicited during these discussions. He or she must be able to create a climate of trust.

5. *Introspection.* Developing a multicultural, empowering classroom and dealing with the emotional topics of diversity may raise personal responses
from the faculty member. It is important for the teacher to be skilled in self-
awareness and be honest about his or her responses to the classroom's emotional climate. Hidalgo (1993) believes teachers must explore how their
own cultural perspectives shape their thinking and actions, beginning this
process by "specific introspective information gathering" (p. 101).
Introspection, therefore, is a process that happens before developing a curriculum on diversity and during the process of teaching as emotions
become evident.

6. *Hunger for knowledge.* Information on diversity and culture is a burgeon-
ing, interdisciplinary body of knowledge found in feminist, multicultural,
and critical pedagogy literature as well as in the literature on cultural studies, communication ethics, language, literacy, and more. Reading it all is
impossible, yet the more the White teacher reads from a variety of sources,
the more he or she begins to comprehend the thinking around the issues.
Information and knowledge also can be gathered by meeting, visiting, talking with, and interviewing non-Whites; watching documentaries and other
video and film presentations; attending conferences; doing research; and
discussing the issues with colleagues, friends, and family members. The
teacher of diversity always must be a student of diversity.

Many other characteristics can be included in this list but, for the purposes of
this book, these six become the foundation on which others can be added. Being an
effective White occupational therapy educator of diversity is challenging, but it is
also exciting and invigorating, bringing a fresh, new perspective to both the educator and the education of occupational therapy students.

Summary

Most White Americans in the United States have high sociocultural status based on
their skin color, resulting in unearned privilege and easier access to things that are
desired and needed in life. This elevated status also results in challenges. Because of
the dominance of White American, middle-class culture in the United States, White
occupational therapy practitioners and educators must recognize the differences in
sociocultural status among various people and be sensitive to the privileges they
possess. To provide culturally competent care, they must examine what it means to
be a White American.

As practitioners and educators, White occupational therapists and occupational therapy assistants must develop characteristics and skills that enable them to
be effective in the workplace with all clients and students. Cultural competency
requires all practitioners know themselves; learn about and respect others who are
different from them; and develop skills for effective, intercultural communication.

This process is a lifelong one for most, and especially challenging for those who experience the privilege of being a White American.

Reflection

1. Consider the color of your skin.

    a. How is your skin color or tone an advantage or disadvantage to you in U.S. society?

    b. List specific instances of the previous question.

    c. Have you ever tried to change your skin tone by darkening or lightening it? Why?

    d. Do you like the color of your skin? Why or why not?

2. Read Peggy McIntosh's (1988) *White Privilege, Male Privilege* (found in the working papers from the Wellesley Center for Research on Women, Wellesley, MA).

    a. Do you believe all the instances she mentions? Why or why not?

    b. Have you experienced them in any way?

    c. Can you add to her list from the list you made above?

    d. Can you add to your own list from McIntosh's?

3. Consider the following:

    a. How does skin color or tone influence how clients are treated within a health care setting?

    b. Describe any instances of the above that you have witnessed or heard about.

    c. Are you affected by any other skin tone or color?

    d. How will this affect your practice?

References

Accreditation Council for Occupational Therapy Education. (2007). Accreditation Council for Occupational Therapy Education (ACOTE) standards and interpretive guidelines. *American Journal of Occupational Therapy, 61.*

Frankenberg, R. (1993). *White women, race matters: The social construction of whiteness.* Minneapolis: University of Minnesota Press.

Hamzeh, Z. H. (Writer/Director). (2003). *The letter: An American town and the "Somali invasion."* [Documentary film]. Swampscott, MA: Hamzeh Mystique Films.

Hidalgo, N. M. (1993). Multicultural teacher introspection. In T. Perry & J. W. Fraser (Eds.), *Freedom's plow: Teaching in the multicultural classroom* (pp. 99–108). Boston: Routledge & Kegan Paul.

Holzman, C. (1995). Rethinking the role of guilt and shame on White women's anti-racism work. In G. M. Enguidanos & J. Adleman (Eds.), *Racism in the lives of women: Testimony, theory, and guides to antiracist practices* (pp. 325–347). New York: Harrington Park.

hooks, b. (1994). *Teaching to transgress: Education as the practice of freedom.* New York: Routledge.

Howard, G. (1993, September). Whites in multicultural education: Rethinking our role. *Phi Delta Kappan, 75*(1), 36–41.

Jacobs, R. N. (1996). Civil society and crisis: Culture, discourse, and the Rodney King beating. *American Journal of Sociology, 101,* 1238–1272.

Kivel, P. (1996). *Uprooting racism: How White people can work for racial justice.* Philadelphia: New Society.

Kozol, J. (1991). *Savage inequalities: Children in America's schools.* New York: Harper Perennial.

Loffreda, B. (2001). *Losing Matt Shepard: Life and politics in the aftermath of anti-gay murder.* New York: Columbia University Press.

McIntosh, P. (1988). *White privilege and male privilege: A personal account of coming to see correspondences through work in women's studies* (Working Paper 189). Wellesley, MA: Wellesley College Center for Research on Women.

McLaren, P. (1997). *Revolutionary multiculturalism: Pedagogues of dissent for the new millennium.* Boulder, CO: Westview.

McLaren, P. (1998). *Life in schools: An introduction to critical pedagogy in the foundations of education* (3rd ed.). White Plains, NY: Longman.

Nakayama, T. K., & Martin, J. N. (Eds.). (1999). *Whiteness: The communication of social identity.* Thousand Oaks, CA: Sage.

Paley, V. G. (1989). *White teacher.* Cambridge, MA: Harvard University.

Pinderhughes, E. (1989). *Understanding race, ethnicity, and power: The key to efficacy in clinical practice.* New York: Free Press.

Roediger, D. R. (2006, July 14). Whiteness and its complications. *Chronicle of Higher Education 52*(45), B6–B8.

Shor, I. (1992). *Empowering education: Critical teaching for social change.* Chicago: University of Chicago.

Singular, S. (1989). *Talked to death: The murder of Alan Berg and the rise of the neo-Nazis.* New York: Berkeley.

Sleeter, C. (1995). Reflections on my use of multicultural and critical pedagogy when students are white. In C. E. Sleeter & P. L. McLaren (Eds.), *Multicultural education, critical pedagogy, and the politics of difference* (pp. 415–434). Albany: State University of New York.

Steele, S. (1990). White guilt. *American Scholar, 59,* 497–506.

Steele, S. (1998/1999). The culture of deference. *Academic Questions, 12*(1), 54–62.

Steele, S. (2002, November). The age of white guilt. *Harper's Magazine,* pp. 33–42.

Steele, S. (2003, July–August). Word for word: The age of white guilt and the disappearance of the black individual. *About Campus, 8*(3), 3–6.

Wander, P. C., Martin, J. N., & Nakayama, T. K. (1999). Whiteness and beyond: Sociohistorical foundations of whiteness and contemporary challenges. In T. K. Nakayama & J. N. Martin (Eds.), *Whiteness: The communication of social identity* (pp. 13–26). Thousand Oaks, CA: Sage.

8

Professional Power

The power and lack of power inherent in the roles of clinician and client and in their cultural group status can affect clinical process and outcome. Practitioners need to understand how these two dimensions of power can affect their clients, themselves, and their work together.

—PINDERHUGHES (1989, P. 109)

Key Points

- Each person is imbued with personal power.

- Occupational therapy practitioners and educators have professional power.

- An aspect of self-awareness is the consciousness that occupational therapists hold power over their clients.

- Many people with whom occupational therapists work struggle with a sense of powerlessness.

- Occupational therapists strive to empower the people with whom they work.

- Participatory power may be the highest form of empowerment that occupational therapists can help clients achieve.

- Participatory power supports client-centered practice and occupational justice.

THE COMPLEXITY OF CULTURAL SELF-AWARENESS spans the awareness and knowledge of not only personal beliefs and values and how these affect the way people view their world but also how people sees themselves as members of subgroups, including their professional selves. Everyone is imbued with some level of personal power. Additionally, occupational therapy practitioners have earned a certain degree of authority. With authority comes power. This chapter begins by looking at the concept of personal power. It then explores the culture of professionalism and the inherent power associated with having professional status, as well as its possible effect on therapeutic relationships that occupational therapists have with their clients. The chapter ends with the participatory power model as a possible approach for practitioner–recipient interaction.

Personal Power

Driscoll (1994) believes that to be successful in a profession, people must "make a name for themselves" (p. 46), and they cannot do that unless they have a certain level of personal power, which she calls *personal currency.* She speaks specifically of women and believes that personal currency "includes three factors working together: physical demeanor and presence, a persuasive communication style, and a strategic understanding of how to work with the media to achieve specific goals"(p. 46). In reading this article, one must consider the context: A business woman has written it for women in business, a profession that demands high performance and competition—a traditionally male realm. Practitioners in occupational therapy, a traditionally female, caring profession, may look at personal power in a different way.

Glasser's (1984) definition of *personal power* is preferable: "[Personal] power is the need to feel good about ourselves, to believe that we matter and that we have worth and recognition in the eyes of others" (cited in Litwack, 2004, p. 52). This internalized awareness moves a person to feel empowered by "discover[ing] how power operates his [or her] life and then tak[ing] reasonable steps to seize upon personal power and channel it in constructive ways" (Lee, 2005, p. 393). A sense of positive personal power is an awareness of agency, that one can make choices that make a difference in one's life. Occupational therapy students, practitioners, and educators experience this sense of power and agency when they choose occupational therapy as a profession, enroll in an academic program, and successfully graduate.

Some believe power is a basic drive and that the "push to exert power is wired in, instinctual" (Person, 2004, p. 64). Most people learn this sense of control and agency very early in life as they learn that a cry, a request, or a pointing finger can result in receiving what they want and need. Watch a young child constantly practicing standing and walking, determined after numerous falls and tumbles, to successfully walk two steps to her parent. That wondrous and satisfied look on the child's face reflects power. It is the look of "I did it! I can do it!" Pinderhughes (1989) states, "A sense of power is critical to one's mental health. Everyone needs it" (p. 110).

Powerlessness

The opposite of personal power is a sense of *powerlessness.* Readers may have felt at some point in their lives that, no matter what they did, their actions didn't make a difference. Many have experienced this feeling but have managed somehow to get through this tough period, either by their own intrinsic sense of worth or from external support from others. The fact that people are able to move beyond this gives them a heightened sense of personal power. But some people, including a percentage of those with whom occupational therapists work, rarely have the opportunity to feel this way. They may have been unloved or abandoned or—because of poverty, oppression, disease, or other sociocultural or health issues—have never developed a full sense of personal power and agency or have lost what they had developed. Kronenberg and Pollard (2005) suggest that *occupational apartheid*—the systematized segregation of groups of people from meaningful occupations—also contributes to a sense of meaninglessness and powerlessness.

Pinderhughes (1989) states that people who feel powerless will discover and develop strategies that will somehow help neutralize the pain associated with this feeling and help them "turn that powerlessness into a sense of power" (p. 124). She identifies several possible strategies, including
- Developing personal mastery through achievement;
- Making themselves feel better by perceiving that they are better than others;
- Inspiring fear;
- Manipulating people and the environment;
- Engaging in self-destructive behavior to get attention and to get others to take responsibility for them by setting limits and nurturing them;
- Responding with withdrawal and evasiveness;
- Accepting the reality of one's powerless position and developing negative behaviors, such as being passive–aggressive, negativistic, or using oppositional behaviors.

Many with whom occupational therapists work feel powerless and vulnerable because of their health condition or status and may respond in one or more of these ways. If they also are part of the nondominant culture, they experience a kind of double jeopardy, which may increase their perception of powerlessness. As health and human services practitioners, occupational therapists generally try to help their clients meet the first bullet above: develop personal mastery through achievement. If a practitioner comes from a privileged background, however, and experiences the power inherent within that privilege, that person may lack the ability to work effectively with clients who seem powerless to them. Pinderhughes (1989) suggests privilege can distance therapists from their clients. Professional power also can achieve this same result, especially if one is unaware of it. Thus, recognizing the power from being part of a professional group and understanding the effect it may have on relationships with clients is important.

Professional Power

What Is a *Profession?*

To understand occupational therapy professionals and what professional power might mean to them, it is important to understand the meaning of a *profession.* That, however, is not an easy task. In today's world, many people call themselves *professionals.* People not only refer to doctors, health care workers, lawyers, and teachers as professionals, but they also refer to the "professional wrestler," "professional artist," and even "professional streetwalker!" So, what distinguishes a professional from a *nonprofessional,* or has the term itself, which Bell describes as a "muddled concept" (as cited in Freidson, 1986, p. 41), become rather meaningless?

In years past, a *trait approach* was used to attempt to isolate distinguishing characteristics of professional work, but several authors suggest this approach is no longer satisfactory (Curry, Wergin, & Associates, 1993; Wilding, 1982). Yet definitions that include agreed-upon characteristics are found in the literature. Some of these definitions of a profession include the following:
- "An occupation which has assumed a dominant position in a division of labor so that it gains control over the determination of the substance of its own work" (Wilding, 1982, p. 5)
- "An occupation with prestige attached to it due to its formal knowledge" (Freidson, 1986, p. 34)
- "An occupation that regulates itself through systematic, required training and collegial discipline; that has a base in technological, specialized knowledge; and that has a service, rather than a profit orientation enshrined in its code of ethics" (Starr, 1982, as cited in Curry et al., 1993, pp. 5–6).

Occupational therapy certainly fits these descriptions. The profession has systematic and required training that is overseen by the Accreditation Council for Occupational Therapy Education (2007), which writes the standards for occupational therapy educational programs for the field to maintain specialized knowledge and quality of education. Additionally, service to others is written within the *Occupational Therapy Code of Ethics,* created by the American Occupational Therapy Association (2005).

Wilding (1982) states that what professions want most are autonomy and control of their own work, which he suggests "results in the exclusion of others, control of entry, and licensing of members" (p. 15). Again, occupational therapy can be recognized in these comments, as well. Wilding goes on to say that

> Professions claim to have expertise which can be used to solve or alleviate situations agreed to be social problems and the claim is accepted. The professions' good faith is accepted too, and so they are given power to tackle the problems in the way they think best. (p. 15)

He feels this is a way of gaining and justifying power and privilege. What, then, does professional power look like, and how might it affect therapeutic relationships?

Inherent Power of Being a Professional

Much has been written about professional power in health care policy and regulation (Frankford, 1997; Jones, 1999; Wilding, 1982), and although that area of study is a fascinating and important perspective of professional power and is in keeping with the topic of cultural self-awareness, this section of the chapter focuses on the aspect of professional power that relates to power relationships between people.

Wilding (1982) believes professionals are granted power by the public—which accepts the "validity and importance" of the activities in which the professional engages (such as occupational therapy assessment and intervention strategies)—and "by the unprotesting powerlessness of the groups upon whom . . . professionals practice their ministrations" (p. 60). Given these statements, the general public expects occupational therapy practitioners to act with authoritative power, especially by the people with whom they work. Occupational therapists are expected to make decisions on who receives services, what kind of services they receive, and when services end. Clients depend on the occupational therapists to be knowledgeable and skilled and to provide the best intervention for each person. Most clients come to occupational therapists in a vulnerable and dependent state, with expectations that the therapist will help them return to an active and productive life, where they can continue to participate in the roles and activities that are meaningful to them. Power is an inherent characteristic in this relationship, with the therapist seen as the expert and the client seeking his or her assistance.

Considering that relationship, professional power, therefore, is a given and must be acknowledged by the occupational therapist. If the therapist is White and part of the dominant societal group, and his or her client is from a nondominant culture, social power also is an important part of the therapeutic relationship, leaving the client in a place of double jeopardy. Pinderhughes (1989) warns therapists to be very careful not to use this power as a means of "aggrandizement, to satisfy their own needs for power and esteem not met elsewhere" (p. 110). She sees this kind of exploitation as "the most infamous of therapy abuses" (p. 110).

Professional power can be a somewhat heady experience. Occupational therapy students work very hard to be successful in their educational programs so they can earn the right to be called a professional, a certified and licensed occupational therapist, or occupational therapy assistant. It is important to take pride in that achievement. Wearing a nametag with credentials or interacting with a client or family for the first time is a rush but frightening at the same time. Novice practitioners sometimes feel they must know all the answers and be in control of the therapeutic interaction as a way to "prove" themselves. Awareness of one's self as a professional is vital, particularly if one also is aware of the responsibility inherent within the role. Part of this responsibility is to recognize the dignity of each client and to treat each person with the respect he or she deserves. Being sensitive to the power differential inherent in the client–practitioner relationship and learning how to work effectively to support clients within those boundaries is a challenge.

> *Being sensitive to the power differential inherent in the client–practitioner relationship is . . . a challenge.*

Participatory Power

There are many ways to ameliorate the power differential between the therapist and the client. The reality, however, is that because of societal and systematic influences, there *is* an undeniable social power difference between the two. It is important to recognize and acknowledge this fact, and then learn strategies that limit its effect.

Previously, I wrote about the importance of the "health care provider to surrender and share some of her authority and control in order to empower clients to have more agency within their health care" (Black, 2005, p. 414). The ability to move from a "power over" model to a "power to" approach (Sumsion, 1999) takes courage and confidence on the practitioner's part. It means letting go of some of the authority that identifies occupational therapists as professionals to share power, but it does not mean diminishing therapists' knowledge and expertise. In fact, therapists' knowledge must be expanded to effectively interact with people within their care in a manner that helps to empower clients within a disempowering health care system.

Although sharing power is an important step in empowering clients, occupational therapists can make another step as professionals to help clients move to a place of greater agency and control regarding their own health. Borrowing a term found in literature related to community governance (Mosson, 2005), adult literacy (Norton, 2000), and struggles for liberation in Central America (Ecumenical Program in Central America and the Caribbean [EPICA], 2002), one needs to begin to think about *participatory power* as a model for interaction with the people and groups with whom one works (see Figure 8.1).

Participatory power, as conceived in venues outside the field of occupational therapy, is the opportunity for people to become engaged in the decision-making

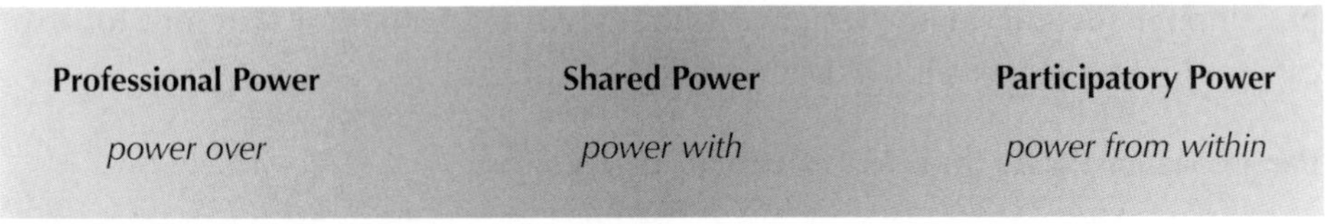

Professional Power	Shared Power	Participatory Power
power over	*power with*	*power from within*

Figure 8.1. Model of participatory power.

process by developing or joining organizations that influence policymakers. Frankford (1997) describes participatory power as a situation in which

> We all participate in its strategies and effects, although simultaneously we live within its grasp in that no individual or collective among us can pull its strings. Power in this sense is participatory by nature in that it stems from and flows through all of our interactions. (p. 191)

Some of the skills of people engaged in this process include listening well and gaining knowledge. Participatory power results in "power-from-within—the belief in oneself to further develop skills, knowledge, and attributes, and to offer them to others" (Norton, 2000). Isn't that what occupational therapy practitioners want for the people with whom they work—the development of a sense of internal power?

One reason we gravitate toward this concept is because it connotes a kind of personal action that "shared power" does not. Inherent within the notion of shared power is the fact that one person has the power and is willing to share it with someone else. There is no clear understanding of how the person who receives the shared power will use it, nor is there a clear expectation. In some ways, it is a gift offered by the person in power (the practitioner) to the person with less power (the client); an important gift to be sure but not a reciprocal situation.

Participatory power, on the other hand, focuses more on equal power, where each member of the group has a voice and the potential to be a decision-maker. It is a true person-centered interactive approach and, if practiced, might potentially result in "communities of health" (Frankford, 1997, p. 210) rather than the typical power-over model often seen today. A main thrust in current occupational therapy practice is to support people to participate in society and their lives. Within the practitioner–client interaction, what better way to do this than to encourage and—within health and cultural expectations and values—to insist on a client's active participation? When practitioners ask clients about their goals, they need to listen closely to what they are told, and if practitioners are using a participatory model, they will help the clients find ways to accomplish them. Within this model, the practitioner's role may include providing education about the client's condition, community resources, environmental adaptations, or sociopolitical realities so that the recipient can make an informed choice. Then, through collaborative efforts, the therapist works with the client to achieve those ends. This model also moves beyond practitioner advocacy of the recipient, although teaching the recipient how to advocate for himself or herself still is extremely important.

Participatory Power and Occupational Justice

Some may view this model as somewhat optimistic in today's health care arena or too challenging for clients who are cultural minorities and have lived a life filled with discrimination and oppression. It is a goal, however, for which practitioners must strive. Townsend and Whiteford (2005) speak of participatory occupational justice and the importance of empowerment-oriented approaches. Providing true opportunities for person-centered voice (ideas, beliefs, concerns) and decision-making will help move occupational therapists and clients toward a participatory power model of interaction that will strengthen not only the practitioner–client interaction but also the larger communities where one works. Helping people participate in meaningful occupations is an aspect of *occupational justice*. Teaching folks to advocate for themselves within regulatory agencies and health care institutions is an aspect of participatory power that strengthens not only the client but also the agencies and communities with which they interact. Recognizing the power practitioners hold and moving from shared power to a participatory power relationship is an aspect of self-awareness that helps practitioners toward cultural competence and culturally competent care.

Reflection

1. Examine power relationships in the workplace.

    a. Diagram the power relationships in your workplace. Include administrators, supervisors, staff, clients, and yourself.

    b. Determine which relationships represent professional power, shared power, and participatory power.

    c. What would this diagram look like with more participatory power?

2. Consider your professional power stance.

    a. Re-examine where you fit in the diagram.

    b. Within which power models do you currently work?

    c. Which power model is most effective for your workplace? Why?

    d. Under which power model are you most comfortable? Why?

3. Develop a model workplace.

    a. Determine whether the workplace will be in a large institution, smaller agency, a client's home, or other community setting.

    b. What authoritative relationships will you develop?

c. How will you set these up?

d. How do you perceive these functioning?

e. Once the model workplace has been achieved, what will be your role?

f. Draw a diagram that illustrates the power relationships.

References

Accreditation Council for Occupational Therapy Education. (2007). Accreditation Council for Occupational Therapy Education (ACOTE) standards and interpretive guidelines. *American Journal of Occupational Therapy, 61.*

American Occupational Therapy Association. (2005). Occupational therapy code of ethics. *American Journal of Occupation Therapy, 59,* 639–642.

Black, R. M. (2005). Intersections of care: An analysis of culturally competent care, Client-centered care, and the feminist ethic of care. *WORK: A Journal of Prevention, Assessment, and Rehabilitation, 24,* 409–422.

Curry, L., Wergin, J. F., & Associates. (1993). *Educating professionals: Responding to new expectations for competence and accountability.* San Francisco: Jossey-Bass.

Driscoll, D. M. (1994). Personal power. *Executive Female, 17*(5), 46–51.

Ecumenical Program in Central America and the Caribbean. (2002). *A letter from the editors. A new woman, a new power in America.* Retrieved, February 6, 2006, from www.epica.org/Library/editors/editors-7.htm

Frankford, D. M. (1997). The normative constitution of professional power. *Journal of Health Politics, Policy, and Law, 22*(1), 185–221.

Freidson, E. (1986). *Professional powers: A study of the institutionalization of formal knowledge.* Chicago: University of Chicago Press.

Jones, I. R. (1999). *Professional power and the need for health care.* Brookfield, VT: Ashgate.

Kronenberg, F., & Pollard, N. (2005). Overcoming occupational apartheid: A preliminary exploration of the political nature of occupational therapy. In F. Kronenberg, S. S. Algado, & N. Pollard (Eds.), *Occupational therapy without borders: Learning from the spirit of survivors* (pp. 58–86). Edinburgh, Scotland: Elsevier/Churchill Livingstone.

Lee, C. C. (2005). A reaction to EGAS: An important new approach to African American youth empowerment. *Professional School Counseling, 8,* 393–394.

Litwack, L. (2004, Spring). Personal power. *Ostomy Quarterly,* pp. 52–53.

Mosson, G. (2005). Power to our neighborhoods! *The Futurist, 39*(1). Retrieved February 4, 2006, from www.wfs.org/trend4jf05.htm

Norton, M. (2000). Challenges to sharing power in an adult literacy education program. In M. Norton & G. Malicky (Eds.), *Learning about participatory approaches in adult literacy education: Six research in practice studies* (pp. 159–191). Edmonton, Alberta: Learning at the Centre.

Person, E. S. (2004). Personal power and the cultural unconscious: Implications for psychoanalytical theories of sex and gender. *Journal of the American Academy of Psychoanalysis and Dynamic Psychiatry, 32*(1), 59–75.

Pinderhughes, E. (1989). *Understanding race, ethnicity, and power: The key to efficacy in clinical practice.* New York: Free Press.

Sumsion, T. (Ed.). (1999). *Client-centered practice in occupational therapy: A guide to implementation.* New York: Churchill Livingstone.

Townsend, E., & Whiteford, G. (2005). A participatory occupational justice framework: Population-based processes of practice. In F. Kronenberg, S. S. Algado, & N. Pollard (Eds.), *Occupational therapy without borders: Learning from the spirit of survivors* (pp. 110–126). Edinburgh, Scotland: Elsevier/Churchill Livingstone.

Wilding, P. (1982). *Professional power and social welfare.* Boston: Routledge & Kegan Paul.

Section B

Cultural Knowledge

9

Exploring Cultural Knowledge

*Traveling and meeting other people and having those experiences are . . .
the best thing. That's how I grow and have become who I am.*

—STUDY PARTICIPANT (BLACK, 2002B, PP. 123–124)

Key Points

- There are multiple areas of information to explore to become culturally competent.
- These areas can be separated into macro-information and micro-information kinds of knowledge.
- *Micro-information* is information that is most personal to the client, while *macro-information* is broader and more societal in nature.
- Knowledge can be gained in many ways, including
  - Written resources
  - Electronic sources
  - Community resources and activities
  - Conferences and workshops
  - Experiential activities: face-to-face interactions with culturally diverse people.
- Acquiring cultural knowledge is a lifelong process.

THE SECOND MAJOR CHARACTERISTIC outlined in the Cultural Competency Model is (cultural) knowledge. There is much to know and learn to become effective in cross-cultural interactions. In the previous section, we emphasized the importance of self-knowledge. This chapter and those included in this section point out additional knowledge practitioners may seek when working with people from different cultures.

What Knowledge Is Necessary?

The literature on cultural competence identifies many areas of knowledge to explore. One obvious area is learning about clients' specific culture (Pedersen & Ivey, 1993) and understanding how people within that culture define health and wellness. Gaining knowledge may mean learning clients' language (Lynch & Hanson, 1998), including gestures and other body language. In an article on early childhood intervention in South Africa, Louw and Avenant (2002) emphasize the importance of understanding the culture's family structure, beliefs about the nature of infants, and child-rearing practices. Understanding sociocultural roles within society and how they limit or support access to health care is important, as is knowing which community agencies are available and supportive of clients' needs. Being culturally knowledgeable also means having a clear and explicit understanding of the field (Pedersen & Ivey, 1993) and knowing how to provide the best possible health care to each client, regardless of his or her cultural background.

The most comprehensive list comes from McPhatter (1997), who identifies the following as a "grounded knowledge base" necessary for cultural competence (pp. 266–270):

- Knowledge of the history, culture, traditions and customs, preferred language or primary dialect, value orientation, religious and spiritual orientations, art, music, and folk or other healing beliefs of clients
- Intimate familiarity about social problems and issues that have different effects on minority group members
- Knowledge of the client's neighborhoods and communities and how they influence a client's life
- Firm understanding of the dynamics of oppression, racism, sexism, classism, heterosexism, and other forms of discrimination
- Knowledge of health and social systems and their effect on disadvantaged groups
- Awareness of diversity of family structure and the often-overlooked functionality of diverse family forms
- Knowledge of culturally relevant interventions employed within the professional structure.

McPhatter's list is broadly based, thorough, and overwhelming in breadth. Many readers may think, "I can't learn all that! Where would I find the time in my busy schedule to research all that information?" Many occupational therapists work in geographical areas with numerous and diverse cultural groups and couldn't possibly know everything necessary to be culturally competent with each group.

How then can competency be achieved? Students often ask this question, and it is important to consider. A somewhat simplistic answer is that very few occupational therapists ever fully achieve cultural competence, but it is a goal for which to constantly strive. As such, developing cultural competence is a lifelong process. Schim, Doorenbos, and Borse (2005) state that "Healthcare providers are not expected to achieve complete cultural competence, but, rather, that they strive to match their competencies to the specific populations, subgroups, and individuals with whom they work" (p. 355).

Even if occupational therapy practitioners accept this statement as truth, the fact is that, to develop cultural competence, they must gain knowledge in at least some of the areas outlined in the list above. The question then becomes, how do I begin researching this information, and what information should I start with?

Micro- and Macro-Knowledge and Information

One way to examine the list by McPhatter (1997) is to organize it into micro-knowledge and macro-knowledge and information. With the client in the center of concentric circles (see Figure 9.1), *micro-knowledge* is the information that, in some ways, is the closest to him or her, including the long list of cultural characteristics outlined in McPhatter's first statement. As one moves outward from the client, from micro- toward *macro-knowledge*, McPhatter's 6th point—"awareness of diversity of family structure"—might be found next. The next ring of knowledge would incorporate "awareness of clients' communities and neighborhoods," as well as other external contextual factors, which is McPhatter's 3rd point.

Near the level of macro-information, knowledge is more societal than personal but affects all people. This would include McPhatter's (1997) 2nd, 4th, and 5th points, such as familiarity of social problems and issues that affect minorities, understanding of the dynamics in all forms of oppression, and knowledge of health and social systems and their effect on disadvantaged groups. An understanding of health disparities fits here as well. In the literature, much overlap occurs in these last three areas.

Having at least a beginning knowledge from these 6 categories leads to McPhatter's 7th point: "knowledge of culturally relevant interventions." Understanding that there are levels of knowledge may lessen the sense of bewilderment and provide some direction in helping plan for cultural competence development

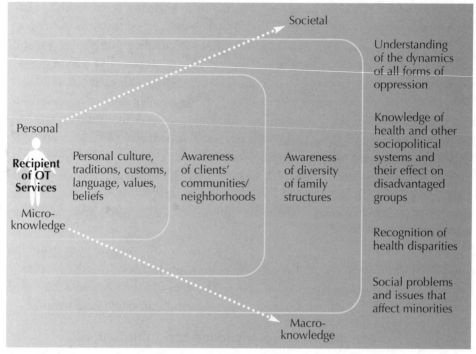

Figure 9.1. Levels of knowledge necessary to deliver culturally relevant occupational therapy interventions.

(see Chapter 16). Knowing *what* one needs to learn, however, does not explain *how, where,* and *when* one learns it. The following section explores these options.

Seeking and Acquiring Knowledge

Students already may have gained much of the macro- and some micro-knowledge in undergraduate and graduate coursework. This is a good place to begin. For practitioners with several years of experience but little formal education in these topics, what they gained in working with diverse clients, as well as with those culturally similar to them, gives them another kind of education that also is beneficial. Both formal and informal education coupled with cross-cultural experiences are important avenues for learning. Chapter 18 addresses educating for cultural competence in an academic setting. This chapter, therefore, focuses more on informal approaches to gaining cultural knowledge.

Written Resources

Researching written resources may be the most familiar and, in some ways, the easiest approach to learning about other cultures. Many books and resources within the different health care fields describe characteristics of various cultural groups and their effect on health and wellness (Julia, 1996; Lattanzi & Purnell, 2006; Spector, 2000). These resources are a good place to begin for foundational information, but readers must remember that not all people from the same cultural group will share all or any of these highlighted characteristics. One may learn specific information about the culture from sources such as these, but a practitioner also must learn the uniqueness of each client. If practitioners assumed that every Cambodian woman, for instance, simply will fall into the categories identified in written descriptions about Cambodian culture, they may stereotype them and not provide culturally competent care, despite their research. If practitioners, however, use the foundational information gathered from one of the books mentioned previously to help them get to know the Cambodian client on a personal level, then that information is useful in helping establish rapport.

Although the information about multiple cultural groups is not replicated in this book, Chapter 12, which introduces the Somali culture, provides an example of the kind of information one might gain from such sources. Other written resources include ethnographies, biographies, or written documentaries (Barnes, 1994; Burns, 1993; Sacks, 1989). One of the most compelling is Fadiman's (1997) *The Spirit Catches You and You Fall Down,* the story of a young Hmong girl with a seizure disorder and her parents' tragic interaction with the committed, yet misguided, health care community in Merced, California. The poignant report clearly explains how cultural *in*competence can have disastrous results.

Training manuals, workbooks, and reports from health care organizations (Campinha-Bacote, 1998; Fleming & Towey, 2002; Health Resources and Services Administration, 2001) provide information about culturally effective approaches for working with diverse groups. Depending on the organization and its focus, these resources may be *culture general* (information that can be used with multiple cultural groups) or *culture specific* (information about one particular group), but all provide additional, important information about working with diverse populations in a health care arena.

The final group of written resources discussed here is professional journal articles, which can contain a plethora of information about cultural groups, information, and competence from other health professions such as nursing, social work, and clinical psychology. More information about these subjects now appears in occupational therapy literature as well. Examples include information about working with specific groups such as Australian Aboriginals (Haig, 1993; Nelson & Allison, 2000; Preston, 1990), Chinese people (Chow, 2001; Jang, 1995), Hispanic individuals (Dickerson & Fisher, 1995), Japanese people (Goto, 1996; Iwama, 2006; Kondo, 2004), immigrants in general (Dyck, 1989), and others.

Other articles address culture and diversity in occupational therapy (Black, 2002a; Bonder, 2001; Fitzgerald, 2004; Iwama, 2004; Paul, 1995), while an increasing number examine aspects of cultural competence in the profession (Black, 2002b, 2005; Forwell, Whiteford, & Dyck, 2001; Odawara, 2005; Wittman, 2002). Making time to read some of these resources not only increases cultural knowledge but also establishes a beginning framework of how these concepts are being explored in the profession.

Electronic Sources

Today's students are much more adept with technology and tend to use electronic sources and the Internet for exploration. Although some of the sources are questionable, the Internet is becoming a much faster and reliable approach to research. While it should not be the only approach to researching different cultures, information retrieved through *Google Scholar* or other online full-text articles and chapters often is very useful.

In addition, the federal government and state governments, as well as health organizations and research institutes, have informative Web sites, including the following:

- *Boston Center for Refugee Health and Human Rights:* www.glphr.org/refugee/library.htm
- *California Endowment Program—Cultural Competence:* www.calendow.org/program_areas/cultural_competence_recent_publications.stm
- *Center for Cross-Cultural Health:* www.crosshealth.com/
- *Cushing/Whitney Medical Library, Yale University:* http://tidbits.med.yale.edu/lib_dev/education/culturalcomp/
- *DiversityRx:* www.DiversityRx.org/html/eslang.htm
- *Ethnomed:* http://ethnomed.org
- *Gay, Lesbian, and Straight Education Network:* www.glsen.org
- *National Center for Cultural Competency:* www11.georgetown.edu/research/gucchd/nccc/
- *U.S. Department of Health and Human Services, Office of Minority Health:* www.omhrc.gov/.

Community Resources and Activities

Communities in the United States rarely are so homogeneous that they have no cultural diversity. Many cities and towns celebrate their diversity through art exhibits, festivals, and educational offerings. Even in Maine, the least ethnically and racially diverse state in the Union (Mills, 2002), hosts Franco-American festivals, multicultural presentations, open gatherings welcoming immigrant populations, gay pride marches, educational forums celebrating Maine's African American history, and many other sources for learning. Taking advantage of these offerings is another viable avenue for learning and often in a personal manner. Attending the festivals, smelling delicious foods from various cultures, watching and listening to people interact, enjoying multiple presentations, talking with folks, and joining in the dancing provides an opportunity to participate in the richness of other cultures in a manner that reading about them does not.

Eating in ethnic restaurants and conversing with the wait staff is another way to experience other cultures. I took a small group of students to a local Somali restaurant, and the experience of ordering food with no menu offerings, washing their hands in the same room where the food was served, being the only people in the restaurant who did not speak the local language, eating unrecognizable food cooked in a manner they were not used to, and having no utensils certainly made a lasting impression. Many students thoroughly enjoyed the experience, and the reflective discussion in the following class offered them an opportunity for more self-analysis, as well as increased knowledge of Somalis.

Local museums also highlight various local cultures, as do churches, synagogues, or temples. This information may seem commonplace, but many people do not take advantage of the resources around them to learn about their culturally different neighbors, but they can be possible resources to plans for developing cultural competency.

Conferences and Workshops

Another effective way to gather knowledge is to attend conferences or workshops on culture and diversity. The American Occupational Therapy Association (AOTA), state occupational therapy associations, other professional organizations, local colleges and universities, places of employment, or local communities all offer such events. The 2007 AOTA National Conference in St. Louis offered more than 30 presentations on issues related to culture and diversity.

Experiential Activities

Although this approach to learning is last on the list, face-to-face interaction with culturally diverse people may be the most exciting and transformative for learners. In a study that examined the meaning of cultural competence and culturally competent care for occupational therapy students (Black, 2002b), one participant described her cross-cultural experiences:

> To actually be there and to have it be part of your experience and to see it and to feel it and to share it, all of a sudden it really hits home. It means something. It's real, not just a vague notion of what it would be. I think it opens your mind. (p. 166)

Experiential learning theory has proven over and over the old adage "experience is the best teacher." Drawing on the works of Russian cognitive theorist Lev Vygotsky, as well as from Dewey, Lewin, Piaget, and other educational theorists,

Kolb (1984) asserts, "learning from experience is the process whereby human development occurs" (p. xi). The accuracy of this statement is clear as one reads the study
participant's words as she talks about how her understanding of people and culture
changes when she has an opportunity to actually interact with them:

> I read a lot and have people tell me about things . . . but until I go out
> and actually see it, it's abstract. But once you're doing it, and once you've
> done it, it becomes real. . . . It's kind of like that 'ah hah' moment. (Black,
> 2002b, p. 167)

Within cultural competence literature, several authors mention but do not
emphasize that cross-cultural experience is important in cultural competence
development (Jones, Bond, & Mancini, 1998; Kramer & Bateman, 1999; Leonard &
Plotnikoff, 2000; Pope-Davis, Prieto, Whitaker, & Pope-Davis, 1993). Pope-Davis,
Breaux, and Liu (1997), however, are among the few who suggest that cross-cultural experiences might be fundamental "because such in vivo experiences may provide the basis for reducing prejudice and racism" (p. 228). They go on to say that
contact between groups is more effective if significant time is spent together.
Research suggests short cross-cultural or simulated activities actually may increase
ethnocentrism and bias (Bruschke, Gartner, & Seiter, 1993; Rothbart & Lewis,
1994). Bruschke and colleagues (1993) attribute this finding to a lack of adjustment
time following a period of culture shock. Based on their examination of the literature, Pope-Davis and colleagues (1997) concluded, "the most valuable experiential
exercise would be one of longer duration involving in vivo contact" (p. 232). Kim's
(1996) study of occupational therapy practitioners supports this finding. She found
that practitioners who practiced in another country for at least 3 weeks developed
higher levels of cultural competence than those without international experiences.
Kim also found that, as the number of months overseas increased, so did the practitioners' cultural self-awareness.

In addition, research supports the transformational nature of cross-cultural
experiences. One participant in Black's (2002b) study states, "things change me
when it directly happens to me. I mean I can read about things and know more, but
[the experience] really impacts me" (p. 169). Not only do such experiences alter
one's understanding, they shift the sense of self—who one is in a multicultural
world. A transformation has occurred, not only in knowledge but also in people.
Mezirow and Associates (2000) clearly explain this in the following statement:

> Transformative learning refers to the process by which we transform our
> taken-for-granted frames of reference (meaning perspectives, habits of
> mind, mind-sets) to make them more inclusive, discriminating, open,
> emotionally capable of change, and reflective so that they may generate
> beliefs and opinions that will prove more true or justified to guide action
> . . . . Transformative learning has both individual and social dimensions

and implications. It demands that we be aware of how we come to our knowledge and as aware as we can be about the values that lead us to our perspectives. (pp. 7–8)

In this statement, Mezirow and Associates articulate the purpose of learning and knowledge in the development of cultural competence, especially the transformative power of cross-cultural experiences.

Summary

Cultural knowledge is a vital characteristic of a culturally competent occupational therapy practitioner. Knowledge can be acquired through formal or informal means, and knowing what information to gather and where to find it is important. Literature indicates that, of the many ways to learn about a person's culture, the most transformative is direct contact with people over time.

This fact has implications for academic programs that are trying to move students toward cultural competence and for practitioners whose days are filled with back-to-back client interventions. Realistically, researching and gaining cultural knowledge is time consuming and, if it involves travel to another country, costly. Students, educators, practitioners, and the agency or institution where one works or studies must make efforts to provide the time and financial resources necessary to support this endeavor.

As stated earlier, developing cultural competence is not easy, but as the United States moves toward a more diverse culture and global context through technology and the ease of international travel, occupational therapy practitioners also must move in this direction to provide the necessary care and intervention.

The following chapters in this section provide both micro- and macro-information necessary for a beginning knowledge base in diversity and culture issues. Chapters 10 and 11 provide overviews on the effect of culture, ethnicity, and race on health conditions, health care access, and health care use. Chapter 12 gives readers a culture-specific look at one refugee population, the Somalis, while Chapter 13 demonstrates how to assess a specific community, in this case, Brownsville, Texas.

Reflection

1. Read a book about another culture, such as *The Spirit Catches You and You Fall Down* (Fadiman, 1997).

   a. With others, discuss what you learned that was most significant to you.

   b. In what ways is this culture different from your own?

   c. What are the similarities between your culture and the one identified in the book you read?

    d. How will you use what you learned in your practice with people who are culturally different from you?

2. Learn about community offerings on culture and diversity.

    a. Contact your local library, city hall, museum, church, etc., to determine what cultural offerings are available.

    b. Choose one and visit or participate with a friend.

    c. Write a journal entry about what this was like. What did you learn? How did you feel? With whom did you interact? Did it spark your interest? Do you want to learn more?

3. Discover your personal learning style.

    a. How do you learn best?

    b. Use that style to gather more information about a culture different from yours.

    c. Go outside your comfort zone to gather knowledge in another way.

References

Barnes, V. L. (1994). *Aman: The story of a Somali girl, as told to Virginia Lee Barnes and Janice Boddy.* New York: Vintage.

Black, R. M. (2002a). Occupational therapy's dance with diversity. *American Journal of Occupational Therapy, 56,* 140–148.

Black, R. M. (2002b). *The essence of cultural competence: Listening to the voices of occupational therapy students.* Unpublished dissertation, Lesley University, Cambridge, MA.

Black, R. M. (2005). Intersections of care: An analysis of culturally competent care, client-centered care, and the feminist ethic of care. *Work, 24,* 409–422.

Bonder, B. R. (2001). Culture and occupation: A comparison of weaving in two traditions. *Canadian Journal of Occupational Therapy, 68*(5), 310–319.

Bruschke, J. C., Gartner, C., & Seiter, J. S. (1993). Student ethnocentrism, dogmatism, and motivation: A study of BAFA. *Simulation and Gaming, 24,* 9–20.

Burns, A. F. (1993). *Maya in exile: Guatemalans in Florida.* Philadelphia: Temple University Press.

Campinha-Bacote, J. (1998). *The process of cultural competence in the delivery of healthcare services: A culturally competent model of care* (3rd ed.). Cincinnati, OH: Transcultural CARE Associates.

Chow, S. M. K. (2001). The Movement Assessment Battery for Children: A comparison of 4-year-old to 6-year-old children from Hong Kong and the United States. *American Journal of Occupational Therapy, 55,* 28–35.

Dickerson, A. E., & Fisher, A. G. (1995). Culture-relevant functional performance assessment of the Hispanic elderly. *Occupational Therapy Journal of Research, 15*(1), 50–68.

Dyck, I. (1989). The immigrant client: Issues in developing culturally sensitive practice. *Canadian Journal of Occupational Therapy, 56,* 248–255.

Fadiman, A. (1997). *The spirit catches you and you fall down.* New York: Farrar, Straus, & Giroux.

Fitzgerald, M. H. (2004). A dialogue on occupational therapy, culture, and families. *American Journal of Occupational Therapy, 58,* 489–498.

Fleming, M., & Towey, K. (2002). *Delivering culturally effective health care to adolescents.* Chicago: American Medical Association.

Forwell, S. J., Whiteford, G., & Dyck, I. (2001). Cultural competence in New Zealand and Canada: Occupational therapy students' reflections on class and fieldwork curriculum. *Canadian Journal of Occupational Therapy, 68*(2), 90–103.

Goto, S. (1996). The assessment of motor and process skills applied cross-culturally to the Japanese. *American Journal of Occupational Therapy, 50,* 798–806.

Haig, N. (1993). The Gardia experience: Implications for occupational therapists working with Australia's indigenous people in Kimberly region. *Australian Occupational Therapy Journal, 40*(4), 157–158.

Health Resources and Services Administration. (2001). *Cultural competence works: Using cultural competence to improve the quality of health care for diverse populations and add value to managed care arrangements.* Merrifield, VA: U.S. Department of Health and Human Services, Author.

Iwama, M. (2004). Guest Editorial—Meaning and inclusion: Revisiting culture in occupational therapy. *Australian Occupational Therapy Journal, 51,* 1–2.

Iwama, M. (2006). *The Kawa model: Culturally relevant occupational therapy.* Toronto, Ontario: Churchill Livingstone.

Jang, Y. (1995). Chinese culture and occupational therapy. *British Journal of Occupational Therapy, 58*(3), 103–106.

Jones, M. E., Bond, L. L., & Mancini, M. E. (1998). Developing a culturally competent work force: An opportunity for collaboration. *Journal of Professional Nursing, 14,* 280–287.

Julia, M. C. (1996). *Multicultural awareness in the health care professions.* Needham Heights, MA: Allyn & Bacon.

Kim, B. M. (1996). *The impact of cross-cultural practice on multicultural competence among occupational therapists.* Unpublished master's thesis, Rush University, Chicago.

Kolb, D. A. (1984). *Experiential learning: Experience as the source of learning and development.* Englewood Cliffs, NJ: Prentice Hall.

Kondo, T. (2004). Cultural tensions in occupational therapy practice: Considerations from a Japanese vantage point. *American Journal of Occupational Therapy, 58,* 174–184.

Kramer, E. J., & Bateman, W. B. (1999). A cultural competence curriculum. In E. J. Kramer, S. L. Ivery, & Y.-W. Ying (Eds.), *Immigrant women's health: Problems and solutions* (pp. 322–329). San Francisco: Jossey-Bass.

Lattanzi, J. B., & Purnell, L. D. (2006). *Developing cultural competence in physical therapy practice.* Philadelphia: F. A. Davis.

Leonard, B. J., & Plotnikoff, G. A. (2000). Awareness: The heart of cultural competence. *AACN Clinical Issues, 11*(1), 51–59.

Louw, B., & Avenant, C. (2002). Culture as context for intervention: Developing a culturally congruent early intervention program. *International Pediatrics, 17,* 145–150.

Lynch, E. W., & Hanson, M. J. (1998). *Developing cross-cultural competencies: A guide for working with children and their families* (2nd ed.). Baltimore: Paul H. Brookes. Retrieved February 2, 2000, from www.pbrookes.com/e-catalog/books/lynch-3319/excerpt.htm

McPhatter, A. R. (1997). Cultural competence in child welfare: What is it? How do we achieve it? What happens without it? *Child Welfare, 76*(1), 255–278.

Mezirow, J., & Associates (2000). *Learning as transformation: Critical perspectives on a theory in progress.* San Francisco: Jossey-Bass.

Mills, D. A. (Ed.) (2002). Race and ethnicity. In *Healthy Maine 2010: Opportunities for all* (pp. 15–32). Augusta: Bureau of Health, Maine Department of Human Services. Retrieved August 20, 2007, from http://www.maine.gov/dhhs/files/hm2010/oppforall/b04raeth.pdf

Nelson, A., & Allison, H. (2000). Values of urban Aboriginal parents. *Australian Occupational Therapy Journal, 47*(1), 28–40.

Odawara, E. (2005). Cultural competency in occupational therapy: Beyond a cross-cultural view of practice. *American Journal of Occupational Therapy, 59,* 325–334.

Paul, S. (1995). Culture and its influence on occupational therapy evaluation. *Canadian Journal of Occupational Therapy, 62*(3), 154–161.

Pedersen, P. B., & Ivey, A. (1993). *Culture-centered counseling and interviewing skills.* Westport, CT: Praeger.

Pope-Davis, D. B., Breaux, C., & Liu, W. M. (1997). A multicultural immersion experience: Filling a void in multicultural training. In D. B. Pope-Davis & H. L. K. Coleman (Eds.), *Multicultural counseling competencies: Assessment, education and training, and supervision* (pp. 227–241). Thousand Oaks, CA: Sage.

Pope-Davis, D., Prieto, L. R., Whitaker, C. M., & Pope-Davis, S. (1993). Exploring multicultural competencies of occupational therapists: Implications for education and training. *American Journal of Occupational Therapy, 47,* 838–844.

Preston, S. (1990). Making rehabilitation work for Australian Aboriginals. In *Book of abstracts of the 10th International Congress of the World Federation of Occupational Therapists* (pp. 179–182). Melbourne, Australia: World Federation of Occupational Therapists.

Rothbart, M., & Lewis, S. (1994). Cognitive processes and intergroup relations: A historical perspective. In P. G. Devine, D. L. Hamilton, & T. M. Ostrom (Eds.), *Social cognition: Impact on social psychology* (pp. 175–183). San Diego: Academic Press.

Sacks, O. (1989). *Seeing voices: A journey into the world of the deaf.* Berkeley: University of California Press.

Schim, S. M., Doorenbos, A. Z., & Borse, N. N. (2005). Cultural competence among Ontario and Michigan healthcare providers. *Journal of Nursing Scholarship, 37,* 354–360.

Spector, R. E. (2000). *Cultural diversity in health and illness* (5th ed.). Upper Saddle River, NJ: Prentice Hall Health.

Wittman, P. (2002). Attaining cultural competence, critical thinking, and intellectual development: A challenge for occupational therapists. *American Journal of Occupational Therapy, 56,* 454–456.

10

Health Disparities

Look. I stretch out my arms. See. I have two of them, as you have. Look at our ears. I have two of them. I have two eyes, two nostrils, one mouth, two feet. I stand erect like you. I am clothed with humanity like you. I think, I reason, I talk, I express my views as you do. Is there any difference between us?

—RICHARD CAIN (CITED IN JOHNSON, 1995, P. 97)

Key Points

- *Health disparities* are population-specific differences in the presence of health outcomes or access to health care. The biggest disparities in health conditions often exist among racial and ethnic-minority populations.

- According to the American Public Health Association (2004), health disparities are differences that occur by gender, race and ethnicity, education level, income level, disability, geographic location, and sexual orientation.

- Disparities often are the result of deficiencies in the health care system and legal and regulatory climate; discrimination, bias, and stereotyping; and uncertainty in clinical communication and decision making.

- To eliminate health disparities, they must first be identified, and then the inequalities in systems and services that perpetuate them must be corrected.

NOWHERE IS THE DIVISION of race or ethnicity and culture more sharply drawn than in the health of people living in the United States. Despite recent improvements and progress in overall national health, disparities in the incidence of illness and death continue to exist among portions of the population (National Center for Cultural Competence, 2005; U.S. Department of Health and Human Services [DHHS], 2004). The U.S. population has been, and remains, two nations: the majority, with adequate quality of health, and the minority, with low quality of health. Ethnicity, race, gender, education level, socioeconomic status, disability, geographic location, and sexual orientation are powerful factors influencing health status, access to health care, and the scope and quality of health care available.

In 2000, DHHS made eliminating health disparities a top priority, including it as one of two overarching goals in its report, *Healthy People 2010*. But the battle to eliminate health disparities is challenging and complex. Multiple factors often are associated and difficult to study independently. The sources of these disparities are complex, are rooted in historical and contemporary inequalities, and involve many participants at several levels. This chapter explores the complex interaction among genetic variations, environmental factors, and specific health behaviors that result in health disparities. It also addresses the challenges of eliminating these inequalities and achieving better health for all Americans.

Background

Demographic changes in the coming decades will magnify the importance of addressing disparities in health status. Because groups currently experiencing poorer health status are expected to constitute an increasingly larger proportion of the U.S. population, the future health of Americans will be improved by addressing the health of these groups. *Healthy People 2010* (DHHS, 2000) targeted two overarching goals: (a) to increase quality and years of healthy life and (b) to eliminate health disparities to improve the health of the nation. The authors of *Healthy People 2010* acknowledged that a comprehensive strategy incorporating research, education, policy changes, and community partnerships would be fundamental to accomplishing these goals.

Health disparities are population-specific differences in the presence of health outcomes or access to health care. The biggest disparities in health conditions often exist among racial and ethnic minority populations. Health disparities include the differences in health status that are due to gender, race or ethnicity, education or income level, disability, geographic location, and sexual identity. These disparities are believed to be the result of the complex interaction among genetic variations, environmental factors, and specific health behaviors. Some health disparities are unavoidable, such as health problems that are related to a person's genetic structure. Other health disparities are potentially avoidable, especially when they are related to factors such as living in low-income neighborhoods or having unequal access to medical care and information. Lack of physicians in rural areas, lack of diversity among health care providers, low health literacy, lack of insurance, and exposure to environmental risks also are contributors to the continuing health disparities in the United States. The health status of racial and ethnic-minority populations lags far behind that of nonminority populations. Racial and ethnic-minority populations in the United States suffer substantially and disproportionately from adverse health conditions and inadequate access to health care services. Many of these health disparities have persisted for years, despite major advances in public health and biotechnology, growing wealth and prosperity, and the overall improvement in the health status of the U.S. population over the past century. Members of minority groups tend to receive lower quality health care across a broad range of diseases and clinical procedures and are more likely to receive less desirable procedures, such as lower limb amputation because of diabetes (Institute of Medicine, 2005). These differences and the resulting health disparities result from socioeconomic, environmental, and systemic gaps in the quality of health and health care among these groups.

Several factors, often working together, contribute to these gaps. Disparities can result from the organization and operation of health care systems and the legal and regulatory climate; discrimination, bias, and stereotyping among providers; and uncertainty in clinical communication and decision making (Institute of Medicine, 2005). Other possible causes include problems in forming patient–physician relationships, difficulty navigating the complex health care delivery system, language problems, and providers' misunderstanding of cultural and folk illnesses and patient health-related beliefs.

Disparities in health are costly to society. For example, premature deaths can have devastating social and economic effects on families. The death rates from cardiovascular disease, breast/cervical cancer, HIV/AIDS, infant mortality, and lack of immunization are 8 times greater for racial and minority populations (Centers for Disease Control and Prevention, 2005; National Center for Cultural Competence, 2005; National Institutes of Health, 2005; Office of Minority Health, 2005d). When people of color have disproportionately high-cost health care problems and deaths, the entire population shares those costs as a part of insurance premiums and other health care costs.

Areas of Disparities

The DHHS selected 6 focus areas in which racial and ethnic minorities experience serious disparities in health access and outcomes. These areas were selected for emphasis because they affect multiple racial and ethnic minority groups at all life stages. Reliable national data have been used to track progress on these goals in a timely fashion (Centers for Disease Control and Prevention, 2005; National Center for Cultural Competence, 2005; National Institutes of Health, 2005; Office of Minority Health, 2005d).

1. *Infant mortality.* Even though the nation's infant mortality rate is down, the infant death rate among African Americans still is more than double that of White Americans. African American and American Indian infants die at a rate 2 to 3 times higher than the rate for White American infants. Among American Indians and Alaskan Natives, the incidence of sudden infant death syndrome is more than 3 to 4 times the rate for White American infants (Centers for Disease Control and Prevention, 2005; National Center for Health Statistics [NCHS], 2005; Office of Minority Health, 2005d).

2. *Cancer screening and management.* The death rate for all cancers is 30% higher for African Americans than for White Americans; for prostate cancer it is more than double. People of diverse racial, ethnic, and cultural heritages are less likely to get medical checkups, receive immunizations, and be routinely tested for cancer compared with the White U.S. population. The 5-year survival rate for African American women diagnosed with breast cancer is 14% lower than the survival rate for White women (Centers for Disease Control and Prevention, 2005; National Center for Cultural Competence, 2005; National Institutes of Health, 2005; Office of Minority Health, 2005d).

3. *Cardiovascular disease.* Racial and ethnic groups have higher rates of hypertension, tend to develop it at an earlier age, and are less likely to obtain treatment to control it. Among males from racial and ethnic groups, stroke is the only leading cause of death for which mortality is higher for Asian American men. Heart disease and stroke are the leading causes of death for all racial and ethnic groups, but heart disease death rates are more than 40% higher for African Americans than for White Americans. Only 50% of American Indians, 44% of Asian Americans, and 38% of Mexican Americans have had their cholesterol checked in the past 2 years (National Center for Cultural Competence, 2005; NCHS, 2005).

4. *Diabetes.* Diabetes is the seventh leading cause of death in the United States. American Indians and Alaska Natives are 2.6 times more likely, African Americans are 2.0 times more likely, and Hispanics are 1.9 times more likely than White Americans to be diagnosed with diabetes. American Indians and African Americans have higher rates of diabetes with related complications, such as kidney disease and amputations, compared to the total population. The rate of diabetes for American Indians is more than twice that for White Americans, and the Pima people of Arizona have one of the highest rates of diabetes in the world. Hispanics living in the United States are almost twice as likely to die from diabetes as non-Hispanic White

Americans. Hispanics also have higher rates of high blood pressure and obesity than non-Hispanic White Americans (National Center for Cultural Competence, 2005; NCHS, 2005).

5. *HIV infection and AIDS.* The death rate from HIV/AIDS for African Americans is more than 7 times that for White Americans. Among African Americans, 56% of new HIV/AIDS cases and 20% of Hispanic groups are a result of intravenous drug usage. African Americans and Hispanics accounted for 66% of adult AIDS cases and 82% of pediatric AIDS cases in 2001. Seventy-five percent of HIV/AIDS cases reported among women and children occurred among minority racial and ethnic groups (National Center for Cultural Competence, 2005; NCHS, 2005; Office of Minority Health, 2005d).

6. *Immunizations.* Children living below the poverty threshold are less likely to have received the full vaccination series than children living at or above poverty. Hispanics and African Americans ages 65 or older are less likely than non-Hispanic Whites to report having received influenza and pneumococcal vaccines. In 2002, 60.6% of White Americans, 36.1% of African Americans, and 23.8% Hispanics had received the pneumococcal vaccination (Centers for Disease Control and Prevention, 2005; National Center for Cultural Competence, 2005).

Additional diseases and conditions that disproportionately affect racial and ethnic minorities include the following (Centers for Disease Control and Prevention, 2005):

- *Mental health disorders.* American Indians and Alaska Natives appear to suffer disproportionately from depression and substance abuse. Members of minority groups have less access to mental health services.
- *Hepatitis.* In 2002, 50% of those infected with hepatitis B were Asian Americans and Pacific Islanders.
- *Syphilis.* Seventy-five percent of primary and secondary syphilis cases diagnosed in 1999 involved African Americans, 16% White Americans, 8% Hispanics, and 1% other.
- *Tuberculosis.* Of all tuberculosis cases reported from 1991 to 2001, 80% affected Asian Americans and Pacific Islanders.

Disparities in Health Care

Access to Care

Barriers to quality care extend well beyond the issues of being underinsured and uninsured. Expense, distance, inconvenient hours, long waits, and the prospect of unfriendly treatment construct a formidable barrier to care (Young, 1994). Facing unpleasant and bewildering circumstances, many individuals abandon their quest to obtain care. In addition to economic status and health knowledge, provider attitudes and behaviors related to race and ethnicity may pose barriers to access and health care use. Immigration status, acculturation level, language, and organizational and other cultural factors also influence access to care, patterns of health care use, and outcomes (Friedman, 1994; M. B. Smith, 1998; U.S. Public Health Service, 1994). Lack of access to routine medical services has been identified as a major factor in the increasing health-related vulnerability of certain racial and ethnic populations, poor people, and women. For example, in a Kaiser Family Foundation (2000) survey, 58% of physicians cited the simple fact that many people from minority groups live in medically underserved areas where there are fewer doctors and other health care providers.

Primary care underpins the health care system, and having a usual source of care raises the chances that people receive adequate preventive care and other important health care. About 30% of Hispanic and 20% of African Americans lack a usual source of health care, compared with about 16% of White Americans. Hispanic children are nearly 3 times as likely as non-Hispanic White children to have no usual source of health care. African Americans and Hispanic Americans are far more likely to rely on hospitals, emergency rooms, or clinics for their usual source of care than are White Americans (Agency for Healthcare Research and Quality, 2000; NCHS, 2005). Members of minority groups are less likely to obtain care in a private physician's office, even when insured at the same level as White individuals (Institute of Medicine, 2005).

In examining health care access issues, one also must consider the legal, regulatory and policy interventions climate in which health care systems operate. Enforcement of federal regulations and statutes that prohibit discrimination in health care are an important strategy to address health care disparities. Complaints to the U.S. Department of Health and Human Services' Office of Civil Rights—the agency in charged with enforcing Title VI of the 1964 Civil Rights Act—have increased in recent years. Yet, the agency has suffered from insufficient resources to investigate complaints of possible violations or to be proactive in their investigation strategies (Institute of Medicine, 2002). The fragmentation of health care financing and delivery can limit access to quality care as well as serve as a potential area for discrimination. The United States has a hodgepodge of private insurance coverage based primarily on employment, along with public insurance coverage for older adults (Medicare), military personnel, veterans, and the poor and disabled (Medicaid) that creates serious gaps in coverage (Institute of Medicine, 2000). Racial and ethnic minorities either are disproportionately enrolled in lower cost health plans or have no insurance, which puts greater per-patient limits on health care spending, available services, and discrimination (Institute of Medicine, 2002).

Managed care regulations to one extent or another provide patient protections, such as avenues for appeal of care denial decisions, improved access to specialty care, required health plans to disclose information about coverage, the banning of physician "gag" clauses, and legal remedies to resolve disputes to enrollees. These regulations, however, apply only to private managed care organizations, not publicly funded health plans (e.g., Medicare and Medicaid). Given that many racial and ethnic minorities are disproportionately represented among the publicly insured who receive care within managed care organizations, the same patient protections that apply to the privately insured also should apply to those in publicly funded plans (Hashimoto, 2001). Financial factors such as capitation and health plan incentives to physicians to limit services pose greater barriers and discrimination to racial and ethnic patients than to White patients insured at the same level. Low payment rates limit the supply of physician and other health care provider services to low-income groups (Institute of Medicine, 2002).

Diagnosis and Treatment

Race and ethnicity influence an individual's chance of receiving certain procedures and treatments. According to the Agency for Healthcare Research and Quality (AHRQ, 2000), African Americans are 13% less likely to undergo coronary angioplasty and one third less likely to undergo bypass surgery than White Americans. Among preschool children hospitalized for asthma, only 7% of African American and 2% of Hispanic children, compared with 21% of White children, were prescribed routine medications to prevent future asthma-related hospitalization. Asian American, Hispanic, and African American residents of nursing homes are all far less likely than White residents to own sensory and communication aids, such as glasses and hearing aids. The length of time between an abnormal screening mammogram and the follow-up diagnostic test to determine whether a woman has breast cancer is more than twice as long for Asian American, African American, and Hispanic women as for White women (AHRQ, 2000).

The 5-year survival rate for African American women diagnosed with breast cancer was 14% lower than the rate for White women in 2000 (NCHS, 2005). Mexican American mothers are 3 times as likely as non-Hispanic White mothers to begin prenatal care in the third trimester or not to receive prenatal care at all (Office of Minority Health, 2005a).

Diabetes and high blood pressure are a greater burden for racial and ethnic groups, as their higher rates of amputations and kidney disease show. Despite being disproportionately represented on waiting lists for kidney transplants, African American patients are half as likely as White patients to receive transplants and wait longer for them (Gaston, Ayres, Dooley, & Diethelm, 1993). African American patients also are less likely to receive hip or total knee replacements or undergo gastrointestinal endoscopy, among other procedures, but are more likely to undergo hysterectomy and amputation of the lower extremity compared to White patients (Gormick, Eggers, & Reilly, 1996).

Any degree of uncertainty a physician may have relative to patients' condition can contribute to disparities in treatment. To make a diagnosis, doctors depend on inferences about severity based on their observations of the illness and of the patient (including race, age, gender, and sometimes socioeconomic status). If information related to the illness is lacking or deemed to be inaccurate, doctors tend to rely on their observations of the patient (which may include unfair assumptions) in making diagnostic decisions. The consequence is that treatment decisions and patients' needs are potentially less well matched (American Medical Student Association, 2004).

Health Insurance Coverage

Access to regular care is contingent on health insurance coverage, private or public, which is directly connected to one's employment or lack thereof. Because many people in this country do not have health insurance, a large number of people have no access to care. Health care costs account for an increasing share of the U.S. economy and are placing a rising burden on federal, state, and local governments and private employers (Gabel, Claxton, Gil, Pickreign, & Whitmore, 2005; Ginsburg, 2005). These costs also contribute to the rising proportion of the population who lack health insurance coverage. The lack of insurance coverage in some groups is dramatic: Hispanics (32%), non-Hispanic African Americans (18%), and American Indians (32%) are more likely to lack health insurance than non-Hispanic White people (12%). People of Mexican origin (37%) are more likely to be uninsured than non-Hispanic African Americans and other Hispanics. Access to health insurance coverage through employment is lowest for Hispanic people (NCHS, 2005).

The growing number of Hispanic immigrants, of which Mexicans are the largest group (31% of all U.S. immigrants in 2004 were from Mexico; Centers for Disease Control and Prevention, 2005), are expected to further increase the percentage of the population with no employer-based health insurance coverage. In 2001 to 2003, the average percentage of the population with no health insurance coverage ranged from 8% in Minnesota to 25% in Texas. Ten percent of children younger than age 18 years had no health insurance coverage in 2003, and children in low-income families were more likely than children in higher income families to lack coverage. People of Hispanic origin and American Indians under age 65 years were more likely to have no health insurance coverage than those of other racial and ethnic groups (NCHS, 2005).

Geographic Access

Although lack of health insurance coverage is a significant problem, the provision of health insurance alone will not ensure equity of access or care. Geography and lack of transportation can result in the underuse of health services. A shortage of physicians and health services providers in certain areas compromises access, especially in rural areas. Many hospitals have closed as a result of ongoing structural and political changes in health care, and the lack of access to hospital and physician care has risen. Many hospitals that historically served ethnic communities have closed, relocated to predominantly White communities, or been privatized (Betancourt, Green, Carrillo, & Ananeh-Firempong, 2003; Coleman-Miller, 2000). When a hospital closes in any area, rural or urban, physicians often leave the area. As a result, remaining physicians have extremely heavy workloads (Friedman, 1994; Randall, 1994; D. B. Smith, 1993). If no providers are available, whether or not an individual has insurance is irrelevant. Patients who are housebound, lack private transportation, or face other transportation difficulties are increasingly vulnerable as available providers become more distant (Friedman, 1994).

Residents of rural areas have less contact and fewer visits with physicians (Intercultural Cancer Council, 2001). With the exception of family practitioners and general practitioners, fewer physicians are in rural areas in all regions of the nation. Only about 10% of U.S. physicians practice in rural areas, despite the fact that one fourth of the population lives in these areas (American Public Health Association, 2004; Gamm, Hutchison, Bellamy, & Dabney, 2002).

Other Disparities

Other areas in which disparities in health care have been documented include the following:

- *Lack of diversity among health care providers.* Lack of diversity among health care providers can be a barrier to communication. Minority group members make up 28% of the U.S. population but only 3% of medical school faculty, 16% of public health school faculty, and 17% of all city and county health officers (Center for the Advancement of Health, 2004).
- *Low health literacy.* People with poor health literacy may have problems communicating with their physicians, reading instructions and labels on medicines, completing medical and insurance forms, and understanding many other aspects of health care. More than half of the people living in the United States struggle with health literacy. Adults with poor health literacy are likely to have 3 times as many prescriptions filled as adults with higher literacy, and diabetes patients with poor health literacy are nearly twice as likely to have poorly controlled blood sugar and serious long-term health complications (American Public Health Association, 2004).

- *Exposure to environmental risks.* People in low-income communities often have less healthy surroundings than people in other communities. Low-income communities often are located in or near polluting industrial areas and have cheaper and older housing, where lead paint and pests are a threat (Environmental Justice & Health Union, 2003). Environmental risk factors ranging from tobacco smoke to chemical waste to dietary habits can cause serious health problems. Research has linked the incidence and severity of cancer, asthma, Alzheimer's disease, autism, birth defects and infertility, and other problems to environmental contaminants (American Public Health Association, 2004).

Socioeconomic Inequalities and Health Inequities

Socioeconomic status plays an important role in the maintenance of health, perceptions of illness, and the pattern of treatment individuals seek. Poverty is a major factor compromising the health status of members of ethnic minorities and women. Poverty is highly correlated with adverse health, primarily because it limits or precludes access to needed health services (Institute of Medicine, 2002; M. B. Smith, 1998).

Health disparities resulting from socioeconomic status begin early in life and have long-lasting effects. A mother's low socioeconomic status is associated with multiple risk factors for adverse birth outcomes, unplanned and unwanted pregnancies, single or adolescent motherhood, smoking, urogenital tract infections, chronic illness in the mother, and inadequate prenatal care (Fiscella & Williams, 2004). Low socioeconomic status also is associated with low birthweight and high infant mortality. In 2002, infant mortality rates were highest for infants of non-Hispanic African American mothers (13.9 deaths per 1,000 live births), Hawaiian mothers (9.6 per 1,000), American Indian mothers (8.6 per 1,000), and Puerto Rican mothers (8.2 per 1,000) and were lowest for infants of mothers of Chinese origin (3.0 per 1,000 live births) and Cuban American mothers (3.7 per 1,000; NCHS, 2005).

Socioeconomic disparities persist into childhood, resulting in increased risk of death from infectious disease, sudden infant death syndrome, accidents, and child abuse for poor children. In 2003, 30% of Hispanic and 34% of African American children were poor, compared with 10% of Asian and 13% of non-Hispanic White children (NCHS, 2005). Lower income children have higher rates of exposure to lead poisoning and second-hand smoke, asthma, developmental delays and learning disabilities, conduct disturbances, and avoidable hospitalizations (Fiscella & Williams, 2004). Poor children are more likely to have untreated dental cavities than children in families with incomes above the poverty level. In 2003, 7% of children under the age of 18 experienced limitations of activities because of the chronic health conditions seen as an outcome of living in poverty. The conditions most often mentioned among preschool children (younger than age 5 years) were speech problems, asthma, and mental retardation or other developmental problems, whereas among school-age children (ages 5–17 years), learning disabilities and attention deficit hyperactivity disorder were the most frequently mentioned (NCHS, 2005).

Adolescents living below the poverty level are at higher risk for pregnancy, sexually transmitted disease, depression, obesity, and suicide. They are more likely to be sexually abused, drop out of high school, or be killed (Gold, Kennedy, Connell, & Kawachi, 2002; Goodman, Slap, & Huang, 2003; McCall, 1991; Rice, Roberts, Handsfield, & Holmes, 1991).

In adulthood, health disparities related to socioeconomic status continue. People living below the poverty level experience higher rates of death and premature chronic morbidity, as well as earlier onset of disabilities such as hypertension, diabetes, cardiovascular disease, obesity, depression, osteoarthritis, oral pathology, and many cancers (Fiscella & Williams, 2004). More than one-fifth of adults 55 to 64 years of age have incomes below the poverty level, so health disparities among the elderly population remain high (Fiscella & Williams, 2004; NCHS, 2005; Von Dem, Luschen, Cockerham, & Siegrist, 2003). In 2003, among people ages 65 years and older, one-fifth of Hispanic people and nearly one-quarter of African Americans were living below the poverty level (NCHS, 2005).

People with low socioeconomic status also are at risk for exposure to environmental toxins, including lead, passive smoking, air pollution, and cockroach excrement (Gunier, Hertz, Von Behren, & Reynolds, 2003; Leaderer et al., 2002; Morland, Wing, Diez, & Poole, 2002). Unhealthy behaviors such as inadequate physical activity, smoking, alcohol use, and poor diet are more prevalent among people of low socioeconomic status (NCHS, 2005). Lack of resources, financial hardship, low literacy, and limited access to health care are all associated with chronic stress and trauma, which add to detrimental effects on health. In addition, low socioeconomic status is associated with poor psychological coping and perceived lack of control and self-efficacy, which in turn are associated with poor health and increased mortality (Fiscella & Williams, 2004).

The social distribution of risk factors may partially explain health disparities among racial and ethnic populations.

The social distribution of risk factors may partially explain health disparities among racial and ethnic populations. People with little education are more likely to have lower incomes, be jobless, and share a household with others of the same status in lower socioeconomic status communities. Even those whose health has not been affected are more likely to have family members with ill health. Low-income children typically attend schools where risk factors are concentrated. Individuals with low-income socioeconomic status are more likely to be exposed to crime, violence, and drug trafficking, and they are less likely to be exposed to successful role models and social networks that facilitate upward mobility (Fiscella & Williams, 2004). The cumulative toll from these risk factors can be destructive to individuals, families, and communities.

The relationship between socioeconomic status and health persists across time and place. It creates social disadvantages across the stages of life and across environments. Whether measured by income, educational achievement, or occupation, socioeconomic status is linked with disparities in health status. Closing the gaps among racial, ethnic, and class groups will require altering the socioeconomic conditions of disadvantaged persons in the United States. Thus, fighting poverty must be part of any overall strategy for eliminating health disparities.

Other Vulnerable Populations

Several other vulnerable populations experience health disparities in physical, psychological, or social health. According to Aday (2001),

> These groups' needs are serious and in many cases debilitating or life-threatening ones; they require an extensive or intensive set of medical and non-medical services; the growth in their numbers and the seriousness of their needs are placing increasing demands on the medical care, public health, and related service delivery sectors; and their complex and multifaceted needs are not adequately met through existing financing or service delivery arrangements. (p. 10)

At-Risk Groups

Lack of material and nonmaterial resources contributes to the vulnerability of at-risk groups to poor health, and the consequences of their poor health make them susceptible to harm and neglect. Although all members of families and communities are potentially vulnerable, the following groups have been identified by Aday (2001) as especially vulnerable:

- *High-risk mothers and infants.* Mothers and infants who are socioeconomically and educationally disadvantaged are the most vulnerable group for poor health. High-risk childbearing is indicative of teenage pregnancies, prospective mothers who fail to receive adequate prenatal care, infants who are born prematurely or are underweight at birth, and mothers of babies who die at the beginning of life. Very young, African American, and poorly educated mothers, less than high school, are much less likely to have adequate prenatal care and more likely to bear low birth weight or very low birth weight infants. The presence or absence of strong social networks can directly affect whether they seek prenatal care or have child care. Environmental and behavioral risks associated with poverty, such as substance abuse or unsafe living conditions, also make this group vulnerable to health disparities (Aday, 2001; NCHS, 2005; Office of Minority Health, 2005e).

- *People who are chronically ill and disabled.* Long-term chronic diseases (e.g., heart disease, cancer, diabetes) present challenges that increase during the course of the disease by lowering people's ability to live with their problems, limiting their abilities to perform activities of daily living and instrumental activities of daily living, and causing associated complications and eventually death. Men are more likely to die from chronic illnesses than women, but elderly women are less able to perform normal daily routines. African American men are more likely to experience serious disabilities and death from chronic illnesses. The growing proportion of children who experience parental divorce; are born to single-parent families; or are raised in low-income, low-education households are attributing to an increasing number of children with behavioral and psychosocial problems (Aday, 2001; NCHS, 2005; Office of Minority Health, 2005e). Long-term deprivation of social support and economic and community resources directly affects the health of people of all ages who are chronically ill and disabled.

- *People living with HIV/AIDS.* Higher proportions of African Americans and Hispanics than White Americans are HIV positive, develop and die of AIDS, and contract the disease through drug use or sexual contact with drug users. Increasing numbers of mothers and children are contracting the disease and face the prospect of being abandoned by their families. Persons living with HIV/AIDS often are physically unable to work after the onset of symptoms, resulting in a loss of income and insurance benefits that are required to obtain adequate medical care. Unstable housing situations for this population also can result in less access and continuity of care as well as poorer functional health status (Aday, 2001; Office of Minority Health, 2005d).

- *People who are mentally ill and disabled.* People with mental illness and those with mental retardation and other cognitive impairments are at risk. Children are more likely to have developmental and behavioral problems. Older adults are more likely to have organic brain syndrome, whereas adults are more likely to have substance abuse disorders, schizophrenia, affective disorders, and anxiety disorders. Mental illness is more prevalent among women, and substance abuse and antisocial personality disorders are more prevalent among men. Stressful life events that require a great deal of change or adaptation, such as marriage or the loss of a spouse, have been found to play in role in producing mental illness. Living in poverty, lacking family and social support, and having limited educational and job

opportunities exacerbate the stress among people with lower socioeconomic status and racial and ethnic minorities (Aday, 2001; Office of Minority
Health, 2005c; NCHS, 2005).

- *People who abuse alcohol and other substances.* These individuals developed
  a long-term physical or psychological dependency on (or addiction to)
  drugs, alcohol, or tobacco. Adolescence is a period that tends to serve as the
  initiation of the use of certain substances and the use of more addictive
  drugs. Native American youths are much more likely to use alcohol, drugs,
  and cigarettes. Other stages of life can give rise to the onset of serious substance abuse problems and dependence. Minority users are more likely
  than White users to develop life-threatening patterns of abuse. The elderly
  population tends to have problems with alcohol abuse or dependence.
  Education and income are both correlates and consequences of substance
  use and abuse. Rates of substance abuse are higher among unemployed
  people; alcohol abuse is higher among those with limited education; and
  smoking is less among those with higher levels of education and income
  (Aday, 2001; Office of Minority Health, 2005d; NCHS, 2005).

- *Suicide- or homicide-prone individuals.* Suicide rates are highest among older
  White and young American Indian men, while homicide rates are highest
  among young African American, American Indian, and Hispanic men. The
  violence-related deaths for these groups are attributable primarily to the
  greater use of deadly weapons, particularly firearms, in their encounters.
  Firearm-related crime rates are higher in communities that are racially segregated or have substantial economic decline. Homicide and suicide rates
  are higher among individuals in abusive family environments. Among elderly people, the high suicide rate is attributed to illness; economic insecurity; and losses associated with loneliness, isolation, and depression. The role
  of social interaction and ties with others through families, friendships, work,
  neighborhoods, and voluntary associations are predictors of suicidal behaviors (Aday, 2001; Office of Minority Health, 2005d; NCHS, 2005).

- *Families experiencing abuse.* This group includes individuals who are intentionally harmed by close family members, friends, or other intimates. Unemployment and associated economic hardship play a major role in cases of
  maltreatment and neglect within families. Social isolation also is a defining
  characteristic of many abusing families. These families are much less likely to
  participate in organized community or religious activities. They tend to have
  little or no friendship networks or social ties. The abused older adult has been
  relocated from his or her own home and is less likely to participate in external activities that would bring them in contact with other people. The rates
  of abuse are highest in families in which poverty and related unemployment

or underemployment and inadequate housing are problematic. Familial violence is exacerbated when the woman involved has less education or occupational skills or the male head of the household is experiencing considerable status insecurity (Aday, 2001; Office of Minority Health, 2005e).

- *Homeless people.* This group includes the multitudes of men, women, and children who have no place to call home on any given night. Homeless children are much more likely to experience physical, mental, emotional, educational, developmental, and behavioral problems. They are less likely to have obtained immunizations and other preventive health care compared to children who are not homeless. Homeless youths are prone to physical, sexual, substance, or other abuse. Homeless women are vulnerable to unwanted pregnancies, adverse birth outcomes, and sexual and physical assault. Traditional social and economic inequities by race and gender contribute to the increasing number of women, children, minorities, and the poor among homeless people. Homeless individuals have no regular or strong social ties with family, friends, or other social networks, which increases their vulnerability to other disabilities and occupational deprivation (Aday, 2001; Whiteford, 2004).

- *Immigrants and refugees.* People who currently live in the United States who voluntarily left their home countries, as well as those who were pushed out by political, military, or economic hardship, are at risk for poor health. Asian and African immigrants make up a substantial proportion of refugees in this country, but the largest numbers of immigrants come from Europe and Mexico. Many refugees experience substantial problems in adjusting to life in the United States because of cultural differences with their home countries and the circumstances associated with their exodus. These groups are much less likely to have formal education; they are unable to read or write their own language, much less English; and they tend to have the most and most serious health problems. Undocumented persons have the most tenuous legal and social status, networks of families or community support, and financial resources. They are likely to be employed in the least desirable, lowest paying jobs. They generally have no job security or health benefits (Aday, 2001; Office of Minority Health, 2005d).

Women With Physical Disabilities

According to the National Study of Women with Physical Disabilities (1997), women with disabilities often are denied reproductive and other types of health care and given substandard care compared to women with uncomplicated care needs. Women with disabilities face numerous barriers in obtaining health information, including low health literacy. Several studies have documented the lack of health insurance among women with disabilities. They are less likely to be employed or married, two of the principal means of access to health insurance. Poverty is another defining characteristic of women with disabilities. The combined effect of unemployment, poverty, and single marital status make women with disabilities much less likely to have private health insurance than women without disabilities. Nearly 15% of women with functional limitations who are ages 45 to 64 have no health care coverage at all. Women with disabilities who do have public or private health insurance often do not have coverage for certain prescription drugs, occupational or physical therapy, assistive devices, medical equipment, medical supplies, or in-home attendant care services.

According to the Center for Research on Women with Disabilities (CROWD; 2005), the most significant health disparities among women with physical disabilities affect those with the following conditions:

- *Osteoporosis.* One-quarter of a convenience sample of women with physical disabilities ages 18 to 83 reported having osteoporosis (Nosek et al., 2006).
- *Diabetes.* One-third of women with physical disabilities reported having diabetes (Nosek et al., 2006, in press).
- *Depression.* Half of the CROWD (2005) sample of women with disabilities had scores in the mildly depressed range or higher on the Beck Depression Inventory (BDI–II; Beck, Rial, & Wickets, 1974). The women with depression were more likely to have a diagnosis of multiple sclerosis, be younger women, and have a shorter duration of disability. Only 44% of the women with scores exceeding the BDI–II cutoff for significant depressive symptomatology had received recent treatment for depression, and Hispanic women were the least likely to report having received treatment (Hughes, Robinson-Whelen, Taylor, Petersen, & Nosek, 2005).
- *Obesity.* In one study, 47.6% of a convenience sample of women with physical disabilities reported having a body mass index of 30 or greater (Nosek et al., 2006). Another study that used National Health Interview Survey (National Center for Health Statistics, 2002) data for women with functional limitations found that 43.2% of women with three or more limitations were obese (Chevarley, Thierry, Gill, Ryerson, & Nosek, 2006).
- *Hypertension.* CROWD (2005) data showed that 56.2% of a convenience sample of women with physical disabilities reported having hypertension (Nosek et al., 2006, in press).

Cultural Considerations

Many factors influence why people use or do not use health services, including the ease of access to services and the willingness to seek help. Culture is at the heart of such factors. For example, in traditional Chinese culture, many diseases are attributed to an imbalance of cosmic forces known as yin and yang. So the goal is to restore the balance, which might be accomplished through exercise or diet and not necessarily through use of the mainstream health system. Each group, with its individual racial, ethnic, gender, and socioeconomic characteristics, has its own way of dealing with the health care system. The help-seeking behaviors of individuals are closely linked to their culture.

Cultural phenomena can present barriers to health care access. For example, health services are unavailable on Sundays, when people who work all week and keep Saturday as a Sabbath could use them. An inability to communicate in English or Spanish is another problem. For homeless, confused, and chronically mentally ill people, coping with organized delivery systems and insurance is a formidable task (Friedman, 1994).

A history of discrimination tends to discourage people from seeking or getting medical care. Mistrust of the health care system for many African Americans stems from memories of the Tuskegee Syphilis Study (Brooks, Fessler, Bastian, & Alarcon, 1999). According to McCormick and colleagues (1996), older Asian Americans harbor a general distrust of Western medicine. Recent Asian immigrants view the system as intimidating and too hard to understand. Although low-income groups grapple with the greatest barriers to care, moderate- and higher income Hispanics and African Americans also face barriers such as lack of confidence in the health system (Boulware, Cooper, Ratner, LaVeist, & Powe, 2003).

Another cultural barrier is language. Hispanics with limited or no English skills often are afraid that they can't communicate well, so they don't seek mainstream health services for fear of being misunderstood (Institute of Medicine, 2005). Lack of language translation services or providers who can speak the patient's language often are reported by Asian Americans and Pacific Islanders (Office of Minority Health, 2000). Even for patients who speak English, differences in the use of language contribute to misunderstanding and distrust. Health care workers may use unfamiliar terms and medical jargon that many African Americans and members of other ethnic groups cannot understand (Dula, 1994). Language barriers not only block health care access but also may cause confusion in diagnosis and intervention.

Cultural differences between providers and patients may present more barriers. Many Hispanics feel more comfortable with Hispanic health care providers who have an understanding or appreciation of their culture (Gomes & McGuire, 2001). A study by Asbury, Walker, Belgrave, Maholmes, and Green (1994) of African Americans in rehabilitation found that the most influential predictor of level of participation was whether the service provider was of the same race or ethnicity as the client. Clients who were of the same ethnic group as the service provider were more likely to participate in rehabilitation on a continuous basis.

Some barriers to care emerge from the failure to develop culturally specific health delivery services. When health care providers neglect cultural concerns, minority and disadvantaged people get the message that their culture, belief system, and health are not valued. Mayeno (1992) advocated for ethnically targeted, comprehensive community-based primary health care services for Asian Americans. She states that comprehensive community-based services have the ability to respond to changing needs in the community; are the first-line source of preventive health care, outreach, and education; and focus on the whole person. This type of holistic service is very important in Asian cultures (Tom, 1992).

Inclusive and comprehensive services also have been called for in Native American communities. Services including the whole realm of self: Mind, body, spirit, and feelings must be at the core of effective health services for Americans Indians. According to Whiterabbit (cited in DHHS, 1995), simply addressing a specific health disease or disorder will not be a catalyst for change. In addition to "talking about how to protect both the mind and body from disease, you must go into lots of issues that are specific to the community, like how loss of land and loss of culture affect attitudes about health" (p. 4).

Migrant workers face additional barriers to access health services—a lack of knowledge and understanding about how to access and utilize services and lack of ability to fully participate in the medical interview. Approximately 300,000 children of migratory farm workers live in the United States. Even though the majority of these children are impoverished and meet one of several criteria for Medicaid enrollment, the transitory nature of their parents' work, language and cultural barriers, and difficulties transporting Medicaid benefits across states pose formidable access barriers to early and periodic screening, diagnosis, and treatment for eligible children (National Conference of State Legislatures, 1996).

Paying for health coverage is not the only cost families consider in whether or not to use health services (Riportella-Muller, Selby-Harrington, Richardson, Donat, & Luchok, 1993). Among the obstacles families face in using health services are problems arranging care for children or other family members, inability to take time off from work, family crises, a parent's own poor health, misperception of the child's need for preventive care, a lack of sense of responsibility for the child's health, a child's chronic illness that makes well-child care secondary, outreach materials that are ineffective (including print materials mailed to parents who cannot read English), scheduling difficulties, and trouble with transportation.

The link between culture and health is a key in reducing health disparities. Understanding and appreciating life histories, cultural attitudes and behaviors, and language can go a long way toward eliminating the distrust of the health care system that is shared by many racial and ethnic populations. At the individual and social levels, overcoming linguistic and cultural barriers is fundamental to providing culturally competent care to all people. Hiring bilingual and bicultural staff members, tailoring interventions on the basis of culturally specific knowledge, modifying services by integrating traditional medicine with Western medicine, and developing appropriate cultural service models and specialized programs are a few steps toward achieving ethnically sensitive health care services.

Increasing the number of trained health care providers from ethnic backgrounds is a strategy that must be pursued (Komaromy et al., 1996). Professionals who are most like the racial and ethnic communities whom they serve need to be recruited and hired to help reduce disparities in health care. All health care professionals must be trained to consider the culture of their clients rather than just their health and human services needs. According to the American Medical Student Association (2004), doctors rated African American patients as less intelligent, less educated, more likely to abuse drugs and alcohol, more likely to fail to comply with medical advice, more likely to lack social support, and less likely to participate in cardiac rehabilitation than White patients, even after patients' income, education, and personality characteristics were taken into account. These findings suggest that, although the relationship between race or ethnicity and treatment decisions is complex, providers' perceptions and attitudes toward patients often are influenced in subtle ways by patient race or ethnicity.

Summary

A disparity is an inequality. All Americans should be able to count on receiving care that meets their needs and is based on the best scientific knowledge available. Instead, they are faced with a health care system that does not provide consistent, high-quality medical care to all people. It is a system characterized by inefficiency, unequal access, gaps in quality and coverage, and inequity. The fragmented nature of the system—with multiple public and private financing and delivery processes— poses many barriers to high performance. The overarching goal of any health care system should be to help all citizens live long, healthy, and productive lives by providing the right care safely, at the right cost, and as efficiently as possible regardless of income, race, ethnicity, health status, geographic location, gender, sexual identity, religious affiliation, or age. People need access to both preventive care and prompt treatment of illness and injuries. In varying magnitudes by condition and population, disparities exist in almost all aspects of health care.

When racial and ethnic minorities, people who are poor, women with disabilities, gay men and lesbians, and people who are transgendered receive lower quality health care than the privileged majority, then disparities exist. Some progress has been made; according to the AHRQ's (2005) *National Healthcare Disparities Report,* disparities in quality of care are decreasing for most racial minorities; however, for Hispanics, the reverse is true. All disparities in access to care that could be tracked were becoming smaller; yet Hispanics and the poor population were falling behind. The single largest access problem faced by all groups, except Asians, is lack of health insurance; the largest problem Asian Americans report is lack of a primary care provider. Minorities and poor people receive lower quality of care and have worse access to care. Differences among groups will always exist. It is wrong, however, when these differences lead to unequal care.

How can people begin to address the disparities in a health care system committed in principle to providing care to everyone? Some ways are to work together, share knowledge and research, find common ground, and set common goals to reduce these disparities. Coordinated actions at the federal, state, and local levels are needed to extend the benefits of regional and local successes nationwide. Patients, providers, purchasers, and policymakers, through collaboration and hard work, can make full access to high-quality care a reality for all.

Occupational therapy practitioners, meanwhile, must attain knowledge and information about diverse communities. They must recognize, understand, and incorporate into their interventions the sociopolitical and ethnoracial variations found within these communities. The health problems of women, gay men and lesbians, ethnic minorities, and the poor would be more adequately resolved if understood within their respective sociopolitical contexts. Practitioners must work in partnership to promote mutual understanding and collaboration with not only the client but also the family or caregiver and the community at large. Concepts such as family systems, communities, cultures, organizational missions, and societal commitments must be foremost in the minds of both researchers and practitioners if they are to change the way health care is practiced with and received by vulnerable populations. When everyone participates, when everyone is accountable, and when the changes are systemic and cultural, the health disparities will close.

Reflection

1. Explore health disparities in your state.

   a. Contact your state's Department of Health and Human Services to acquire information about health disparities in your state.

   b. List all disparities that you identify.

   c. Prioritize and choose one or two issues that your class, your program, or your state occupational therapy association could work toward resolving.

   d. Develop a simple project that would address these disparities.

2. Explore health disparities in your community.

    a. Determine how you can learn about health disparities in your community that are related to occupation or occupational therapy.

    b. Develop a service learning project for students that addresses health disparities in your community.

References

Aday, L. A. (2001). *At risk in America: The health and health care needs of vulnerable populations in the United States* (2nd ed.). San Francisco: Jossey-Bass.

Agency for Healthcare Research and Quality. (2000, February). *Addressing racial and ethnic disparities in health care: Fact sheet.* Rockville, MD: Author. Retrieved December 12, 2005, from www.ahrq.gov/research/disparit.htm

Agency for Healthcare Research and Quality. (2005). *National healthcare disparities report.* Rockville, MD: Author.

American Medical Student Association. (2004). *Cultural competence in medicine.* Retrieved June 13, 2004, from www.amsa.org/programs/gpit/cultural.cfm

American Public Health Association. (2004). *Health disparities: A general overview.* Retrieved December 12, 2005, from www.nphw.org

Asbury, C. A., Walker, S., Belgrave, F. Z., Maholmes, V., & Green, L. (1994). Psychosocial, cultural, and accessibility factors associated with participation of African-Americans in rehabilitation. *Rehabilitation Psychology, 39,* 113–121.

Beck, A. T., Rial, W. Y., & Rickets, K. (1974). Short form of depression inventory: Cross-validation. *Psychological Reports, 34,* 1184–1186.

Betancourt, J. R., Green, A. R., Carrillo, J. M., & Ananeh-Firempong, O. (2003). Defining cultural competence: A practical framework for addressing racial/ethnic disparities in health and health care. *Public Health Reports, 118,* 293–302.

Boulware, I. E., Cooper, L. A., Ratner, L. E., LaVeist, T. A., & Powe, N. R. (2003). Race and trust in the health care system. *Public Health Reports, 118,* 358–365.

Brooks, K., Fessler, B. J., Bastian, H., & Alarcon, G. (1999). Sociocultural issues in clinical research. *Arthritis Care and Research, 45*(2), 203–207.

Center for the Advancement of Health. (2004). Facts of life: Issue briefings for health reporters. *CFAH, 8*(3). Retrieved May 31, 2006, from www.cfah.org/factsoflife/vol8no3.cfm

Center for Research on Women With Disabilities. (2005). *Health disparities between women with physical disabilities and women in the general population.* Retrieved December 22, 2005, from www.bcm.edu/crowd/?PMID=1331.

Centers for Disease Control and Prevention. (2005). *Disease burden and risk factors.* Rockville, MD: Office of Minority Health, U.S. Department of Health and Human Services. Retrieved January 5, 2006, from www.cdc.gov/omh/AMH/dbrf.htm

Chevarley, F., Thierry, J., Gill, C., Ryerson, B. A., & Nosek, M. A. (2007). *Health and well-being for women with disabilities: Analysis of data from the 1994–1995 National Health Interview Survey on Disability.* Manuscript in preparation.

Coleman-Miller, B. (2000). A physician's perspective on minority health. *Health Care Financing Review, 21,* 45–56.

Dula, A. (1994). The life and death of Miss Mildred: An elderly Black woman. *Clinics in Geriatric Medicine, 10,* 419–430.

Environmental Justice & Health Union. (2003). *Environmental disparities and racial disparities.* Retrieved October 31, 2006, from www.ejhu.org/disparities.html.

Fiscella, K., & Williams, D. R. (2004). Health disparities based on socioeconomic inequities: Implications for urban health care. *Academic Medicine, 79,* 1139–1147.

Friedman, E. (1994). Money isn't everything: Non-financial barriers to access. *Journal of the American Medical Association, 271,* 1535–1538.

Gabel, J., Claxton, G., Gil, I., Pickreign, J., & Whitmore, H. (2005). Health benefits in 2005: Premium increases slow down, coverage continues to erode. *Health Affairs, 24,* 1273–1280.

Gamm, L., Hutchison, L., Bellamy, G., & Dabney, B. J. (2002). Rural healthy people: Identifying rural health priorities and models for practice. *Journal of Rural Health, 18*(1), 9–14.

Gaston, R. S., Ayres, I., Dooley, L. G., & Diethelm, A. G. (1993). Racial equality in renal transplantation. *Journal of the American Medical Association, 270,* 1352–1356.

Ginsburg, P. B. (2005). Competition in health care: Its evolution over the past decade. *Health Affairs, 24,* 1512–1522.

Gold, R., Kennedy, B., Connell, F., & Kawachi, I. (2002). Teen births, income inequality, and social capital: Developing an understanding of the causal pathway. *Health Place, 8,* 77–83.

Gomes, C., & McGuire, T. G. (2001). Identifying the sources of racial and ethnic disparities in health care use. In Institute of Medicine, *Unequal treatment: Confronting racial and ethnic disparities in health care* (p. 4). Washington, DC: National Academy of Sciences.

Goodman, E., Slap, G. B., & Huang, B. (2003). The public health impact of socioeconomic status on adolescent depression and obesity. *American Journal of Public Health, 93,* 1844–1850.

Gormick, M. E., Eggers, P. W., & Reilly, T. W. (1996). Effects of race and income on mortality and use of services among Medicare beneficiaries. *New England Journal of Medicine, 335,* 791–799.

Gunier, R. B., Hertz, A., Von Behren, J., & Reynolds, P. (2003). Traffic density in California: Socioeconomic and ethnic differences among potentially exposed children. *Journal of Exposure Analysis and Environmental Epidemiology, 13,* 240–246.

Hashimoto, D. M. (2001). The proposed Patients' Bill of Rights: The case of the missing equal protection clause. *Yale Journal of Health Policy, Law, and Ethics, 1,* 77–93.

Hughes, R. B., Robinson-Whelen, S., Taylor, H. B., Petersen, N., & Nosek, M. A. (2005). Characteristics of depressed and non-depressed women with physical disabilities. *Archives of Physical Medicine and Rehabilitation, 80,* 473–479.

Institute of Medicine. (2000). *Crossing the quality chasm: A new health system for the 21st century.* Washington, DC: National Academies Press.

Institute of Medicine. (2002). *Unequal treatment: Confronting racial and ethnic disparities in health care.* Washington, DC: National Academies Press.

Institute of Medicine. (Ed.). (2005). *Confronting the nation's health disparities*. Washington, DC: National Academies of Sciences.

Intercultural Cancer Council. (2001). *Rural poor and the medically underserved and cancer*. Retrieved October 31, 2006, from http://iccnetwork.org/cancerfacts/ICC-CFS6.pdf

Johnson, V. (1995). *Heart full of grace: A thousand years of Black wisdom*. New York: Simon & Schuster.

Kaiser Family Foundation. (2000). *Racial and ethnic disparities in access to health insurance and health care*. Los Angeles: UCLA Center for Health Policy Research. Retrieved January 5, 2006, from www.healthpolicy.ucla.edu

Komaromy, M., Grumbach, K., Drake, M., Vranizan, K., Lurie, N., Keane, D., & Bindman, A. (1996). The role of Black and Hispanic physicians in providing health care for underserved populations. *New England Journal of Medicine, 334,* 1305–1310.

Leaderer, B. P., Belanger, K., Triche, E., Holford, T., Gold, D. R., Kim, Y., et al. (2002). Dust mite, cockroach, cat, and dog allergen concentrations in homes of asthmatic children in the northeastern United States: Impact of socioeconomic factors and population density. *Environmental Health Perspectives, 110,* 419–425.

Mayeno, L. (1992). Primary care recommendations for health care system reform. In *Partners in human service: Shaping health care and civil rights policy for Asian and Pacific Islander Americans, final report* (pp. 20–23). Washington, DC: U.S. Department of Health and Human Services.

McCall, P. L. (1991). Adolescent and elderly White male suicide trends: Evidence of changing well-being? *Journal of Gerontology, 46,* 43–51.

McCormick, W. C., Uomoto, J., Young, H., Graves, A. B., Vitaliano, P., Mortimer, J. A., et al. (1996). Attitudes toward use of nursing homes and home care in older Japanese-Americans. *Journal of the American Geriatrics Society, 44,* 769–777.

Morland, K., Wing, S., Diez, R. A., & Poole, C. (2002). Neighborhood characteristics associated with the location of food stores and food services places. *American Journal of Preventive Medicine, 22,* 23–29.

National Center for Cultural Competence. (2005). *Rationale for cultural competence in primary care*. Washington, DC: National Center for Cultural Competence, Georgetown University Center for Child and Human Development, University Center for Excellence in Development Disabilities. Retrieved December 22, 2005, from http://gucchd.georgetown.edu/nccc/cultural6.html

National Center for Health Statistics. (2002). *Summary health statistics for U.S. adults: National Health Interview Survey*. Hyattsville, MD: Author.

National Center for Health Statistics. (2005). *Health, United States, 2005 with chartbook on trends in the health of Americans*. Hyattsville, MD: Author.

National Conference of State Legislatures. (1996). *State's legislatures' role in multicultural health: Project summary*. Washington, DC: Author.

National Institutes of Health. (2005). *Addressing health disparities: The NIH program of action*. Retrieved December 22, 2005, from http://healthdisparities.nih.gov/whatare.html

National Study of Women With Physical Disabilities. (1997). *Final Report 1992–1996: National study of women with physical disabilities*. Houston, TX: Baylor College of

Medicine, Center for Research on Women with Disabilities, Department of Physical Medicine and Rehabilitation.

Nosek, M. A., Hughes, R. B., Petersen, N., Taylor, H. B., Robinson-Whelen, S., Byrne, M., & Morgan, R. O. (2006). Secondary conditions in a community based sample of women with physical disabilities over a one-year period. *Archives of Physical Medicine and Rehabilitation, 87*(3): 320–327.

Office of Minority Health. (2005a). *Hispanic/Latino profile.* Retrieved May 31, 2006, from www.omhrc.gov/minoritypopulations/Hispanic/Latino

Office of Minority Health. (2005b). *Men's health 101.* Retrieved May 31, 2006, from www.omhrc.gov/healthtopics/menhealth

Office of Minority Health. (2005c). *Mental health 101.* Retrieved May 31, 2006, from www.omhrc.gov/health topics/mental health

Office of Minority Health. (2005d). *Minority populations.* Retrieved May 31, 2006, from www.omhrc.gov/minoritypopulations

Office of Minority Health. (2005e). *Women's health 101.* Retrieved May 31, 2006, from www.omhrc.gov/healthtopic/womenhealth

Randall, V. R. (1994). Racist health care reform: Reforming an unjust health care system to meet the needs of African Americans. *Health Matrix, 3,* 155–156.

Rice, R. J., Roberts, P. L., Handsfield, H. H., & Holmes, K. K. (1991). Sociodemographic distribution of gonorrhea incidence: Implications for prevention and behavioral research. *American Journal of Public Health, 81,* 1252–1258.

Riportella-Muller, R., Selby-Harrington, M. L., Richardson, L. A., Donat, L. N., & Luchok, K. J. (1993, June 29). *Barriers to the use of preventive health care services for children: The case of Early and Periodic Screening, Diagnosis, and Treatment program.* Paper presented at the 10th annual meeting of the Association for Health Services Research, Washington, DC.

Smith, D. B. (1993). The racial integration of health facilities. *Journal of Health Politics, Policy, and Law, 18,* 850–854.

Smith, M. B. (1998, March). Race, ethnicity, class, and culture. *Closing the Gap Newsletter,* p. 2.

Tom, C. (1992). Health care reform: Beyond financial barriers to access to care. In *Partners in human service: Shaping health care and civil rights policy for Asian and Pacific Islander Americans, final report* (pp. 9–11). Washington, DC: U.S. Department of Health and Human Services.

U.S. Department of Health and Human Services. (1995, July). Recognizing the link between Indian culture and health. *Closing the Gap Newsletter,* p. 4.

U.S. Department of Health and Human Services. (2000). *Healthy People 2010.* Washington, DC: Author. Retrieved August 4, 2004, from www.healthypeople.gov/publications

U.S. Department of Health and Human Services. (2004). *The initiative to eliminate racial and ethnic disparities in health: HHS fact sheet.* Retrieved December 22, 2005, from www.omhrc.gov/healthdisparities/index.htm

U.S. Public Health Service. (1994). *Improving minority health statistics: Report of the Public Health Task Force on Minority Health Data.* Washington, DC: U.S. Department of Health and Human Services, Office of Minority Health

Von Dem, K. O., Luschen, G., Cockerham, W. C., & Siegrist, J. (2003). Socioeconomic status and health among the aged in the United States and Germany: A comparative cross-sectional study. *Social Science and Medicine, 57,* 1643–1652.

Young, L. J. (1994). Toward an ethic of care and community in education and medicine. In A. Dula & S. Goering (Eds.), *"It just ain't fair": The ethics of health care for African Americans* (pp. 244–263). Westport, CT: Praeger

Whiteford, G. (2004). When people cannot participate: Occupational deprivation. In C. H. Christiansen & E. A. Townsend (Eds.), *Introduction to occupation: The art and science of living* (pp. 221–242). Upper Saddle River, NJ: Prentice Hall.

11

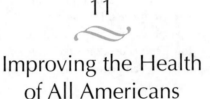

Improving the Health
of All Americans

*E*ducation must not simply teach work—it must teach life.

— W. E. B. DuBois (cited in Johnson, 1995, p. 86)

Key Points

- After years of rising health care costs, medical technology innovations, and ongoing health disparities, the U.S. health system continues to fail in providing quality care to all Americans.

- Health data describe the well-being or ill health of the population, which enables health care professionals to develop interventions for preventing and controlling disease in populations and evaluate the effect of these interventions. Health status data include a variety of measures, including the nature and extent of mortality, morbidity, and disability in people and populations and their knowledge, attitudes, and behaviors concerning health and health care.

- Life expectancy and the overall health of the nation continue to improve for a large number of Americans. But the prevalence of chronic conditions has increased, together with their associated pain and resultant disability.

- Of particular concern in recent years is the incidence of obesity among the U.S. population, which is a risk factor for many chronic diseases and disabilities, including heart disease, hypertension, and diabetes.

- Socioeconomic and cultural differences among racial and ethnic groups will likely continue to influence future patterns of disease, disability, and health care use.

- The health care delivery system is poorly organized to meet the challenges involved in eliminating health discrepancies.

THE UNITED STATES SPENDS MORE ON HEALTH CARE per capita than any other country. In 2004, national health care expenditures totaled $1.7 trillion. Much of the spending has been for care that controls or reduces the effect of chronic diseases and conditions affecting an aging population. Hospital care accounted for 31% of this expenditure. Inpatient care has become more complex, with more cardiac procedures being performed, especially for older adult patients. New types of health care providers, including ambulatory surgery centers and end-stage renal disease facilities, have emerged to provide services previously available only in hospitals (National Center for Health Statistics [NCHS], 2005).

Because of inefficiencies in the health care system, the high level of spending has not benefited all sectors of the population. For example, in 2004, the percentage of people living below the poverty level who reported their health status as fair or poor was more than 3 times higher than for people living above the poverty level. Levels of fair to poor health were twice as high among Hispanic people and African Americans as among White people. Most of the rise in health care spending has been linked to innovations in pharmacological treatment options and new treatment procedures. Many of these innovations have been successful in improving survival rates and have given physicians new approaches for treating patients, but their cost-effectiveness has not been established (Thorpe, 2005). The least costly drugs or procedures are sometimes more effective than the innovative approach (Gabel et. al., 2005). Innovations in medical treatment have paradoxically contributed to the shortfall of quality care in the U.S. health care system.

Americans should be able to rely on receiving care that meets their needs and is based on the best scientific knowledge. Instead, continuing health disparities among different U.S. subpopulations reflect the fact that the U.S. health care system does not provide consistent, high-quality medical care to all people. It is a system characterized by inefficiency, unequal access, gaps in quality coverage, and inequity. The fragmented nature of the system, with multiple public and private financing and delivery processes, poses many barriers to high performance. Following years of rising health care costs, expensive medical technology innovations, and ongoing health disparities, the U.S. health care system continues to fall short in its ability to provide consistent, quality care.

The overarching goal of any health care system should be to help all citizens live long, healthy, and productive lives by providing the right care safely, at the right cost, and as efficiently as possible regardless of income, race, ethnicity, health status, geographic location, or age. People need both access to preventive care and prompt treatment of illness and injuries. This chapter presents health data, illustrating the effects of an inefficient health care system and the measures necessary to improve health care delivery in the United States.

Health Data Sources

To assess and understand the health of the nation and to develop approaches to sustain it, U.S. government agencies collect and disseminate health data. National disease prevention and health promotion initiatives such as Healthy People have improved the monitoring and reporting of changing health status and emerging risks to health and service delivery. The Healthy People reports, of which the latest is *Healthy People 2010* (U.S. Department of Health and Human Services, 2000), describe the initiatives and objectives intended to achieve improved health for all Americans and the data used to support them.

Health status describes the myriad components of the well-being or ill health of the population so that health care professionals can develop interventions for preventing and controlling disease and evaluate the effect of these interventions. Health status includes a variety of measures, such as the nature and extent of mortality, morbidity, and disability in people and populations, as well as their knowledge, attitudes, and behaviors concerning health and health care. *Health data* encompass all major areas of health statistics, including population and health status, health resources, health care utilization, and health care expenditures, as well as program management data. In support of its mission to protect the health of the nation's population, the U.S. Public Health Service gathers a wide variety of timely and reliable data, including epidemiological and statistical information. To meet these needs, the U.S. Public Health Service uses a variety of data collection, analysis, and dissemination activities. Health data come from a variety of sources—vital records, censuses, birth certificates, industrial records, hospital records, death certificates, registries, and surveys.

The NCHS is one component of the Centers for Disease Control and Prevention and serves as the federal government's designated agency for general purpose health statistics. The NCHS obtains information on the health of the U.S. population through several mechanisms, such as the National Vital Registration System, the Behavioral Risk Survey, the National Health Interview Survey, the National Health and Nutrition Examination Survey (NHANES), and record-based surveys of health care providers, including hospitals, physicians' offices, and nursing homes. Some of the information is collected annually and some only periodically.

In addition to the NCHS, the following centers and agencies (frequently known by their acronyms) collect data from surveys that include items on race and ethnicity: the Center for Chronic Disease and Health Promotion; the Alcohol, Drug Abuse, and Mental Health Administration (ADAMHA); the National Institute on Drug Abuse (NIDA); the National Institute of Mental Health (NIMH); the Agency for Health Care Policy and Research (AHCPR); and others, such as the Indian

Health Service (IHS), the National Institutes of Health (NIH), and the Health Resources and Services Administration (HRSA).

Although improvements have been made, several gaps and issues remain in the availability of data on the health status of racial and ethnic-minority populations in the United States. Getting information about ethnic and gender health is not easy. No clearinghouse for statistics lists comprehensive data by race, ethnicity, gender, or socioeconomic status. In terms of race and ethnicity, a wide variety of health data are available for White and African American populations but considerably fewer national data are available for other ethnic populations. Some sources cite figures for Whites and Blacks; others list African Americans, Hispanics (who may be Black or White), and Whites; others list African Americans, Americans Indians (or Native Americans), Asians/Pacific Islanders, Hispanics, and Whites. Few tables list any further breakdown by ethnicity. Very limited data are available on the Asian and Pacific Islander populations. National data tend to mask the diversity among Chinese, Japanese, Korean, and most recent immigrants from Southeast Asia. Any people of Cuban, Mexican, Puerto Rican, South or Central American, or other Spanish culture or origin, regardless of race, are reported as Hispanics or Latinos. Similarly, national data on the total Native American population are limited, nor is there a plethora of health data by tribal affiliation. To complicate matters further, the definition of race and ethnicity has changed over time and self-reported ethnicity has been found to change from year to year.

U.S. Health Status and Determinants

Life expectancy and the overall health of the nation continue to improve for a large number of Americans as a result of an increased focus on preventive medicine, advances in technology, and health education. Over the past century, notable achievements in public health have included the control of infectious diseases, implementation of vaccination programs, fluoridation of water, and improvements in motor vehicle safety. The U.S. population has experienced increased longevity and a sharp decline in deaths from cardiovascular diseases. On the other hand, the prevalence of chronic conditions has increased, together with their associated pain and disability. Progress in some areas, such as infant and cause-specific mortality, morbidity from chronic conditions, and prevalence of risk factors including smoking and lack of exercise, has not been as rapid as one would like to see. And these improvements have not been equally distributed by income, race, ethnicity, education, and geography (NCHS, 2005).

The 29th annual *Health, United States* report (NCHS, 2005) describes the health status of the nation as improving. In 2004, life expectancy reached an all-time high of 77.6 years, with 74.9 years for men and 80.1 years for women. The infant mortality rate was 6.9 infant deaths per 1,000 live births. The age-adjusted death rate for the total population declined 43%, to 831 deaths per 100,000. This reduction was driven largely by a decline in mortality from heart disease, stroke, and accidents and unintentional injury.

Even though the overall death rates declined, racial, ethnic, and educational disparities in mortality persisted. Infant mortality rates were highest for infants of non-Hispanic African American mothers (13.9 deaths per 1,000 live births), Hawaiian mothers (9.6 per 1,000), American Indian mothers (8.6 per 1,000), and Puerto Rican mothers (8.2 per 1,000). Infant mortality increased among infants of mothers ages 20 years and older as the mother's level of education decreased (NCHS, 2005).

Health data sources also have tracked changes in health insurance coverage. The United States has a hodgepodge of private insurance coverage based primarily on employment, along with public insurance coverage for older people (Medicare), military service members, veterans, and the poor and disabled population (Medicaid). Nearly 46 million U.S. residents have no insurance, and the numbers keep growing. The likelihood of being uninsured varies substantially among the states, ranging from 8% in Minnesota to 25% in Texas (NCHS, 2005). In 2004, 10% of children in the United States were without health insurance (NCHS, 2005). Those with insurance struggle to pay higher premiums, deductibles, and copayments. Working families are experiencing more out-of-pocket costs for doctor's visits, escalating prices for prescriptions, and increased delays in getting medical care. Some are declining to obtain care altogether. Employers are responding to increasing costs by shifting more and more health care costs onto their workers through larger copayments and deductibles (Gabel et al., 2005; Ginsburg, 2005). Insurance coverage problems can produce more expensive care, as well as preventable pain, suffering, and deaths.

Health Behaviors and Risk Factors

Health behaviors and risk factors have a significant effect on health outcomes. For example, cigarette smoking increases the risk of lung cancer, heart disease, emphysema, and other respiratory diseases. Heavy and chronic use of alcohol and illicit drugs increases the risk of disease and injury. Among adolescents ages 12 to 17 years in 2004, 12% smoked cigarettes, and 18% used alcohol (NCHS, 2005). Seat belt use is another important health behavior; in 2004, 22% of male high school students and 15% of female students rarely or never used a seat belt. Regular physical activity lessens the risk of diseases and enhances mental and physical functioning, but only one-third of adults ages 18 years and older engaged in regular leisure-time physical activity in 2004 (NCHS, 2005).

Of particular concern in recent years is the incidence of obesity among the U.S. population, which is a risk factor for many chronic diseases and disabilities, including heart disease, hypertension, and diabetes. Nearly one-tenth of adults, and about one-fifth of adults older than age 65, had diabetes in 2004, and a substantial proportion of the population experienced conditions such as arthritis, headache, and back pain that are exacerbated by obesity and can affect quality of life (NCHS, 2005). The rising number of children and adolescents who are overweight and obese raise further concerns about the future health of the U.S. population. Sixteen percent of adolescents ages 12 to 17 and 26% of children ages 6 to 11 were overweight (NCHS, 2005). Of adults age 20 or over, 67% are overweight or obese, and 32% were obese in 2004 (NHANES, 2005). The prevalence of overweight and obesity among adults ages 20 to 74 increased from 47% to 65%. The prevalence of obesity among adults doubled from 15% to 31% (NHANES, 2005).

Health Indicators for Specific Populations

Efforts to improve Americans' health will be shaped by racial and ethnic demographic changes. There are continuing differences in the burden of illness and death experienced by African Americans, Hispanic Americans, Native Americans and Alaskan Natives, and Asian Americans and Pacific Islanders as compared with the U.S. population as a whole. Racial and ethnic minorities tend to receive lower quality health care than do White Americans, even when access-related factors are controlled. Racial and ethnic minorities may experience a range of barriers to accessing care, such as language, geography, and cultural unfamiliarity. Financial and institutional arrangements of health systems, as well as the regulatory and policy environment in which they operate, may have negative effects on some groups' abilities to attain quality care (Agency for Healthcare Research and Quality [AHRQ], 2005; Institute of Medicine, 2000; NCHS, 2005). Socioeconomic and cultural differences among racial and ethnic groups will likely continue to influence future patterns of disease, disability, and health care use.

So, what is the current health status of Americans? The following sections summarize the health status and trends of the U.S. population.

Men and Women

Of the 143 million male residents of the United States in 2004, 11% had fair to poor health, and 11% had activity limitations attributable to one or more chronic health conditions (Lethbridge-Cejku, Rose, & Vickerie, 2006). Twenty-four percent smoked cigarettes, 69% were overweight, and 28% had hypertension (NCHS, 2005). The leading causes of death for men were heart disease, cancer, and accidents or unintentional injuries (Anderson & Smith, 2005). Of the 148 million female residents in 2004, 13% were in fair to poor health, and 13% had activity limitations attributable to one or more chronic health conditions (Lethbridge-Cejku et al., 2006). Nineteen percent smoked cigarettes, 62% were overweight, and 33% had hypertension (NCHS, 2005). The leading causes of death for women were heart disease, cancer, and stroke (Anderson & Smith, 2005).

Older People

Of the 35.9 million residents ages 65 and older in 2004, 26% were in fair to poor health, and 35% had activity limitations caused by chronic health conditions. Ten percent of older men and 8% of older women smoked cigarettes. Of this population, 76% of men ages 65 to 74, 67% of men ages 75 and older, 71% of women ages 65 to 71, and 60% of women ages 75 and older were overweight. Eighteen percent of individuals ages 65 to 74 years and 16% of those ages 75 and older had a diagnosis of diabetes. A large number lived with hypertension—60% of men ages 65 to 74 and 69% of men ages 75 and older, as well as 73% of women ages 65 to 74 and 83% of women ages 75 and older (NCHS, 2005). Only about 3% of the population ages 65 to 74 and 3% ages 75 and older did not have a usual place of care (Adams & Barnes, 2006). The leading causes of death for people ages 65 and older were heart disease, cancer, and cerebrovascular diseases (Anderson & Smith, 2005).

White Americans

In 2004, 236 million U.S. residents were White. Life expectancy was 78 years, with 75.4 for males and 80.5 for females (NCHS, 2005). Nine percent were in fair to poor health, and 12% lived with activity limitations attributable to one or more chronic health conditions (Adams & Barnes, 2006). Of the adult population, 24% of men and 20% of women smoked cigarettes, 70% of men and 57% of women were overweight, and 24% of men and 23% of women had hypertension (NCHS, 2005). Sixteen percent of those younger than age 65 had no health insurance. The portion of the population without a usual source of health care was 14% for adults (Lethbridge-Cejku et al., 2006) and 5% for children (Bloom & Dey, 2006). The leading causes of death for White Americans were heart disease, cancer, and stroke (Anderson & Smith, 2005).

African Americans

Life expectancy among the 38 million African Americans living in the United States has improved. From 1970 to 2003, the overall gap in life expectancy between African Americans and White Americans narrowed from 6.9 years to 5.3 years (Hoyert, Heron, Murphy, & Kung, 2006). In 2004, African Americans had a life expectancy at birth of 72.7 years, 69.0 for men and 76.1 for women. Twelve percent were in fair to poor health, and 13% had activity limitations attributable to one or more chronic health conditions. Twenty-seven percent of men and 18% of women were smokers, 62% of men and 77% of women were overweight, and 36% of men and 42% of women had hypertension (NCHS, 2005). Five percent of children and

14% of adults had no usual source of health care (Adams & Barnes, 2006). The leading causes of death were heart disease, cancer, stroke, and diabetes (Anderson & Smith, 2005).

Mexican Americans

Ten percent of Mexican Americans were in fair to poor health in 2003, and 6% lived with activity limitations attributable to one or more chronic health conditions (Adams & Barnes, 2006). Of this population, 21% of men and 10% of women were smokers, 70% of men and 69% of women were overweight, and 17% of men and 19% of women had hypertension (NCHS, 2005). Thirty-eight percent of those younger than age 65 were without health insurance. Thirty-two percent of adults and 11% of children had no usual source of health care (Adams & Barnes, 2006).

Hispanic Americans

Hispanic Americans made up 40 million of the U.S. population in 2004. Seven percent had activity limitations attributable to one or more chronic health conditions, and 10% were in fair to poor health (Adams & Barnes, 2006). Twenty-one percent of men and 11% of women smoked cigarettes (NCHS, 2005). Of those younger than age 65, 35% did not have health insurance, and 28% of adults did not have a usual source of health care (Adams & Barnes, 2006). The leading causes of death for Hispanics were heart disease, cancer, and accidents or unintentional injuries (Anderson & Smith, 2005).

American Indians and Alaska Natives

Among American Indians and Alaska Natives, 13% were in fair to poor health, and 17% had activity limitations attributable to one or more chronic conditions in 2004. Thirty-three percent of the men and 31% of the women were smokers. Only 18% of the adults did not have a usual source of health care, but 35% of those younger than age 65 had no health insurance (Adams & Barnes, 2006). The leading causes of death were heart disease, cancer, and accidents and unintentional injuries (Anderson & Smith, 2005).

Asian Americans and Pacific Islanders

Of the 13 million Asian Americans and Pacific Islanders in 2003, 6% were in fair to poor health, and 5% had activity limitations attributable to one or more chronic health conditions. Six percent of women and 17% of men were smokers (NCHS, 2005). Eighteen percent of adults had no usual source of health care, as well as 8% of children (Adams & Barnes, 2006). The leading causes of death were cancer, heart disease, and stroke (Anderson & Smith, 2005).

Improving the U.S. Health Care System

Despite improvements in the health of Americans, the U.S. health system is falling short in addressing disparities in health care among racial, ethnic, and socioeconomic groups. According to the *National Healthcare Disparities Report* (AHRQ, 2005), disparities in quality of care are decreasing among members of racial minorities overall; however, for Hispanics, disparities are rising. The single largest access problem faced by all groups except Asian Americans and Pacific Islanders is lack of health insurance; the largest problem Asian Americans and Pacific Islanders reported is lack of a primary care provider (AHRQ, 2005). Minorities and the poor receive lower quality care and have the worst access to care. People living in poverty are more likely to be in fair or poor health and to have disabling conditions and are less likely to have used many types of health care services (NCHS, 2005).

The health care delivery system is poorly organized to meet the challenges involved in eliminating health discrepancies. The system is complex and uncoordinated, resulting in delays in provision of services and increasing the risk of substandard care. Health care organizations, hospitals, and physician groups typically operate as separate entities without access to complete information about the patient's condition, medical history, and medications and services provided by other professionals (Institute of Medicine, 2000).

The current U.S. health care delivery system relies solely on internal quality improvement programs, which raises questions about responsibility and accountability, whereas traditional quality assurance programs tend to focus on individual practitioners or facilities, have a more regulatory cast, and are imposed from the outside (Lohr, 1997). Quality measurements and assessments should involve both processes of acquiring quality assurance and outcomes for the entire system. A focus on only one will not improve the state of care in this country. These cumbersome processes waste resources, leave unaccountable voids in coverage, and lead to loss of information and data. They also fail to build on the strength of all health professionals involved to ensure that care is appropriate, timely, safe, and culturally appropriate.

Summary

Despite the shortcomings of the U.S. health care delivery system, all Americans can have the quality and services they want and deserve. A high-quality performance system must maximize its capacity to improve. It must have a motivated, skilled, and culturally prepared health care workforce that meets the needs of the population and the tools necessary to integrate new technologies and research into patient care, and it must constantly assess and reassess itself to become cost-effective and culturally appropriate. The U.S. health system must determine better ways to finance, organize, and deliver care. It has to address the needs of its populations, the process of providing care, and the effectiveness of that care. Everyone loses when this system is ineffective, expensive, and inequitable.

Reflection

1. How would you describe the overall state of health care in the United States?

2. Discuss possible ways to promote an illness prevention agenda for the nation.

3. Develop your own set of goals and objectives to improve the health of your community, school, or clinical site. Collect information from government data sources, public forums, Internet commentary, individual interviews, and the literature.

References

Adams, P. F., & Barnes, P. M. (2006). *Summary health statistics for the U.S. population: National Health Interview Survey, 2004* (Vital and Health Statistics Series 10, No. 229). Hyattsville, MD: U.S. Department of Health and Human Services, National Center for Health Statistics.

Agency for Healthcare Research and Quality. (2005). *National healthcare disparities report.* Rockville, MD: Author.

Anderson, R. N., & Smith, B. L. (2005). Deaths: Leading causes for 2002. *National Vital Statistics Report, 53*(17). Hyattsville, MD: U.S. Department of Health and Human Services, National Center for Health Statistics.

Bloom, B., & Dey, A. N. (2006). *Summary health statistics for U.S. Children: National Health Interview Survey* (Vital and Health Statistics Series 10, No. 227). Hyattsville, MD: U.S. Department of Health and Human Services, National Center for Health Statistics.

Gabel, J., Claxton, G., Gil, I., Pickreign, J., Whitmore, H., Finder, B., et al. (2005). Health benefits in 2005: Premium increases slow down, coverage continues to erode. *Health Affairs, 24,* 1273–1280.

Ginsburg, P. B. (2005). Competition in health care: Its evolution over the past decade. *Health Affairs, 24,* 1512–1522.

Hing, E., Cherry, M. S., & Woodwell, B. A. (2006, June 23). *National ambulatory medical care survey, 2004 summary* (Advance Data from Vital and Health Statistics No. 374). Hyattsville, MD: U.S. Department of Health and Human Services, National Center for Health Statistics.

Hoyert, D. L., Heron, M., Murphy, S. L., & Kung, H. C. (2006). *Deaths: Final data for 2003* (National Vital Statistics Reports. Vol. 54). Hyattsville, MD: U.S. Department of Health and Human Services, National Center for Health Statistics.

Institute of Medicine. (2000). *Crossing the quality chasm: A new health system for the 21st century.* Washington, DC: National Academy Press.

Johnson, V. (1995). *Heart full of grace: A thousand years of black wisdom.* New York: Simon & Schuster.

Lethbridge-Cejku, M., Rose, D., & Vickerie, J. (2006). *Summary health statistics for U.S. adults: National Health Interview Survey* (Vital and Health Statistics Series 10, No. 228). Hyattsville, MD: U.S. Department of Health and Human Services, National Center for Health Statistics.

Lohr, K. N. (1997). How do we measure quality? *Health Affairs, 16*(3), 22.

National Center for Health Statistics. (2005). *Health, United States, 2005 with chartbook on trends in the health of Americans.* Hyattsville, MD: U.S. Department of Health and Human Services, National Center for Health Statistics.

National Health and Nutrition Examination Survey. (2005). *Prevalence of overweight and obesity among adults in the U.S.: 2003–2004.* Retrieved May 29, 2006, from www.cdc/gov/nchs/products/pubs/pubd/hestats/obese03_04/overweight-adult_03.htm

Thorpe, K. E. (2005). The rise in health care spending and what to do about it. *Health Affairs, 24,* 1436–1445.

U.S. Department of Health and Human Services. (2000). *Healthy People 2010.* Washington, DC: Author. Retrieved August 4, 2004, from www.healthypeople.gov/publications

12

The Somalis:
Culture and Health Beliefs
of a Refugee Population

The Saints of God speak the same language.

—SOMALI PROVERB (CITED IN LEWIS, 1998, P. V)

Key Points

- The majority of Somalis in the United States have sought asylum from their war-torn country and hold refugee status.

- One difference between immigrants and refugees is that *immigrants* choose to go to another country, whereas *refugees* are forced to leave their own country. Many refugees long to return to their native land.

- All Somalis are Muslim, and most are Sunni Muslims.

- Many values Somalis hold are similar to those of many Americans.

- Gender roles are clearly defined in Somalia; boys are taught to secure a livelihood for their family and protect them, and girls are taught to maintain the home and children and help the family's economy through animal husbandry.

- Health beliefs are founded in the Islamic faith.

- Somalis use a combination of traditional healing practices and Western medicine.

WHEN OCCUPATIONAL THERAPISTS PROVIDE SERVICES to people who are culturally different from themselves, it is important that they seek information from a variety of sources. Books and other resources are available that discuss various cultural groups and their customs, values, beliefs, and understandings about health, wellness, and illness. Several books have been found to be useful (e.g., Julia, 1996; Lattanzi & Purnell, 2006, Spector, 2004; University of California, San Francisco Nursing Press, 1996). Because these resources are readily accessible, and because of the limited scope of this text, we provide only this chapter as an example of information about a particular cultural group that has received scant attention in the literature.

Refugee vs. Immigrant Status

One cannot begin to know Somali people until one understands what it means to be a refugee. Immigrants are people who choose to live in another country. Although they may make this decision because of adverse conditions in their native land (e.g., famine, civil war), people who immigrate do so out of choice. A *refugee*, however, is "one who flees for safety, especially to a foreign country" (*Merriam-Webster Dictionary*, 1995, p. 439). This simple definition does not explain the complexity of this state of being. Refugeeism is a problem of forced displacement (United Nations High Commission on Refugees [UNHCR], 2000).

According to the UNHCR, women and children make up more than 80% of the world's refugee population (cited in Langer, 2002). Many refugees have fled war and oppression, some have played roles in the resistance in wars, and many have witnessed the deaths of family members and friends or have been injured themselves (Langer, 2002). Initially, refugees may find asylum in refugee camps in their own country, where they are known as *internal refugees* (Cernea & McDowell, 2000). From there, they may migrate to a neighboring country or to a country farther away. Unlike immigrants, the majority of refugees would not have willingly left their countries if they had been safe there. If possible, many refugees would like to return.

Because of their horrifying experiences, refugees have a very difficult time trusting people and political systems. Daniel and Knudsen (1995) characterize this attitude as putting "trust on trial" (p. 1); refugees mistrust their world and in response are mistrusted. Many refugees also struggle with posttraumatic stress disorder (Summerfield, 1995), as well as depression, frustration, isolation, and terror (Langer, 2002). These conditions usually result not from a specific traumatic event but rather from an "enduring, cumulative process that continues during exile because of distinct new events, both in the native country and the country of exile" (Van der Veer, 1995, p. 152).

Somalis living in the United States experience many of these problems. Somali women often arrive in the host country as the head of the household, a role forced on them because the men in their families died in the civil war. Additionally, they rarely have other family members living close by and are solely responsible for their children. They arrive in the United States facing numerous problems, usually unable to speak English and often illiterate in theirs. In addition, they must learn to manage cultural differences. Most refugees are recipients of relief programs that provide care and maintenance but are never sufficient to restore their livelihoods (Cernea & McDowell, 2000). Despite their difficulties, however, many Somali refugees live quite successfully in the United States. As more health care providers are beginning to work with Somalis, it is important to have a greater understanding of their history and culture.

Historical Background

Somalia is located on the east coast of Africa, in an area called the Horn of Africa, and was first created when Britain, Italy, France, and the Abyssinian empire partitioned and colonized that strip of land in the 19th century (see Figure 12.1 for a map). Initially, the British colonized the northern section of the country and the Italians the southern section (Gardner & El Bushra, 2004). In 1960, these areas united to form the Somali Republic. In 1969, General Mohammed Siad Barre overthrew a democratically elected but corrupt government in a military coup, leading to years of civil unrest and war. By the early 1980s, the country's economy was collapsing, and by 1989 an estimated 50,000 people in the northwest had been killed by their own government (Gardner & El Bushra, 2004). Widespread human rights abuses led to a decrease in U.S. military assistance and a suspension of the UNHCR and World Food Programme assistance (UNHCR, 2000). In 1991, President Siad Barre was overthrown, but violence, famine, and population displacement continued to intensify. In the next decade, an estimated 500,000 people, 300,000 of whom were children, died in the war and subsequent famine. About 1.5 million Somalis fled the country at that time (Gardner & El Bushra, 2004), and between 1980 and 1993 4,589 Somalis were granted refugee admission to the United States (Morency, VanHise, & Cote, 2002). Currently, the largest Somali population in this country lives in Minnesota.

The Somali People

Somalia's population is mostly rural. Nearly 80% are pastoralists, agriculturalists, or agropastoralists. Except for a small number of Somalis who rely on fishing, the rest of the population are urban dwellers. In the past few years, civil war and famine have changed urban demographics as hundreds of thousands of displaced Somalis have poured into the cities seeking sanctuary and relief.

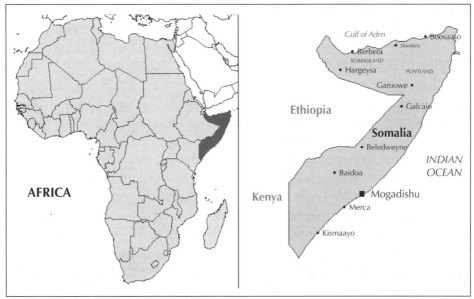

Figure 12.1. Maps of Africa and Somalia.

Ethnically and culturally, Somalia is one of the most homogeneous countries in Africa, yet Somalia has its minorities: People of Bantu descent live in farming villages in the south, and Arab enclaves are in the coastal cities. A small number of Europeans, mostly Italians, live on farms in the south. But the great majority of the people are ethnic Somalis who speak dialects of the same language, Somali, and who practice the same religion, Islam. In a land of sparse rainfall, more than half of the population raise camels, cattle, sheep, and goats. There are farmers, mostly in the south and northwest, and in recent years a new urban group of government workers, shopkeepers, and traders has emerged, but it is the nomadic way of life, with its love of freedom and open spaces, that is celebrated in Somali poetry and folklore (Cultural Orientation Project, 2000).

Somalia had about 6.3 million people in 2001, 44% of which were younger than age 14 because of cultural expectations for large families and the decimation of older men in the war (Gardner & El Bushra, 2004). Almost 250,000 registered Somali refugees are in other African countries, and an estimated 1,000,000 are in the wider diaspora. Somalia is a poor country, with a gross national product per capita equivalent to $200 and one of the lowest rates of literacy in the world (17.1%). Of literate Somalis, 65% are male; 22% of adult men and 12% of adult women are literate (Gardner & El Bushra, 2004). All literacy figures have dropped since 1985.

Despite these disadvantages, or perhaps because of them, Somalis are a hard-working, strong, and proud people. They often choose work that benefits or serves others (Morency et al., 2002). They are warm, humorous storytellers, with an oral tradition that allows them to argue well in addition to spinning tales. Work and leisure are both seen as valuable, as long as they do not interfere with religious duties.

Values

Many Somali values are similar to those of U.S. society. Somalis believe strongly in independence, democracy, egalitarianism, and individualism. Like Americans, Somalis value generosity. Unlike Americans, however, Somalis generally do not express their appreciation verbally.

Somalis respect strength and often challenge others to test their limits. Somali justice is based on the notion of "an eye for an eye." Somalis are a proud people—excessively so, some would say—and their boasting can stretch the truth more than a little. Saving face is very important to them, so indirectness and humor are often used in conversation. Somalis also are able to see the humor in a situation and to laugh at themselves. Although Somalis can be opinionated, they generally are willing to reconsider their views if presented with adequate evidence. Somalis have a long history of going abroad to work or to study and are known for their ability to adjust to new situations (Cultural Orientation Project, 2000).

Religion

Virtually all Somalis are Muslims. Most are Sunni Muslims and believe in following the examples and sayings of the prophet Mohammed. Like most Muslims, they follow the five pillars of Islam (Abdullahi, 2001):
1. Believing in the oneness (monotheism) of Allah and in Mohammed as the messenger
2. Saying prayers five times a day
3. Fasting in the month of Ramadan
4. Offering alms
5. Making the *hajj*, or pilgrimage to Mecca, when possible.

Ablution (washing the face, arms, legs, and private parts) is a requirement before praying, and women are not required to pray during their menstrual periods (Morency et al., 2002).

The beliefs and spiritual practices of Somalis as Muslims are based in the teaching of the *Koran*. Because there is no organized clergy or hierarchy, all Muslims are expected to know the religious rituals and laws well enough to be an active participant in all practices. They follow these practices in their homes or in mosques. The experts in the religion are referred to as *wadaad* or *sheikh* (Abdullahi, 2001).

Food and Dress

Abdullahi (2001) discusses the many reasons why Somali cuisine is not well known. He describes it as a "knowledge system" learned through apprenticeship, and it often is not eaten by European tourists. Additionally, it is kept somewhat secret; Somalis do not cook or eat on the street; it is against their culture to eat in public "because of a cultural stipulation that eating alone when others are not doing likewise is selfish" (Abdullahi, 2001, p. 109). A Somali proverb states "A man killed by his sword is better than a man killed by his gluttony" (Aden, 1995).

Somali cuisine is typical of the Horn of Africa, influenced mainly by East African, Indian, and Arabic foods. It can be divided into rural and urban fare, with rural foods being simpler, with fewer vegetables and fruit. Generally, Somalis eat many cereal-based products such as rice, spaghetti, sorghum, corn, and beans; fresh vegetables and fruit; and fresh meat including mutton, goat, beef, fish, and chicken (Abdullahi, 2001). They use a wide variety of spices to flavor their food. Pork and meat from horses or donkeys is forbidden *(haaraan)* by the religion, and other consumed meats must be *halal* (i.e., butchered according to Muslim practice; Abdullahi, 2001) or kosher (Morency et al., 2002). Somalis also eat a variety of soups and stews, usually with meat, and their cuisine is known for its large variety of breads.

Restaurants in Somalia often are traditional in style, usually with no printed menus available, and the waiters tell diners what is available for that day. More expensive restaurants may have printed menus, and the food may be spicier (Abdullahi, 2001). Because of their Muslim beliefs, Somalis tend neither to make nor drink alcoholic beverages. Soda and fruit drinks are popular, and they may drink strong coffee or sweet tea.

A Somali custom is to eat food with the hands, and it is considered rude to eat with utensils if everyone else is eating with their hands (Abdullahi, 2001). Within the United States, however, it is usual to see Somalis eating with fork and spoon, as is the custom in this country. If eating from a common platter with the hands, etiquette requires that people wash their hands before eating and that they eat only from the area of the platter directly in front of them. Belching or making other eating-related noises is considered bad manners (Abdullahi, 2001). After people have finished eating, they wash their hands again and wipe their hands and mouth on a towel. Somalis often express their gratitude to Allah after a meal (Abdullahi, 2001).

Somali men living in the United States often wear Western clothing. They are expected to cover their body from knees to waist and may wear pants or a kilt, Western shirts and jackets, or sometimes shawls (Morency et al., 2002). Women usually wear a scarf, called a *maser* (McGown, 1999), to cover their hair and may develop complex knots in them for style. They must be covered from neck to ankle, with only their hands and feet showing, but may choose Western clothes over flowing skirts and tops (see Figure 12.2). Somali women are not expected to wear the *hijab,* the veiled dress that covers a woman from head to toe (Abdullahi, 2001; Morency et al., 2002).

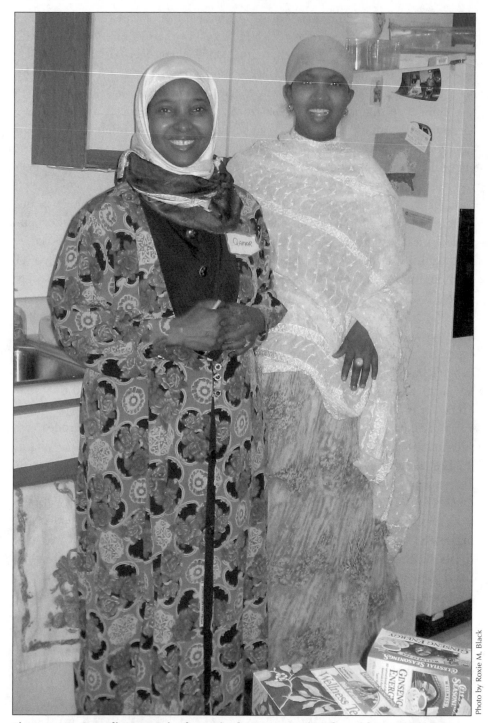

Photo by Roxie M. Black

Figure 12.2. Somali women in the United States wearing the wide range of dress acceptable in their culture.

Language and Communication

Most of Somalia's population traces its descent to one ethnic group and so speaks the same language. Somali, which did not have a written version until as recently as 1972, is the official language of Somalia; the Somali script uses the Roman alphabet. English is widely used in the north and Italian in the South (JourneyMart.com, 2002). Most Somalis speak Somali, but many also speak Arabic, and educated Somalis usually speak either English or Italian as well. Swahili also is spoken in coastal areas near Kenya. Somali has adopted many Arabic words, including modern phrases to deal with modern institutions, such as government and finance, and older Arabic terms to discuss international trade and religion. Somali also contains old Qahtani words common to Cushitic and Semitic languages (Cultural Orientation Project, 2000).

Before independence in 1960, English and Italian served as the languages of administration and instruction in Somalia's schools, and Arabic was used for unofficial transactions or personal correspondence. After the Somali script was adopted in 1972, Somali became the language of government and education. As a result, young Somalis currently have very little exposure to English or Italian until they go to college. Those who are middle aged and educated, however, often have some proficiency in English, Italian, Arabic, or Russian. In the past few years, private English classes have flourished in Somalia (Cultural Orientation Project, 2000).

Gender Roles

Somalia is a patriarchal society, with more value given to boys than to girls, although all children are seen as blessings from God (Gardner & El Bushra, 2004). Traditionally, families prefer a balance of male and female children. Men take the dominant roles in society, religion, and politics, yet "Somali women, whether nomadic or urban, have never been submissive, either to natural calamities or to social oppression" (Hassan et al., 1995, quoted in Gardner & El Bushra, 2004, p. 9). There is a strict division of labor, but Somali women have played an important part in the economy even though their sphere of influence has traditionally been the home. In pastoral or nomadic groups of Somalis, women's roles have included domestic tasks such as child care, food preparation, and other household chores, but they also have had an important role in animal husbandry, which is the mainstay of the national economy (Gardner & El Bushra, 2004). Women always were allowed to possess wealth and to trade in villages and towns (Abdullahi, 2001). Since the war, women and girls in Somalia are valued more highly than in the past, not necessarily because of a shift in values but because of their increased economic importance. Many women's roles have now shifted to that of primary breadwinner because husbands and brothers have been killed or maimed in the war (Gardner & El Bushra, 2004).

Children learn their respective and complementary gender roles early in life. A young boy in Somalia is taught early on how to secure a livelihood for his family and how to protect them. His socialization prepares him for marriage and supporting a family (Abdullahi, 2001). Boys are encouraged to be strong, not cry, and not show emotions, although girls may. Boys are socialized to be adventuresome and brave, whereas girls are supposed to be more cautious, home bound, and obedient.

Although Islam has championed women's rights for years (Abdullahi, 2001), in 1975, progressive law reform ensured women's equal rights with men and made discrimination illegal (Gardner & El Bushra, 2004). Very little was done, however, to educate pastoral or nomadic groups, the majority of whom are illiterate, so the reforms had little effect on these groups.

Marriage and Family

In Somalia, marriage is viewed as a relationship between two families or clans. However, young people can select their own mates with the active involvement of their families. Girls are married at a very young age (typically around ages 13 or 14) to ensure their virginity. The family of the young man usually pays a bride price and offers gifts to the girl's family (Abdullahi, 2001). Polygamy was practiced as long as a man could maintain the entire family (generally never more than four wives), provide for them, and protect them from harm. Somali culture teaches respect and deference between in-laws (Abdullahi, 2001). Divorce is a legal and simple option for dissolution of a marriage; usually, the man repeats the divorce formula in front of a man of God *(wadaad)* and witnesses. A woman, supported by her family, can petition for divorce in front of a judge *(qadi)*. No stigma is attached to divorce in Somalia, but there are economic repercussions, resulting in a rather low incidence of divorce.

Somali society is organized into large extended clan families that are determined by paternal lineage (Morency et al., 2002). Being a high-context society, Somalis define *family* as including both immediate and extended family members. They are raised to respect their parents and to seek advice and blessings from them. Older parents with grown and married children are viewed as the center of the extended family and often are sought out to provide advice and the final say in decision making (Abdullahi, 2001). Children of both sexes are expected to take care of their elderly parents if there is a need. Somalis deeply value family and loyalty to others. A woman's status is enhanced by the number of children she has, and it is common for a Somali family to have seven or eight children.

Favored Occupations

Despite the battering the general populace received during the war, traditional crafts have survived in Somali society. Among the different clans, traditional music, folk songs, tribal dances, and narrative poems passed down by word of mouth keep the old cultures alive. Arts and crafts were designed to be part of tribal rituals to appease dead ancestors; gods; and evil spirits, or *jinn*. Somalia is famous for its native crafts, such as gold and silver jewelry, finely woven cloth, basketry, and woodcarvings. Palm leaves are woven into baskets, mats, and trays for winnowing rice and grains. Leatherwork also is a popular craft, one that had many buyers in happier times (JourneyMart.com, 2002).

Beliefs About Health, Wellness, and Illness

Many Somali customs and beliefs are founded in their Islamic faith and the *Koran*. As a result, Somalis value cleanliness, bathing and washing often and as part of their prayer rituals and following defecation (O. Ahmed, personal communication, November 29, 2006).

Traditional Healing

Somali "traditional doctors" are usually older men in the community who learned their skills from older family members. They treat infectious diseases, hunchback (kyphosis), facial droop or paralysis, and broken bones. Treatment techniques include fire burning (applying to the skin a heated stick from a certain tree), herbal teas, and prayer. Traditional doctors also help cure illnesses caused by spirits *(jinn)*. Somalis believe that when the spirits residing within each individual become angry, illnesses such as fever, headache, dizziness, and weakness can result. The cure involves a healing ceremony that includes reading from the *Koran*, eating special foods, and burning incense. Somali beliefs also include the "evil eye"; a person can give someone else the evil eye on purpose or inadvertently by praising that person, which brings harm or illness to the person praised. Somali mothers cringe when doctors tell them their babies are big and healthy out of fear that the evil eye will cause something bad to happen to the child (T. Lewis, Ahmed, & Hussein, 1996).

Maternal and Child Health

In Somalia, childbirth most often takes place at home, attended by a midwife. The new mother and baby stay at home for 40 days after birth, with female relatives and friends helping to care for them. Newborn care includes warm water baths; massages with sesame oil, myrrh, incense, and balsam; and passive stretching of the baby's limbs. Breastfeeding is common up to age 2 years, usually supplemented with animal milk (camel, goat, or cow). The animal milk is offered from a cup rather than a bottle. Diapering is not common in Somalia. When the baby is awake, the mother holds a small basin in her lap and at regular intervals holds the baby in a sitting position over the basin. At night, a piece of plastic is placed between the mattress and the bedding, and the bedding and plastic are cleaned daily. Somali mothers say that infants are toilet trained very quickly (T. Lewis et al., 1996).

Circumcision

Circumcision is an old traditional ritual that is seen as a purification (Abullahi, 2001). Both boys and girls in Somalia are circumcised before the age of 5. Circumcision is viewed as a rite of passage and necessary for marriage; uncircumcised people are seen as unclean. Male circumcision may be performed by a traditional doctor or by a medical doctor or nurse in a hospital. Female circumcision is usually performed by female family members but is also available in some hospitals. The most common procedure in Somalia for female circumcision, known as "infibulation" (and known in the West as female genital mutilation), involves removal and suturing of most genital tissue, leaving a posterior opening (T. Lewis et al., 1996). Because of the unsanitary conditions where this procedure is performed and the very small opening left (about the size of a bean; Abdullahi, 2001), girls often contract serious infections that leave them with significant scarring and may lead to death. According to Abdullahi (2001), this form of surgical intervention is waning somewhat in favor of the milder form including removal of the clitoral prepuce and a partial clitoridectomy. Female circumcision is not a religious or Islamic ritual, as some people believe, but a cultural expectation (F. Hussein, personal communication, March 5, 2004) that "resolutely hinders or minimizes impregnation until such a time when it is socially permissible" (Abdullahi, 2001, p. 135). Despite this strong assertion, however, some believe that it is not a deterrent to sexual immorality (Shandall, 1967).

The controversy surrounding the practice of female circumcision includes questions of human rights violations (Althaus, 1997; Cook, Dickens, & Fathalla, 2002) versus the "medicalization" of the procedure, making it a safer practice (Shell-Duncan, 2001). It also is a public health concern in the United States as more and more African refugee and immigrant women arrive (Toubia, 1994). Because the practice is unfamiliar to most U.S. physicians, many gynecologists and obstetricians have had to learn new procedures to help circumcised African immigrant and refugee women through childbirth (Bacon, Gilson, Vill, & Curet, 1993) and other gynecological conditions, while developing cultural sensitivity to treat these patients in an accepting and nonjudgmental manner.

Mental Health Issues

There are few mental health data for Somali people because of the absence of culturally validated and appropriate assessment tools (Bhui et al., 2006). Somalis do suffer from mental health symptoms but often believe that their problems are associated with spirit possession, particularly devil possession (I. M. Lewis, 1998). The identification of spirit possession becomes a "refuge of the weak and injured: it is utilized by those who seek redress but find other means of effective action blocked or culturally inappropriate" (I. M. Lewis, 1998, p. 108). Mental distress also may be seen as caused by being cursed, by sorcery, or by being the recipient of the evil eye. Because Somalis believe that health and illness are within God's power to withhold or bestow (Lewis, 1998), they accept and endure most symptoms in a somewhat fatalistic manner.

Yet it is recognized that war-related experiences, the process of the refugeeism and migration, and other traumatic experiences have resulted in multiple mental health symptoms, including what Westerners would identify as posttraumatic stress disorder and common mental disorders (Bhui et al., 2002, 2006; Guerin, Guerin, Diiriye, & Yates, 2004; McCrone et al., 2005). Somalis may have above-average mental health needs but below-average access to services. Somalis do not seek out mental health services until they judge their problems to be severe. According to Guerin et al. (2004), Somalis identified mental illness as when "someone is mad or insane, or when they go around throwing stones, yelling, hitting, eating from dumpsters, and walking naked" (p. 60). If this is their conception of mental illness, it is no wonder they resist seeking services. As a result, however, mild anxiety and depression often are not treated. In addition, Somalis may seek out *Koran* readings, counseling by community members and elders, and complementary and alternative therapeutic approaches to deal with their mental health concerns rather than approaching a hospital, doctor, or mental health professional.

Death

It is considered uncaring to tell a terminally ill Somali or his or her family that the person is dying. It is acceptable to describe the extreme seriousness of an illness, however. When death is impending, a special portion of the *Koran* is read at the patient's bedside (T. Lewis et al., 1996).

Medical Care

Somalis believe that "illness is ultimately in God's power" (I. M. Lewis, 1998, p. 109). Despite this belief, most Somalis, especially those from cities, have had at least some experience with Western medicine. The most common illnesses for which Somalis seek help in Western hospitals are diarrhea, fever (usually malaria), and vomiting. Patients almost always receive an antibiotic at the hospital. Families also may bring their children to the hospital to treat a cold and will receive oral medication (T. Lewis et al., 1996).

Implications for Occupational Therapy Practice

Medical Care and Providers

Because Somalis are accustomed to getting medication when they go to a Western-style hospital, even for a cold, they expect to receive medicine from any medical visit. T. Lewis and colleagues (1996) report that in their experience with Somalis in Seattle, families often were very unhappy when they traveled a long distance, waited to be seen in a clinic, and were subsequently sent home with instructions that the patient would get better by himself or herself. Therefore, occupational therapy practitioners must carefully try to elicit how the client and his or her family understand the illness or disability experience and must clearly explain how occupational therapy might support them in their recovery.

Circumcision

Circumcision is an important and sensitive issue for Somali women seeking health care. Female circumcision has been debated in the Western world as a potentially harmful cultural practice. Many Somali women, however, view circumcision as normal, expected, and desirable (T. Lewis et al., 1996). Although occupational therapy practitioners do not deal with the medical aspect of this condition, showing cultural sensitivity around this issue when treating female clients who have been circumcised will help practitioners maintain open communications.

Religious and Social Customs

Other barriers to health care access are similar to those for other Muslim cultures. For example, because of prohibitions against interactions between adult men and women, Somali women have a strong preference for working with female interpreters and health care providers. Practitioners need to honor this preference whenever possible.

Somalis perceive mental health issues differently from Western health professionals. Because they believe that God controls all aspects of their health, Somalis may accept and endure symptoms until they are very severe before seeking out mental health support. Occupational therapists must learn how Somali clients interpret their mental health symptoms and work within their cultural belief systems when collaborating on interventions.

Because of the daytime fast during the month of Ramadan, clients consume medications, food, and liquids only after sundown. Occupational therapists must take this tradition into consideration when planning feeding, eating, and kitchen activities. Additionally, Somalis do not eat pork or gelatin products, and occupational therapists should ask clients about any other dietary restrictions.

Summary

Somali culture is very different from Western cultures. Therefore, occupational therapy practitioners cannot assume that they understand the clients' values and beliefs, whether cultural or religious, or their interpretation of health care practices in the United States. To develop the level of understanding necessary for culturally competent care, practitioners must be aware of their own responses to their Somali clients, seek out as much information about their clients as they can, and interact with a respectful and open-minded attitude. If practitioners can provide culturally competent care, both client and practitioner will be enriched by the experience.

Reflection

Choose a cultural group from your community or state. Research that group through library databases, the Internet, and community information.

1. Find an agency that works with that cultural group and learn about the agency's goals.

2. Go to a restaurant, store, or other public venue owned by members of this cultural group, and describe in your practice journal what you learned.

3. Seek out a member of the group to interview or converse with regarding his or her occupational interests, activities, and health beliefs.

4. Interview occupational therapists or other health professionals in your local hospitals or health agencies to learn about the health behaviors of members of this cultural group.

5. Put together a reflective report about what you have learned about the cultural group from your activities. Describe what your occupational therapy practice will look like when you have a member of this group as a client.

References

Abdullahi, M. D. (2001). *Culture and customs of Somalia.* Westport, CT: Greenwood Press.

Aden, A. H. (1995). *From the soul of nomads: Proverbs and sayings of the Somali.* Paris: UNESCO.

Althaus, F. A. (1997). Special Report. Female circumcision: Right of passage or violation of rights? *International Family Planning Perspectives, 23*(3). Retrieved July 29, 2007, from http://agi-dc.org/pubs/journals/2313097.html

Bacon, C. A., Gilson, G. J., Vill, M. D., & Curet, L. B. (1993). Female circumcision: Obstetric issues. *American Journal of Obstetrics and Gynecology, 169,* 1616–1618.

Bhui, K., Abdi, A., Abdi, M., Pereira, S., Dualeh, M., Robertson, D., et al. (2002). Traumatic events, migration characteristics, and psychiatric symptoms among Somali refugees: Preliminary communication. *Social Psychiatry and Psychiatric Epidemiology, 38,* 35–43.

Bhui, K., Craig, T., Mohamud, S., Warfa, N., Stansfeld, A., Thornicroft, G., et al. (2006). Mental disorders among Somali refugees: Developing culturally appropriate measures and assessing socio-cultural risk factors. *Social Psychiatry and Psychiatric Epidemiology, 41,* 400–408.

Cernea, M. M., & McDowell, C. (Eds.). (2000). *Risks and reconstruction: Experiences of resettlers and refugees.* Washington, DC: World Bank.

Cook, R. J., Dickens, B., & Fathalla, M. (2002). Female genital cutting (mutilation/circumcision): Ethical and legal dimensions. *International Journal of Gynecology and Obstetrics, 79,* 281–287.

Cultural Orientation Project. (2000). *Somalis: Their history and culture.* Retrieved November 15, 2006, from www.culturalorientation.net/somali/sart.html

Daniel, E. V., & Knudsen, J. C. (Eds.). (1995). *Mistrusting refugees.* Berkeley: University of California Press.

Gardner, J., & El Bushra, J. (Eds.). (2004). *Somalia, the untold story: The war through the eyes of Somali women.* London: CIIR & Pluto Press.

Guerin, B., Guerin, P., Diiriye, R. O., & Yates, S. (2004). Somali conceptions and expectations concerning mental health: Some guidelines for mental health professionals. *New Zealand Journal of Psychology, 33*(2), 59–67.

JourneyMart.com. (2002). *Somalia: People and society.* Retrieved November 15, 2006, from www.journeymart.com/Dexplorer

Julia, M. C. (1996). *Multicultural awareness in the health care professions.* Needham Heights, MA: Allyn & Bacon.

Langer, J. (Ed.). (2002). *Crossing the border: Voices of refugee and exiled women.* Nottingham, UK: Five Leaves.

Lattanzi, J. B., & Purnell, L. D. (2006). *Developing cultural competence in physical therapy practice.* Philadelphia: F. A. Davis.

Lewis, I. M. (1998). *Saints and Somalis: Popular Islam in a clan-based society.* Lawrenceville, NJ: Red Sea Press.

Lewis, T., Ahmed, B., & Hussein, K. (1996). *Voices of the Somali community.* Retrieved November 15, 2006, from http://ethnomed.org/voices/Somali.html

McCrone, P., Bhui, K., Craig, T., Mohamud, S., Warfa, N., Stansfeld, S. A., et al. (2005). Mental health needs, service use and costs among Somali refugees in the UK. *Acta Psychiatrica Scandinavica, 111,* 351–357.

McGown, R. B. (1999). *Muslims in the diaspora: The Somali communities of London and Toronto.* Toronto, Ontario: University of Toronto.

Merriam-Webster Dictionary. (1995). Refugee. Springfield, MA: Merriam-Webster.

Morency, A., VanHise, K., & Cote, L. (2002). The Somali culture. In R. Black (Ed.), *The Maine diversity manual.* Lewiston: University of Southern Maine, Master of Occupational Therapy Program.

Shandall, A. A. (1967). Circumcision and infibulation of females: A general consideration of the problem and a clinical study of the complications in Sudanese women. *Sudan Medical Journal, 5*(4), 178–212.

Shell-Duncan, B. (2001). The medicalization of female "circumcision": Harm reduction or promotion of a dangerous practice. *Social Science Medicine, 52*(7), 1013–1028.

Spector, R. E. (2004). *Cultural care: Guides to heritage assessment and health traditions* (6th ed.). Upper Saddle River, NJ: Prentice Hall Health.

Summerfield, D. (1995). Addressing human response to war and atrocity. In R. J. Kleber, C. R. Figley, & B. P. R. Gersons (Eds.), *Beyond trauma: Cultural and social dynamics* (pp. 17–29). New York: Plenum Press.

Toubia, N. (1994). Female circumcision as a public health issue. *New England Journal of Medicine, 331*, 712–716.

United Nations High Commission for Refugees. (2000). *The state of the world's refugees: Fifty years of humanitarian action.* Geneva, Switzerland: Author.

University of California, San Francisco Nursing Press. (1996). *Culture and nursing care: A pocket guide.* San Francisco: Author.

Van der Veer, G. (1995). Psychotherapeutic work with refugees. In R. J. Kleber, C. R. Figley, & B. P. R. Gersons (Eds.), *Beyond trauma: Cultural and social dynamics* (pp. 151–170). New York: Plenum.

13

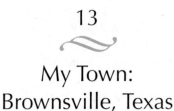

My Town:
Brownsville, Texas

"On the Border by the Sea"

—MOTTO OF BROWNSVILLE, TEXAS

Key Points

- Communities are the battlefields on which health threats will be met.
  Understanding all the perspectives about your community—its history,
  assets, talents, experiences, businesses, cultures, institutions, and physical
  resources—will help you develop sustainable and culturally appropriate
  community infrastructure to support health improvement.

- Knowing your community, inside and out, is the first step in discovering
  its similarities with and differences from the dominant culture.

- My town (S. W.)—Brownsville, Texas—is a diverse and changing
  community, and through the dedicated efforts of elected officials,
  employees, and residents, will continue to see improvements in
  appearance, health, and quality of life.

HOW WE CONCEPTUALIZE OUR COMMUNITIES powerfully influences what occupational therapy practitioners see and do in practice. We generally are taught to think of a community as a neighborhood of people—the people within a city or county or people with a shared racial, ethnic, gender, or sexual orientation identity (Fazio, 2001). But this conceptualization of a community does not provide as complete a picture as could be useful in our thinking and acting in practice. Within this limited frame of reference we may overlook the influence of history, geography, institutions, experiences, and cultures that shape health needs at a community level.

As occupational therapists move more into community and population-based practice, especially in diverse communities, they must shift their conceptualization of community. This shift entails moving from the community as a social and demographic entity with which one interacts to a multidimensional system of which one is a part. Walter (2002) refers to community as multidimensional to describe the way in which various dimensions or ingredients incorporating diversity, caring, trust, talents, history, and resources that characterize community—such people and organizations or a sense of purpose and values—are integrally related with one another, forming the whole: "To develop an understanding of community, we need to articulate, visualize, and examine the unique qualities exhibited by each of these dimensions and how they come together to make up the complex and dynamic 'system' of community" (p. 70).

Conceptualizing community as a multidimensional system enables therapists to see themselves and others as part of a dynamic system that is continually being created and re-created by an unfolding history and changing physical environment. Everything within a community is related, influenced by and influencing all the dimensions, including occupational therapy services (Issel, 2004; Siegel, Howard, Adams, & Wasongarz, 2003; Walter, 2002). Therefore, it is important to know the degree to which the community has acculturated to mainstream U.S. society or retained its traditional ways. Are health care providers seen as outsiders within the community in which they work? Are bisexual people included in gay and lesbian communities? Does a business see the people it works with or serves as part of its community? These questions are handled in different ways by different communities and at different times.

Just as occupational therapists learn about traits that are characteristic of a particular cultural group or individual, they also must see each community as a unique multidimensional system. Understanding the community from the perspective of multiple stakeholders with diverse interests is necessary to help not only individuals but also the community as a whole to deal with health problems and issues within their environment. Learning about a community guides and informs health professionals' decisions related to program prioritization and development (Issel, 2004). Learning about a community is a procedure that should be used to collect data, develop relationships with key people in the community, and market services to community groups and the target population. Learning about a community can make practitioners a part of the community, not just an outsider, and will help them understand the people they will serve (Hancock & Minkler, 2002). This chapter demonstrates how occupational therapy practitioners, educators, and students can explore and understand the multidimensional community they're trying to reach. So, let me tell you about my town.

My Town

Like a quilt rich in colors, textures, and patterns, my (S. W.) town of Brownsville, Texas, is made up of many ethnic, racial, religious, and cultural groups. This diversity lends strength and uniqueness to the fabric of my community and society. With a broad history and the range of experiences that the various parts of the population bring, everyday life in my town comes with a need for increased efforts at understanding and valuing differences as well as similarities.

Geography

Brownsville is Texas's southernmost international seaport and the largest city in the lower Rio Grande Valley. It is the county seat of Cameron County and is located across the Rio Grande from Matamoros, a city in the Mexican state of Tamaulipas (its sister city). Brownsville is about 25 miles inland from the Gulf of Mexico at an elevation of approximately 33 feet above sea level (see Figure 13.1). Visitors from all over the United States and Canada are drawn to Brownsville because of its resort-like atmosphere and warm, fun-loving people.

My town's semitropical climate is recognized as one of the most delightful in the nation. The city has an average temperature of 74 degrees and an average rainfall of 25.55 inches. The average relative humidity is 75.25%. The comfortable year-round climate provides for an abundance of recreational fun and activities. Visitors can take in the sights of Matamoros and South Padre Island only minutes away (Brownsville Chamber of Commerce, 2006).

Demographics

General Characteristics

In 2000, my town had 139,722 residents, and by 2005 the population had increased to 171,528; our sister city of Matamoros had a population in excess of 750,000 in 2005. Racially, my town was 81% White, 0.2% African American, 0.4% Native American, 0.3% Asian, 17% other race, and 1% who are of two or more races. In terms of ethnicity, however, my town was 91% Hispanic or Latino. Thirty-one percent of residents were foreign born. There were 47,000 households in the city of

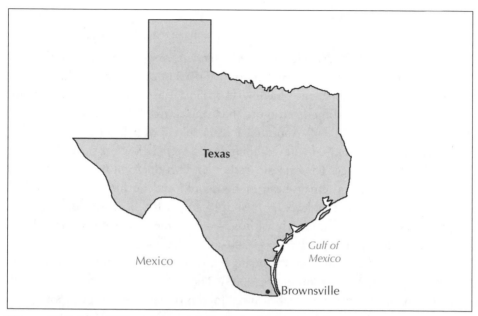

Figure 13.1. Map of Texas. Brownsville is in the lower right corner.

Brownsville in 2005. The average household size was 3.6 people, and the average family size was 4.0 people. Families made up 84% of the households and included 55% married-couple families, 28% other family types, and 16% nonfamily households. Most of the nonfamily households were people living alone, but some were formed by people who were unrelated to the householder (City of Brownsville, Texas, 2007; U.S. Census Bureau, 2005)

My town's population is young. The median age in Brownsville in 2005 was 25.5 years, well below the state and national averages, and 63% of the population was younger than age 34 years. Of the town's population, 12.5% were younger than age 5 years, 61% were ages 18 to 64 years, and 7.6% were age 65 years or older. There were 47.7% male residents and 52.3% female residents (U.S. Census Bureau, 2005).

Social Characteristics

Of the population 25 and older in 2005, 60.0% had graduated from high school, and 14.4% had a bachelor's degree or higher. Among residents who reported having a disability, 3% were 5 to 20 years old, 13% were 21 to 64 years old, and 50% were 65 and older. Eighty-seven percent of the population spoke a language other than English in the home. Veterans made up 5.5% of the civilian population. Of the population 15 years and older, 61% of the men and 50% of the women were married (U.S. Census Bureau, 2005).

Economic Characteristics

The median income of households in Brownsville in 2005 was $24,207. Seventy-eight percent of the households received earnings, and 9% received retirement income other than Social Security. Twenty-five percent of the households received Social Security, and the average income from Social Security was $9,220. (Some households received income from more than one source.) The per capita income for the city was only $10,669. About 43% of people lived below the poverty level, and 55% of related children younger than age 18 were below the poverty level, as were 38% of people ages 65 years old and older. Forty percent of all families and 63% of families with a female head of household and no husband present had incomes below the poverty level. Fifty-six percent of the Brownsville population older than age of 16 was in the labor force, and their mean travel time to work was 19 minutes (City of Brownsville, Texas, 2007; U.S. Census Bureau, 2005).

Brownsville is the 6th-fastest growing manufacturing area in the United States (Brownsville Chamber of Commerce, 2006). The city's industries include agriculture, electronics, apparel, metal fabrication, food processing, and much more. With its proximity to Mexico, the North American Free Trade Agreement (NAFTA) has consolidated Brownsville's role as a gateway for U.S.–Mexico commerce. Brownsville/Matamoros is the third largest border employment center known as *maquiladoras,* or assembly plants for export goods. Brownsville is the only location along the U.S.–Mexico border that provides five modes of transporting goods: deep-water vessel, barge (down the Gulf Coast through the Intercoastal Waterway and the Ohio and Mississippi Rivers), rail, truck, and air.

The shrimping industry pumps an average of $60 million a year into Brownsville's economy and indirectly contributes to the creation of thousands of jobs throughout the community. Home to over 190 shrimp boats, the Port of Brownsville has the 5th-highest overall shrimp harvest in the United States. The Brownsville shrimp fleet, along with that of the nearby town of Port Isabel, makes the area the Shrimp Capital of the United States (Brownsville Chamber of Commerce, 2006; U.S. Census Bureau, 2005).

Housing Characteristics

In 2005, Brownsville had a total of 53,000 housing units, 11% of which were vacant; 72% were single-unit structures, 24% were in multiunit structures, and 4% were mobile homes. Thirty-five percent of the housing units were built since 1990. Of the 47,000 occupied housing units, 63% were owner occupied and 37% were renter occupied. Nine percent of households did not have telephone service, and 14% did not have access to a car, truck, or van for private use. Thirty-four percent had two vehicles, and another 12% had three or more (U.S. Census Bureau, 2005).

The median monthly housing costs in 2005 for owners with mortgages was $941, for owners without mortgages $361, and for renters $505. Forty-seven percent of owners with mortgages, 21% of owners without mortgages, and 51% of renters in Brownsville spent 30% or more of household income on housing (U.S. Census Bureau, 2005).

History

My town's earliest recorded history begins with the exploration and subsequent colonization of the area by Spain after the conquest of Mexico. Colonization north of the Rio Grande River began in 1748, when General José de Escandón was appointed by Spain to colonize Tamaulipas, where Brownsville was later located. In 1835, Texas declared her independence from Mexico, resulting in a war that was won by the Texans at the Battle of San Jacinto in 1836. Texas claimed the Rio Grande River as her southwestern boundary. As a result of this claim, Mexico lost nearly half of what had been the State of Tamaulipas, which caused many disputes that lasted throughout the 9 years that Texas was an independent republic (City of Brownsville, Texas, 2007; Garza & Long, 2007; Kearney & Knopp, 1995).

In 1845, when Texas joined the United States, a dispute broke out over the location of the international border. Texas claimed the border of the Rio Grande, while Mexico claimed it was the Nueces River. This disagreement led to the first battle of the Mexican–American War that was fought at Palo Alto and Resaca de la Palma. General Zachary Taylor arrived in the area and took up a position across from Matamoros to defend the settlement at Fort Taylor. Fort Taylor later was renamed Fort Brown in honor of Major Jacob Brown, killed directing his defenses against Mexican forces. At the end of the Mexican–American War, the Treaty of Guadalupe Hidalgo was signed, and the area where Brownsville is now located was confirmed as being U.S. territory. When the city of Brownsville was founded in 1848, it was named after Fort Brown (Garza & Long, 2007).

Brownsville became the county seat of the new Cameron County in January 1849, and a post office went into operation. Within a short time, the town's population had increased because of the arrival of refugees from Matamoros and 40 miners on their way to the gold fields of California. Despite a cholera epidemic in the spring of 1849 that reportedly killed nearly half the population, the town continued to grow. The 1850 census showed a population of 519, two-thirds of whom were from the Atlantic seaboard states. Most of the remainder were Mexican, Irish, French, English, and German. The culture of the town reflected the characters of its inhabitants, many of whom absorbed the customs and practices of the Mexicans. A large percentage of the residents were fluent in several languages, including Spanish, English, French, and German (Adams & Knopp, 1997; Bay, 1980; Garza & Long, 2007).

Brownsville was originally incorporated by an act of the Third Legislature of the State of Texas in 1850, but this charter was dissolved soon after because of an argument between the United States and Mexico over the ownership of land being sold. By 1853, however, Brownsville was issued a new charter and has continued as an incorporated city ever since. During the Civil War, Brownsville was a major smuggling port through which the Confederate States of America exported large quantities of cotton and other products into Mexico. The last battle of the Civil War, the Battle of Palmito Ranch, was fought on a field located a short distance from Brownsville on May 12 and 13, 1865, nearly 5 weeks after Confederate General Robert E. Lee had surrendered at Appomattox, Virginia, ending the Civil War.

In 1875, the town established the Brownsville public school system and, by 1884, it had two banks, three churches, two ice houses, a cotton gin, and a population of nearly 5,000. The local newspaper, the *Cosmopolitan,* was renamed the *Brownsville Herald* (a paper still serving the city today). In 1904, the first commercial citrus orchard was planted in the area by H. G. Stillwell, Sr., which opened the citrus fruit culture of the valley. In 1908, the city launched its own electric-lighting system, waterworks, and sewerage system, and the first international car bridge connecting Brownsville and Matamoros opened a year later (there are three international car bridges today; Adams & Knopp, 1997; Chilton, 1997; Miller, 1982).

Before 1900, nearly half of all those born in the city were the product of interracial marriages, and both Anglo and Mexican customs were widely practiced and respected. The new residents to town, mostly Protestant and White, were reluctant to assimilate, and as a result ethnic divisions between people of Mexican descent and the Anglo populace began to widen. Racial tensions were not confined to Anglos and Mexicans; the Brownsville Raid of 1906 involved Black troops stationed at Fort Brown. Many of the new Anglo immigrants saw their Mexican neighbors as "racially inferior" and ignorant of the American way of life, whereas Mexican Americans, the majority of whom worked as common laborers, became increasingly resentful of the inequality in income, positions, and land ownership. The animosities grew even worse during the Mexican Revolution (1910–1921), when border raids by Mexican bandits wreaked havoc among the Rio Grande Valley populace (Garza & Long, 2007; Kearney & Knopp, 1995).

From 1865 to 1916, much time was spent in reconstruction and maintenance of law and order. It was necessary for U.S. government troops, state militia, and Texas Rangers to be kept in the area to protect the citizens of Brownsville from raids by bandits, Mexican revolutionaries, and American outlaws who found it easy to plunder along the Rio Grande and then escape across the river. By the early 1900s, however, Brownsville was enjoying increased prosperity and population, and in 1904, the St. Louis, Brownsville, and Mexico Railroad was completed and a telephone system established.

After the turn of the 20th century, the political structure of the city and its environs shifted. Cliques of merchants, lawyers, and large landowners dominated politics in South Texas. In Brownsville, Democratic political boss James B. Wells controlled the political scene. His power rested largely on meeting the needs of his constituents from both the Anglo elite and the Hispanic majority. With the demographic changes and the rising tide of racial hostility, Wells lost control of Brownsville in 1910. A new Anglo elite, made up of mostly recent arrivals, emerged, and a new social order based on de facto segregation became the rule (Anders, 1982; Garza & Long, 2007).

During the 1920s, my town underwent a new period of prosperity, and the Gateway International Bridge was constructed in 1928. The first paved streets in Brownsville, which consisted of wooden block paving, were laid in 1912. The Brownsville International Airport was inaugurated in 1928, and the Port of Brownsville was completed in 1936 (Chilton, 1997). The Junior College of the Lower Rio Grande Valley (later renamed Texas Southmost College) admitted its first class in 1926. In 1945, Fort Brown was decommissioned, and in 1948 the city and college acquired the land. Following the introduction of cotton to the area on a large scale in the late 1940s, the port of Brownsville became the world's leading exporter of cotton (Kearney, 1989).

Between 1950 and 1960, the population increased to 48,040, and by 1970 the town had 52,522 inhabitants. The Brownsville area attracted more than 100 industrial firms that offered 13,600 jobs. Between 1969 and 1979, much of the population growth came from immigration from Mexico, but the area also saw a growing number of retirees (known as Winter Texans) from the North and Midwest. Although approximately 80% of the population in the 1990s was of Mexican descent, Anglos still owned most of the city's wealth (Adams & Knopp, 1997).

The past several decades, however, have seen a growing Hispanic middle class, and Hispanics have begun to play a larger part in political and community affairs. In 1989, the University of Texas system took over Pan American University at Brownsville after considerable lobbying from the local leaders. It was renamed The University of Texas–Pan American–Brownsville, and in September 1991 it was again renamed the University of Texas at Brownsville and began a partnership with Texas Southmost College. Brownsville was declared an American City in 2001. On December 24, 2004, Brownsville had its first instance of measurable snow in 109 years, with 1½ inches, and the first recorded white Christmas. Despite the recent wave of growth, the city faces a variety of problems, including substandard housing in the *colonias,* (residential areas along the Texas–Mexican border that may lack some of the basic living necessities, such as potable water, sewer systems, electricity, paved roads, and safe and sanitary housing), high unemployment, and increasing health disparities (Texas Secretary of State, 2007).

Education

Most of Brownsville is served by the Brownsville Independent School District (BISD). The BISD's total enrollment in 2003–2004 was 45,986 students in 50 schools. It is the 17th largest school district in Texas. A portion of northern Brownsville is served by the Los Fresnos Consolidated Indpendent School District. In addition, Brownsville residents are allowed to apply to magnet schools operated by the South Texas Independent School District, as well as to BISD magnet schools. Each BISD high school has a magnet school within the school (e.g., Homer Hanna High School, a BISD high school, has the district's medical magnet program). The city has about 12 private and parochial schools, as well as two charter schools. At the postsecondary level are the University of Texas at Brownsville and Texas Southmost College, South Texas Vocational Technical Institute, and the University of Texas School of Public Health at Brownsville (Brownsville Chamber of Commerce, 2006).

City Government

Brownsville has a council–manager style of government. The mayor and 6 city commissioners (two at-large and four district) serve staggered 4-year terms, with elections for 1 at-large and 2 district seats held every 2 years. General elections are held on the first Saturday of May in odd-numbered years.

Arts and Culture

The Brownsville area is full of well-established art galleries and museums that display not only art of the region and Mexico but also exhibits from all over the world. The Brownsville area is served by numerous local television affiliates and radio stations. Local attractions include the Gladys Porter Zoo, the Camille Lightner Playhouse, a historical downtown featuring buildings more than 150 years old, the Port of Brownsville, and the Children's Museum of Brownsville (see Figure 13.2). Sunrise Mall is the only shopping mall in the city of Brownsville. Since being remodeled in 2000, the mall has become the primary mall in the Brownsville–Harlingen metropolitan area.

My town has been referenced in a number of songs. It is the hometown of the heroine in the song "Delta Dawn." Bob Dylan performed another song, called "Brownsville Girl" (cowritten with Sam Shepard). It is mentioned in "Matamoros Banks" by Bruce Springsteen and in "Texas Women" by Hank Williams, Jr. Jim White recorded "That Girl From Brownsville, Texas." John Darnielle of the Mountain Goats wrote about Brownsville in "It's All Here in Brownsville" that appeared on the band's *Full Force Galesburg* album. Brownsville Bay is referenced in the song "Somewhere Between Texas and Mexico," recorded by Pat Green.

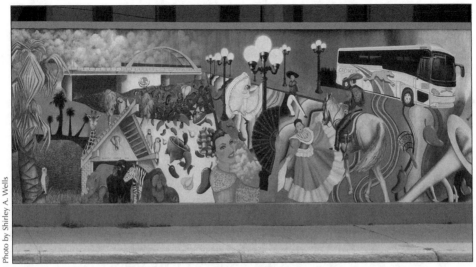

Photo by Shirley A. Wells

Figure 13.2. A mural in downtown Brownsville, Texas, showcases the town's cultural diversity.

Judge Reynaldo G. Garza (1915–2004) of Brownsville was first appointed to the U.S. District Court in 1961 by President John F. Kennedy and to the U.S. Court of Appeals by President Jimmy Carter in 1978. Garza's biography, *All Rise: The First Mexican–American Federal Judge,* was written by Louise Ann Fisch (1996), a Brownsville native. (And I had the privilege of providing occupational therapy services to Judge Garza from 2002 to 2003 prior to his death.)

The U.S. Ambassador to Mexico, Antonio Oscar Garza, was born in Brownsville. Federico Pena, former U.S. Transportation Secretary, former U.S. Energy Secretary, and former mayor of Denver, Colorado, was raised in Brownsville. Actor Kris Kristofferson was born in Brownsville on June 22, 1936, while actress Elka Walker, best known for "The Real World" series, was born in Brownsville on February 2, 1978.

Charro Days is my town's international celebration. Since 1938, it has celebrated the relationship between Brownsville and Matamoros and encompasses a variety of music and bicultural ambience, bubbling with the sounds of traditional mariachis, modern-day Tejano music, and the myriad regional Mexican dances. This event occurs in conjunction with the Sombrero Festival (2½-day event that celebrates Brownsville) during the last week of February (Acosta, 2001; Sombrero Festival Committee, 2007). These festivals celebrate the people, the cultures, and the unique geographic location of two nations. It has never strayed from its simple yet elegant mission: "Let us tell people what we have, and let us continue to be good neighbors."

Health Status

Brownsville is served by three hospitals: Valley Regional Medical Center, which has completed a new state-of-the-art hospital; Valley Baptist Medical Center, to which Brownsville has made major renovations and expansions; and Brownsville Surgical Hospital. The city has one free-standing rehabilitation facility, the South Texas Rehabilitation Hospital; about four nursing homes; and several outpatient rehabilitation centers serving children and adults (City of Brownsville, Texas, 2007).

The health problems of Brownsville are shaped by many factors, including language and cultural barriers, lack of access to care, and lack of health insurance. My town has among the highest incidences of tuberculosis (17.1%) and obesity-related type 2 diabetes (27.8%). Restrepo and colleagues (2007), in a study of the Cameron County–Mexico border, found that tuberculosis and diabetes were more likely to affect Hispanics of Mexican origin. Rates of sexually transmitted diseases and AIDS also are high. The leading causes of illness and death include heart disease, cancer, diabetes, and unintentional injury or accidents (Center for Health Statistics, Texas Department of State Health Services, 2006d). *Curanderismo* (Mexican–American folk healing that is holistic in nature and treats the mind, body, and spirit) continues to be practiced among the population and remains an important link to the past (Manning, 2007).

My town was designated a Health Professional Shortage Area (HPSA) and a Medically Underserved Area (MUA) in March 2002 (Center for Health Statistics, Texas Department of State Health Services, 2006a, 2006c). The U.S. Department of Health and Human Services assigns HPSA status to geographic areas, population groups, and facilities with an acute shortage of health care personnel (primary care medical and osteopathic doctors, dentists, and mental health professionals) and MUA status to areas or populations having a shortage of personal health care services. In September 2006, Brownsville had 58 occupational therapists, 20 occupational therapy assistants, 83 physical therapists, 483 direct patient care physicians, 258 primary care physicians, and 1,772 registered nurses to serve its population (Center for Heath Statistics, Texas Department of State Health Services, 2006b).

Summary

Brownsville has experienced enviable growth, and the demand for services has grown as well. A new fire station will be built to serve the Port of Brownsville area and the Navigation District. A new emergency medical services facility for the north side of town is in its planning stages. Landfill improvements will improve Brownsville's capacity for growth in all areas—industries, housing, and population, and more than $5 million in infrastructure improvements are planned. The

Brownsville/South Padre Island International Airport continues its growth and role as a vital component in the city's economy.

Although my town does not resemble most large urban communities, it has warmth, character, and a strong sense of community. Through the dedicated efforts of elected officials, employees, and residents, improvements continue to be made in the city's appearance and quality of life. From every aspect, Brownsville is a city with unlimited potential and a wealth of opportunity in the years to come. With this knowledge about my town, I am able to plan culturally appropriate occupational therapy services for not only for today but also tomorrow.

Reflection

Research the history and culture of your town. Answer the following questions:

- Has your town acculturated to mainstream America or retained its traditional ways?
- What are the unique qualities of your town?
- How would describe your town?
- What are the health care needs of your town?
- How do you envision your town in the future?

References

Acosta, T. P. (2001). *Charro days: Handbook of Texas online.* Retrieved January 21, 2007, from www.tsha.utexas.edu/handbook/online/articles/CC/lkc2.html

Adams, W., & Knopp, A. K. (1997). *Portrait of a border city: Brownsville, Texas.* Austin, TX: Eakin.

Anders, E. (1982). *Boss rule in South Texas: The progressive era.* Austin: University of Texas.

Bay, B. (1980). *Historic Brownsville: Original townsite guide.* Brownsville, TX: Brownsville Historical Association.

Brownsville Chamber of Commerce. (2006). *Brownsville, Texas: Climate and location.* Retrieved January 21, 2007, from www.brownsvillechamber.com/climate.htm

Center for Health Statistics, Texas Department of State Health Services. (2006a, October). *Health professional shortage areas in Texas.* Retrieved January 15, 2007, from http://www.dshs.state.tx.us/chs/hprc/hpsa.shtm

Center for Health Statistics, Texas Department of State Health Services. (2006b, October). *Health Professions Resources Center.* Retrieved January 15, 2007, from http://dshs.state.tx.us/chs/hprs

Center for Health Statistics, Texas Department of State Health Services. (2006c, October). *Medically underserved areas (MUAs) and populations (MUPs).* Retrieved January 15, 2007, from www.dshs.state.tx.us./hprc/mua.shtm

Center for Health Statistics, Texas Department of State Health Services. (2006d). *Texas selected health facts, 2002*. Retrieved January 15, 2007, from www.dshs.state.tx.us/chs/

Chilton, C. S. (1997). *Port of Brownsville: 60 years of services*. Brownsville, TX: Port of Brownsville.

City of Brownsville, Texas. (2007). *Brownsville: On the border by the sea*. Retrieved January 21, 2007, from www.ci.brownsville.tx.us/demographics.asp

Fazio, L. S. (2001). *Developing occupation-centered programs for the community: A workbook for students and professionals*. Upper Saddle River, NJ: Prentice Hall.

Fisch, L. A. (1996). *All rise: Reynaldo G. Garza, the first Mexican American federal judge*. College Station: Texas A&M University.

Garza, A. A., & Long, C. (2007). *Handbook of Texas online*. Retrieved January 21, 2007, from www.tsha.utexas.edu/handbook/online/articles/BB/hdb4.html

Hancock, T., & Minkler, M. (2002). Community health assessment or healthy community assessment: Whose community? Whose health? Whose assessment? In M. Minkler (Ed.), *Community organizing and community building for health* (pp. 139–156). New Brunswick, NJ: Rutgers University.

Issel, L. M. (2004). *Health program planning and evaluation: A practical, systematic approach for community health*. Boston: Jones & Bartlett.

Kearney, M. (1989). *A brief history of education in Brownsville and Matamoros*. Brownsville: University of Texas–Pan American.

Kearney, M., & Knopp, A. K. (1995). *Boom and bust: The historical cycles of Matamoros and Brownsville*. Austin, TX: Eakin.

Manning, V. (2007, July 22). Curanderismo survives among generations of practitioners, patients. *The Brownsville Herald*, pp. 1, 9.

Miller, M. V. (1982). *Economic change along the U.S.–Mexican border: The case of Brownsville, Texas*. Austin: University of Texas at Austin, Bureau of Business.

Restrepo, B. I., Fisher-Hoch, S. P., Crespo, J. G., Whitney, E., Perez, A., Smith, B., et al. (2007). Type 2 diabetes and tuberculosis in a dynamic bi-national border population. *Epidemiology and Infection, 135*, 483–491.

Siegel, B., Howard, B., Adams, A., & Wasongarz, D. (2003). *Addressing health disparities in a community setting: An analysis of best practices in community-based approaches to ending disparities in health care*. New York: New School University.

Sombrero Festival Committee. (2007). *Mission statement*. Retrieved July, 26, 2007, from www.somberofestival.com

Texas Secretary of State. (2007). *What is a colonia?* Retrieved July 26, 2007, from www.sos.state.tx.us/border/colonias/faqs.shtml

U.S. Census Bureau. (2005). *The 2005 American community survey*. Retrieved January 26, 2007, from http://factfinder.census.gov/servlet/

Walter, C. L. (2002). Community building practice: A conceptual framework. In M. Minkler (Ed.), *Community organizing and community building for health* (pp. 68–83). New Brunswick, NJ: Rutgers University.

Section C

Cross-Cultural Skills

14

Skillful Attitudes and Active Engagement:
The Concept of Willingness

*I*t is not enough to have a goal in mind. People must believe that they have
the capabilities and opportunities needed to achieve their goal. Indeed, such
beliefs are often more fundamental than the actual skills and circumstances
they represent.
                                                                —FORD (1992, P. 123)

Key Points

- One important cross-cultural skill is an attitude of willingness.
- Willingness is a volitional act: Having the will to do something means making a choice.
- The volitional aspect of cultural competence involves one's values, personal causation, and interests.
- Three levels of willingness may exist: unreflective willingness, cautious willingness, and committed willingness.
- Developing an attitude of willingness leads to active engagement.
- Cultural competence is not passive.

IN MUCH OF THE LITERATURE ON CULTURAL COMPETENCE, the key characteristic of culturally competent skill is usually viewed as effective cross-cultural communication, which is the focus of Chapter 15. Through my (R. B.) experience and earlier research, I have identified another and perhaps more compelling aspect of skill development in becoming culturally competent: the development of an attitude of willingness.

Some may state that *attitudes* are not skills but rather dispositions or mental positions people take in relation to something else (*Merriam-Webster Dictionary*, 1995). I argue, however, that attitudes are learned and developed much like any other skill. People shift attitudes in their lives, whether about favorite teams (sometimes depending on whether they win or lose) or about something more important, such as their views about a certain group of people after they have grown to know and understand them better. With increased knowledge and experience, people's attitudes about things, people, and places change. Therefore, certain attitudes can be developed as skillful attitudes. Within the context of cultural competence and culturally competent care, this chapter discusses the implications of an attitude of willingness as a necessary skill.

An Attitude of Willingness

I first became aware of the concept of willingness when analyzing data from an earlier study on cultural competence (Black, 2002). Much of the material in this chapter is taken from that research. In that study, I asked occupational therapy students to identify important characteristics of a culturally competent person, and throughout the transcripts of the interviews, the words *willing* and *willingness* kept appearing in multiple ways across participants. The following are a few of the ways the study participants talked about this concept:

- Willingness to seek out what the differences are
- Willingness to find out what is really going on
- Willingness to accept and experience
- Willingness to listen
- Willingness to understand their situation
- Willingness to let go of assumptions
- Willingness to learn
- Willingness to be open, and listen, and understand
- Willingness to admit you don't know anything.

While reflecting on this concept of willingness to do something, I recognized that the students were talking about making a conscious choice: They were talking about a volitional act. Occupational therapists and occupational therapy assistants understand the importance of volition as part of the theoretical construct surrounding occupational performance. Kielhofner (2002) defined *volition* as "a pattern of thoughts and feelings about oneself as an actor in one's world which occur as one anticipates, chooses, experiences, and interprets what one does" (p. 19). One might infer from this definition that a culturally competent person maintains an attitude or disposition that allows him or her not only to be open to certain experiences but also to choose them. Many study participants stated that a person who is culturally competent chooses to have an open mind, chooses to be self-reflective, and chooses to attempt interactions beyond his or her comfort zone.

Volitional Aspect of Cultural Competence: An Application of Kielhofner's Theory

Having the will to do something connotes having and making a choice; thus, choosing to participate in cross-cultural interactions is a volitional act. It is important, therefore, to examine the concept of volition as part of this discussion. Gary Kielhofner (2002) is an occupational therapy theorist who, along with his colleagues, developed the Model of Human Occupation, a theoretical practice model for occupational therapy practitioners. He has examined the concept of volition quite extensively in his work, and his ideas have guided my thinking about the concept of willingness. Kielhofner conceptualizes volitional thoughts and feelings as pertaining "to what one holds important (values), perceives as personal capacity and effectiveness (personal causation), and finds enjoyable (interests)" (p. 44). Volition, and therefore an attitude of willingness, results from the dynamic interplay between these three concepts.

Values

According to Kielhofner (2002), "*Values* refer to what one finds important and meaningful to do" (p. 15, italics added). Personal values develop from societal and family values. At this point in U.S. history, being sensitive to and having skills in cross-cultural interactions is a developing sociocultural value. It is generally expected that people will be "politically correct" or culturally sensitive in their verbal interactions with others. Herbst (1997) defines the term *politically correct* in the following way:

> *Politically correct* describes the efforts of those seeking to deal politically with such social and political issues as (1) bias related to race, ethnicity, religion, sexual orientation, gender, and age; (2) prejudice against the physically or mentally impaired or those of a stature outside the perceived norms; and (3) neglect of the natural environment. . . . A main goal of those involved with such issues has been to advance the principle of equality. (p. 183)

Because of the increased awareness of and sensitivity to difference, many people in the United States realize that they should not talk to other people in a denigrating manner. However, even after adopting that societal value and knowing which offensive terms to avoid, many are still at a loss when it comes to the appropriate way to interact with those who are culturally different.

The American Occupational Therapy Association developed a *Code of Ethics* and a statement of core values (AOTA, 1993, 2005) that include professional beliefs and values related to diversity issues to guide occupational therapy practice. Even though there may be societal and professional expectations for certain behaviors, however, not everyone within the profession will adopt these values and beliefs if they conflict with personal beliefs and values.

In my study of occupational therapy students (Black, 2002), many of the participants expressed how they valued culturally competent care. One student, when questioned about a clinical interaction she had described in which the therapist respectfully questioned an Asian family whose body language was hard to understand, stated, "I think it's a valuable experience." When asked why, she stated, "I felt satisfied that I got something out of it." For this participant, meaning was derived from the fact that she was learning from the experience.

Other students in the study talked about particular values they had learned as children. One participant stated, "It's how I was raised and the values I was taught [such as] to appreciate and be open minded to everyone, and [that] people are individuals." Another student added, "I've been brought up with the understanding that there's a variety of ways to live and no one way is the right way." For both of these participants, the values they learned early in life contributed to their choice to engage in cross-cultural experiences. These examples of how students valued being open minded, respecting the uniqueness of individuals, and learning about others support Kielhofner's (2002) premise that one's values contribute to one's volition.

Personal Causation

Another aspect of volition, personal causation, correlates with a sense of personal agency and relates to an awareness of how effective people perceive themselves to be when interacting within their environment. Kielhofner (2002) identified two dimensions of personal causation: personal capacity and self-efficacy. *Personal capacity* is the awareness people hold of their abilities, including physical, intellectual, and social abilities, whereas *self-efficacy* is their perception of how they can use their abilities to effect change in the world around them. As Kielhofner describes it,

> Persons who feel capable and effective will seek out opportunities, use feedback to correct performance, and persevere to achieve goals. In contrast, individuals who feel incapable and lack a sense of efficacy will shy away from opportunity, avoid feedback, and have trouble persisting. Consequently, personal causation influences how one is motivated toward doing things. (p. 46)

In other words, people who feel successful at a task will be motivated to try again, and those who do not perceive themselves as capable will tend not to reattempt a task. Many occupational therapists and occupational therapy assistants have seen this exemplified in the clinic or classroom.

How does this notion apply to the idea of someone choosing to engage in cross-cultural interactions? One way to interpret Kielhofner's (2002) definition within the context of culture is that people must have a positive awareness of themselves as sociocultural beings who have the confidence to approach others and learn from each interaction. If that confidence has not developed from childhood, it may result from later interactions. For example, one study participant related that she had feared African Americans because she had had little contact with them and had learned stereotypes from the media (Black, 2002). She not only was not confident in her interactions with African Americans; she actually was afraid to interact with them. While waiting at a bus stop one day, a young African American man came up to her and told her he liked her shirt. She became frightened and moved away. He courageously followed her and gently told her that he only wanted to compliment her on her shirt, and then he walked on. Her response was,

> Although I felt silly, it really helped me out. It was very brave of him, too.
> He didn't have to do that, but in a small way he had educated me—at
> least, enlightened me on my ignorance. And that is always the first step.

This was a defining moment for this participant. Using Kielhofner's terminology, she used the feedback this stranger provided to assess and correct her performance. During my interview with her, she went on to relate her later successes in cross-cultural interactions. Although this participant believes she still had a lot to learn, she does feel that her interactive skills are much more effective than those she possessed at the time of her interaction with the man at the bus stop. Her sense of personal causation had improved, as had her willingness to engage with African American people.

Another student in the study described a school trip to Paraguay with a team working with children and their parents on dental hygiene. She didn't speak the language and knew little about the culture entering the project; nevertheless, she described how the experience resulted in very positive outcomes:

> I think the fact that we were able to communicate and click and get
> through to people who have come from such a completely different
> background . . . [made it] a wonderful experience. It is also such a feeling
> of accomplishment.

This participant's sense of efficacy was high as a result of this positive interaction, even though she had initially evaluated her personal capacity as low because of her inability to speak the language and lack of knowledge about the culture. The positive experience resulted in a strong sense of personal causation.

Interests

The third component of volition is one's interests: "Interests are what one finds enjoyable or satisfying to do" (Kielhofner, 2002, p. 53). They can be simple pleasures, such as reading to a grandchild, or a grand passion, like composing a symphony. Enjoyment from a task may arise from the sensory pleasures, from intellectual fulfillment, from aesthetic satisfaction, or from a "sense of association and fellowship experienced" (p. 55) when interacting and engaging in activities with others. People make choices or have the will to do something based on their interests.

Study participants often spoke of the enjoyment they experienced when interacting with someone different from themselves (Black, 2002). When asked what an international experience was like, one participant replied, "It felt good. I remember being very excited." Another student spoke of her experience working in a Japanese company with several Japanese coworkers: "I enjoyed it. I had been with these people for a long time, so I was very comfortable with them." When describing her experience with the Deaf culture and with friends who were East Indian, a third participant stated, "I think it feels wonderful. It makes you feel a little bit more worldly." For this participant, some of the enjoyment she felt derived from her sense of increased sophistication and knowledge that broadened her worldview. These words clearly demonstrate the feeling of joy these participants shared, which contributed to their interest in and willingness to engage in cross-cultural interactions.

Kielhofner (2002) believes that it is the dynamic interaction among one's values, interests, and sense of personal causation that contributes to one's volition. This notion was evident in the value study participants placed on effective cross-cultural interactions (Black, 2002). Most participants indicated that their sense of personal causation was enhanced by their cross-cultural interactions and that these experiences were enjoyable and piqued their interest. All of these factors contributed to their motivation and willingness to choose to interact with people who were culturally different from themselves.

Levels of Willingness

Kielhofner's (2002) discussion of volition makes it clear that being willing or choosing to embrace the attitudes, knowledge, and skills necessary to become culturally competent is complex. His theory describes what volition is and how it might occur. It does not, however, account for why the participants in my study often identified the concept of willingness (Black, 2002). A deeper analysis of the data suggested that three different levels of willingness may exist, which I have labeled (a) *unreflective willingness,* (b) *cautious willingness,* and (c) *committed willingness.*

Unreflective Willingness

Sometimes people choose to behave in a particular way because it is what is expected of them. With the "political correctness" movement beginning in the mid-1980s (Wilson, 1998) and an increased sensitivity to difference, many people in this country have recognized the need and expectation to be respectful and use inclusive and nondisparaging language when talking about and with people from nondominant groups. As with other kinds of learning, however, some people respond to the lessons and behave by rote, not really thinking about why they behave in this way or really engaging in the learning in an active manner. These people choose to interact with others effectively because they are expected to and feel that they should. They are "doing the right thing" not because of any internal drive but because of external societal expectations. I call this level of choice *unreflective willingness.*

Only a few of the occupational therapy students in the study demonstrated unreflective willingness in cross-cultural interactions (Black, 2002). One participant told of hearing someone tell ethnic jokes. When I questioned her about this, she said, "You're supposed to respect other people . . . and part of being a professional is respect for others and their differences, especially when you're a teacher." This participant recognized that the expected behavior of a professional is to respect others, which means that one does not tell ethnic jokes. She had learned that lesson well. But she did not add anything else to her statement indicating that she had an internal awareness of the oppression, injustice, and hurt inherent in such an act. This participant might choose not to tell this kind of joke, but her decision seemed to be grounded in the behavioral expectations for someone in a professional role rather than in a reflective stance regarding the meaning of the act.

Another participant was talking about how she might react to someone from the Middle East:

> I don't pretend to know more about the Arab countr[ies], but I know women aren't treated as well and are expected to obey the men. So I accept that. Over here I would, too, especially if I was working with them [in a clinical setting]. You know, I'm not going to change it, [but] I don't have to respect it.

Applying cultural relativism is another way that some show unreflective willingness to engage in cross-cultural exploration. This student had learned the concept that each person has his or her own culture that should be respected as unique, but she had not yet reflected on the moral or ethical conflicts that might arise from some cultural practices and customs.

Students and practitioners at this level of willingness are moving in a positive direction, but they have much work to do to develop a level of cultural competence that emerges from their own personal values and attitudes. At this level, people may have acquired some cultural knowledge but still need to develop the areas of self-awareness and skill.

Cautious Willingness

About half of the study participants demonstrated a willingness to learn and behave in more competent interactive patterns but were still hesitant because they either were afraid of making mistakes or lacked confidence in their abilities (Black, 2002). This level of willingness I have labeled *cautious willingness*. The following statement exemplifies this concept:

> I think I am not as culturally competent as I would like to be, because I don't know more about what it means to confront difference . . . 'cause I don't know enough about the difference, the minority, the different cultures.

Although this participant was unsure of her ability and her knowledge, she later indicated that she had a clear understanding of power, inequality, and issues of difference. She also demonstrated beginning skill in cross-cultural interactions when she reported her interaction with an African American man at a party:

> I didn't know him very well. Everyone else was White. I asked him, "Do you feel funny that you are the only Black person?" I didn't know if that was an appropriate thing to ask him or not. And he said, "Yeah."

She went on to explain that she may have been more empathic because she was Jewish and often was in the minority as well. This woman had a significant amount of awareness and self-reflection, sensitivity, and knowledge, but she was somewhat lacking in skill. People with this level of willingness need more practice with cross-cultural interactions to improve their skill, confidence, and sense of self-efficacy, but they are making good progress toward becoming culturally competent. They choose to interact with others because of an internal drive to connect and an interest in people.

Committed Willingness

The final level of willingness is what I call *committed willingness*. The participants who exhibited this level of commitment not only were willing to interact with others but sought out opportunities to do so (Black, 2002). They realized that they might make cultural mistakes and that they still had a lot to learn, but they were eager to work with differing cultures and to learn from their mistakes as part of the process. They had a "bring it on!" mentality and attitude that was contagious. One participant expressed her committed willingness as follows:

> It's like accomplishing [something]. Look what I've come from! Look what I've learned! This is what it has been preparing you for. Oh, wow!

There's a sense of excitement because you realize that there's so much more out there than just . . . backing away. That's the beginning. That's opening a door to a whole new world!

Another expressed it this way:

[Experiences] are exciting, and good, and hard, too. For myself, traveling and meeting other people . . . are the best thing. I feel like I grow and have become who I am by knowing people with different experiences. A lot of stuff I've done in my life I never would have done if I hadn't met people who were different than me.

A third participant observed the following:

You have to be face to face with the person . . . on a daily basis. That's what I mean by exposure. You have to thrust yourself in there. You may get the door slammed in your face, but then you try again. You keep going and going. If you are willing, if you really are committed to understanding their culture, you will come back.

The willingness of these students to interact with others arose from a strong commitment that clearly embodies Kielhofner's (2002) dynamic interaction among values, interests, and sense of personal causation. Although these participants still had much to learn, their motivation and drive to become more culturally competent increased the likelihood that they would attain this goal, and their excitement over the process could only enhance that development.

Active Engagement

Developing an attitude of willingness leads people to engage in the behaviors necessary for competent cross-cultural interactions. Being culturally competent is not a passive position. The participants in this study made it very clear that it involves active engagement. One has to *do* something to make a difference. Thinking about it, learning about it, and wishing one could do something make no impact on the world. However, even attempting to interact with someone different gives one a sense of agency that increases one's sense of personal causation and efficacy. As a student said, "just trying to do something" is moving toward cultural competence; she gave the examples of trying to speak Spanish to a Mexican client, buying and reading a book to educate herself about her own culture, and initiating a conversation with people who were culturally different from herself. In each of these instances, she attempted to do something; she didn't just sit back and let things happen to her. Another student echoed this notion using phrases like

- "Get out there."
- "Really get your foot in the door."
- "Keep going and going."

- "Make a point of going over, of approaching them."
- "Make the effort."
- "Have to thrust yourself in there."

What the study participants suggested is a somewhat simple process: Develop an attitude of willingness, make positive choices, and move to action. Part of that action is the development of good cross-cultural communication skills and one's own personal plan for competence. The next two chapters will provide additional information in these two areas.

Reflection

1. Consider your attitude regarding people who are different from yourself.

   a. Are there particular groups of people you look forward to interacting with?

   b. Are there others you prefer not to interact with? Reflect on why you feel this way.

   c. To what extent are you willing to change your attitude if necessary?

   d. What sustains your lack of willingness?

   e. What would you have to do to overcome this attitude?

   f. What would you need to learn?

   g. What behaviors would you have to change?

2. If you are willing to interact with others, what level describes you?

   a. Do you exhibit unreflective willingness?

   b. Are you at the level of cautious willingness?

   c. Do you see yourself at the level of committed willingness?

   d. Would you rather see yourself at another level?

   e. What steps will you take to move there?

References

American Occupational Therapy Association. (1993). Core values and attitudes of occupational therapy practice. *American Journal of Occupational Therapy, 47,* 1085–1086.

American Occupational Therapy Association. (2005). Occupational therapy code of ethics (2005). *American Journal of Occupational Therapy, 59,* 639–642.

Black, R. M. (2002). *The essence of cultural competence: Listening to the voices of occupational therapy students.* Unpublished doctoral dissertation, Lesley University, Cambridge, MA.

Ford, M. E. (1992). *Motivating humans: Goals, emotions, and personal agency beliefs.* Thousand Oaks, CA: Sage.

Herbst, P. H. (1997). *The color of words: An encyclopedic dictionary of ethnic bias in the United States.* Yarmouth, ME: Intercultural Press.

Kielhofner, G. (2002). *A model of human occupation: Theory and application* (3rd ed.). Baltimore: Lippincott Williams & Wilkins.

Merriam-Webster Dictionary. (1995). Attitude. Springfield, MA: Merriam-Webster.

Wilson, J. K. (1998). *The myth of political correctness.* Durham, NH: Duke University Press.

15

Cross-Cultural Communication and the Power of Language

L anguage is an integral part of human behavior. Speakers use language to convey their thoughts, feelings, intentions, and desires to others. We learn about people through what they say and how they say it; we learn about ourselves through the ways that other people react to what we say; and we learn about our relationships with others through the give-and-take of communicative interactions.

—BONVILLAIN (1997, P. 1)

Key Points

- Language has power.
- Communication is controlled by those who are part of the dominant discourse.
- Speakers from sociocultural groups exhibit differences in the ways they speak and use words.
- Social status and differentiation correlate with differences in speech patterns, and differences in language are used as indicators of social segmentation.
- People who are disempowered do not feel they have a voice in the matters of their lives.

- Often, within health care contexts, clients feel disempowered and silenced.

- Professional jargon does not communicate well, and its use tends to separate health care professionals from the people with whom they work.

- Occupational therapists must be aware that language has power and that the words they use, the linguistic style of their speech, and the way they use their voice influence the people around them.

FOR OCCUPATIONAL THERAPISTS, being able to communicate and establish rapport with clients is very important in client-centered care. But communication and rapport often are difficult to establish in work with clients who are culturally different from oneself. Effective cross-cultural communication is one of the skills of cultural competence. According to Trenholm and Jensen (2004), "Whenever we interact with others who have been taught a different set of understandings about the world, we are engaging in cross-cultural communication" (p. 374). Thus, women communicating with men, an 80-year-old person speaking with a 20-year-old person, a lesbian interacting with a heterosexual person, a child with cerebral palsy interacting with an occupational therapist without disability, a homeless man interacting with a businessman on the street, and two people from different nationalities or cultures talking with each other are all examples of engagement in cross-cultural communication.

Because groups and individuals hold differing worldviews, beliefs, and values, and because people often are unaccustomed to difference, cross-cultural communication is difficult; "one of the reasons we avoid those who are different is that cross-cultural communication usually takes extra effort" (Trenholm & Jensen, 2004, p. 377). Yet occupational therapy practitioners must engage in such communication, because they cannot avoid the people who are their clients. They must learn to interact well with people who differ culturally. To deliver culturally competent care and to work effectively with colleagues, they must develop skill in cross-cultural communication.

Language has power. Occupational therapists and occupational therapy assistants must be aware of the words they choose to use when dealing with one another and with their clients. They cannot establish rapport or effectively communicate and work with people from different cultural backgrounds if their language is not understandable; if they do not interpret clients' nonverbal language accurately; or if the words they use unintentionally anger, hurt, or oppress clients. Being aware of and sensitive to not only one's own words and language but also those of one's clients is essential for culturally competent practice.

Power of Language

Many have observed that whoever does the naming has the power. Wolf (1982), for example, believed that naming things, acts, and ideas is the "ability to bestow meanings" (p. 386). He went on to say that

> Control of communication allows the managers of ideology to lay down
> the categories through which reality is to be perceived. Conversely, this
> entails the ability to deny the existence of alternative categories to assign
> them to the realm of disorder and chaos, to render them socially and
> symbolically invisible. (p. 386)

Historically in the United States, the naming has been done by those who have been dominant and those in powerful positions. The English language that has developed here from its European roots was developed by those in power and has helped maintain the social hierarchy that was discussed in Chapter 6. Learning and having control of language are defined as *literacy,* and according to Bennett (1991), "literacy is intricately tied up in the maintenance of vested interests in an already existing structure of power" (p. 14).

When discussing the concept of literacy, Gee (1989) identifies the importance of discourse as "a socially accepted association among ways of using language, of thinking, and of acting that can be used to identify oneself as a member of a socially meaningful group or social network" (p. 18). Several important points can be made about discourses: (a) *Discourses* involve a set of values and viewpoints from which one must speak and act; (b) any discourse puts forth certain concepts, viewpoints, and values at the expense of others, resulting in the diminishing or marginalization of other discourses; and (c) "discourses are intimately related to the distribution of social power and hierarchical structure in society. Control over certain discourses can lead to the acquisition of social goods (money, power, status) in a society" (p. 18). Therefore, those who engage in the dominant discourses are empowered within a particular society, and those who hold sociocultural power have access to the dominant discourses.

> *Each person has a unique way of speaking that reflects his or her gender, class, geographic location, race, and ethnicity.*

Not everyone in the United States, however, has immediate access to the dominant discourses that Gee (1989) identified. Children acquire their first and foremost language from their family or caregivers. This language as discourse is socioculturally defined. *Sociolinguistics* is a method of studying communication behavior that believes a dynamic relationship exists between language and social factors. Two complementary processes recognized within the discipline of sociolinguistics are that social status and differentiation among people correlate with differences in speech patterns and that differences in language are used as indicators of social segmentation. As Bonvillain (1997) puts it, "Speakers of socially ordered groups exhibit differences in frequency of use of certain sounds, words, and grammatical features" (p. 131). Each person has a unique way of speaking that reflects his or her gender, class, geographic location, race, and ethnicity. In addition, most people in a given social group are aware of these speech differences and know where their language places them within the social structure. For example, women's speech patterns tend to differ from those of many men, and in a patriarchal society, those differences in language have been given a value that places women and men with feminine speech patterns within a lower social status than that of the majority of men. Therefore, many women, to appear more authoritative or powerful, learn to modulate their voices so as not to sound too feminine. Several characteristics contribute to differences in language and power, including the words one chooses to use, one's linguistic style, and one's use of voice.

Words

The words one chooses to use hold cultural, societal, and personal meaning for both the user and the person addressed. Tanno (1997) states that words and labels convey volumes about assumptions and perceptions. Many words indicate bias and prejudice, serving to demean and maintain people in oppressed positions. Herbst's (1997) reference book identifies more than 850 ethnic and racial terms and expressions that indicate bias in today's society. He states that "all of the words here will—in one of their senses, in some ways or context—restrict, misrepresent, or distort how people are known" (p. ix). Every American has grown up knowing, hearing, and sometimes using some of these words. People may not mean to be prejudiced or to show bias toward someone from another group, but because they live in a society that harbors institutional racism, sexism, homophobia, and all the other *isms,* it is difficult not to make unintended verbal mistakes. Sometimes the slurs are intentional, but often people use biased language without being aware of the hurt it causes, mainly because it has become part of the accepted vernacular or the dominant discourse. How many of us have referred to elder women as "cute little old ladies" without considering the fact that this language diminishes these women and negates the wisdom and experience that are the result of many years of life? Biased language is so much a part of American English that most of us do not even realize we are using it.

In the health care arena, professionals make an effort to use words carefully so as not to label people. The use of "person-first language" is an effort to use words that indicate that one recognizes that people happen to have or are living with particular conditions rather than labeling and identifying them by their conditions (American Psychological Association, 2001). Examples of person-first language include the following:
- "The woman with the hip fracture" rather than "the hip in room 203";
- "The young man with cerebral palsy" rather than "that CP boy";
- "The man with schizophrenia" rather than "the schizophrenic."

This subtle difference in the use of language makes a significant difference in a person's self-esteem and sense of self, as well as in the way that person is viewed by others.

Linguistic Style

Another unique feature of language use is *linguistic style,* or the manner in which one incorporates features such as pronunciation, intonation, grammatical variants, and choices of vocabulary (Bonvillain, 1997). All people learn to express themselves in different and individualized ways according to the cultural norms that teach and reinforce differentiated roles related to age, gender, race, ethnicity, class, and other characteristics. A person may speak English, but the style in which he or she speaks immediately identifies his or her place in society. Although there are many ways this feature could be represented, for the purposes of this chapter I have chosen only two examples: (a) gender differences and (b) Black English.

Linguistic Differences Related to Gender

Differences between the speech of White American men and women have been studied for years. Although the significant number of women currently in the work-place may have altered some of these differences, specific speech patterns and styles continue to be identified as more masculine or feminine. No patterns are exclusive of either gender, but particular styles are culturally associated with and often stereo-typed for each. Bonvillain (1997), summarizing the differences in pronunciation between men and women, observes that pronunciation relates to class differentiation and that

> Women are socialized to behave with propriety and politeness (reflected by middle-class speech), and given a system of gender stratification in which men are privileged and in which men who act like women are strongly criticized, men consciously or unconsciously strive toward speech norms that reject styles associated with women. Because women model their behavior on middle-class styles, men covertly prefer working-class speech. (p. 172)

The polite style of feminine speech puts women at a disadvantage in the workplace, where more masculine modes of conversation and interaction are valued.

Women generally use more dynamic intonation than men. *Intonation* is "a complex combination of rhythm, volume, and pitch overlaying entire utterances" (Bonvillain, 1997, p. 173). Women tend to use "a wider range of pitches within their repertory and a more rapid and marked shift in volume and velocity" (p. 173). Research on gender differences in intonation indicates that dynamic patterns are interpreted as indicating emotionality and natural impulses, which are ascribed to women, whereas use of narrow intonational ranges is taken to indicate control and restraint, seen as more masculine qualities (McConnell-Ginet, 1983). The more controlled (masculine) speech patterns are given more cultural value in U.S. socie-ty, whereas the more expressive, dynamic patterns used more often by women have identified women as more unstable and unpredictable, substantiating and main-taining cultural stereotypes of women.

In summarizing the research on grammatical variants, Bonvillain (1997) notes that it has been inconclusive regarding gender differences; however, choice of vocabulary generally has been found to differ in men and women. Women use more specific terms than men when denoting colors (e.g., using terms like *magenta* and *turquoise*), and women use more modifiers such as adjectives and adverbs in their speech. Although this last characteristic also has been given the negative connotation of superficiality, Bonvillain (1997) comments that many of the modifiers are affective in nature (e.g., words such as *wonderful* or *lovely*). This increased expressiveness signifies that women in our culture have been allowed to display emotions and emotional thought more readily than men, which is reflected in their language.

One additional and interesting area of vocabulary difference is women's tendency to use hedge words in discourse. Bonvillain (1997) defines *hedge words* as "words or expressions that covertly comment on assertions in one's statements" (p. 178). The following are examples:

- I've been *sort of wondering whether* I should go.
- *I'm no expert on this subject,* but I think . . .
- I don't do too badly, *for a woman.*
- *I'm not sure I can do that,* but I'll give it a try.

This style of speaking signals a speaker's uncertainty about the validity of her statements or her abilities and makes her appear indecisive, ineffective, and weak. Many women speak in this manner, even those in positions of power or leadership. McIntosh (1985), in her fascinating essay *Feeling Like a Fraud,* reports that even successful women, when placed in the center of the public's attention, often feel fraudulent and use hedge words or phrases. Perhaps, in this new millennium, as more women rise to power and authority, they will use this language style less.

In summary, the linguistic styles of White American men and women not only indicate their sociocultural status but also serve to maintain the difference in status by supporting stereotypical cultural roles. Gleaned from this information, the message to women is to be aware of their mode of discourse and how it affects those around them. With awareness, they can then choose to continue to verbally present themselves in the usual manner, to adopt a more culturally valued style of speaking, or to vary their verbal style depending on context. Any choice can be seen as positive, as long as the speaker is aware of the effect she makes on others.

Many female occupational therapists assume a professional voice and style that tend to diminish gender differences in speaking. A linguistic style and discourse accepted by all other health professionals may help a woman to be perceived as an equal with the men on the health care team.

Linguistic Style Associated With Black English

Many African Americans speak a variety of English known as *Black English, Black English Vernacular,* or *Ebonics.* Some use their own dialect in all their communications, whereas others use it only in familiar contexts such as with family or friends.

Some African Americans do not use it at all. Wherever it is used, Black English is never regarded as part of the dominant discourse. Some of the differences from *Standard English,* or the accepted and expected language of the dominant group in the United States, are in structure and linguistic style.

Grammatical differences include the following: Black English reduces the final consonants in words, such as in *las' night* rather than *last night;* sometimes omits the past tense ending of *–ed;* and often omits the final *–s* when it indicates a possessive form. This language form also uses the contraction and deletion of the verb *to be* in a particular stylistic form (Bonvillain, 1997). The following are some examples:

- Why you *be running* in the street so much?
- She *fold* that *baby* little shirt.
- I *jus* now saw him *runnin* away.
- He *fas* in *everythin he do.*

Although this usage does not reflect Standard English format, linguists have determined that it does maintain its own grammatical rules. Nevertheless, because this style of speaking is not part of the dominant discourse, people who speak it often are devalued and stereotyped.

Consider the word *standard* in the phrase *Standard English.* If something is the standard, it becomes the yardstick by which everything else in that category is measured. If something competes with that standard and does not measure up to it, it is then seen as substandard—diminished, devalued, or less than that with which it is compared. Black English fits into a substandard category. In addition, African Americans' historical status as an oppressed minority has resulted in the tendency of many White Americans to "perceive Black English as a mass of random errors committed by Blacks trying to speak English" (Labov, Cohen, Robins, & Lewis, 1968, p. 366). Those who believe this think of African Americans as less intelligent or less educated than most people.

African American children who are more comfortable speaking Black English often are stigmatized by their teachers and White classmates and may become quiet or even silent in school where Standard English is the expected norm. Some of these children become angry and hostile in an environment that does not seem to understand them or meet their needs. They run the risk of being misjudged and labeled by teachers, the majority of whom are not African American and who then may place them in special education settings or lower their expectations for success for these students (Kozol, 1992). Orvando (1997) reports that, historically, speakers of Black English have been misperceived as language deficient and cognitively impaired. Perhaps this biased thinking is one of the many factors that limit the numbers of African American students found in occupational therapy academic programs.

Whether or not an African American child who speaks Black English should be taught Standard English in school is controversial. Many authors, however, support the idea that even though their native discourse should be honored and encouraged in a variety of settings, African American children should be taught Standard English to empower them to be more successful in the dominant culture (Delpit, 1995). Smitherman (1984) observes that "both linguistic forms have been demanded for Black survival—Black language for use in the Black community where *talking proper* is negatively equated with *talking White*, White language for use in attempts to get admitted to the White American mainstream" (p. 108). Smitherman's comment is important: Within a sociocultural context, one must speak in a particular way to have access to the dominant discourse.

In summary, a person's linguistic style has an effect on the perception and reality of his or her social status. In an occupational therapy practice context, practitioners will be judged and evaluated by their supervisors, colleagues, and clients on the basis of their speech. White American women must be aware of their linguistic style and how it affects others' perceptions of them as professionals. White American men and women also must be sensitive to their responses to the linguistic style of their clients, particularly if the clients are people of color. Are occupational therapists making assumptions about clients' abilities based solely on their manner of speech? Are clients inadvertently being treated differently because they speak English in a nonstandard manner or with an accent? Although occupational therapists probably cannot, and should not, try to change their manner of speaking and linguistic style for each person with whom they communicate, establishing rapport with clients, colleagues, and supervisors will be easier if they have an awareness of how others perceive them because of the way they speak. It also is vitally important for them to be aware of how they perceive those who speak differently than themselves.

Voice

The term *voice* is defined in the *Merriam-Webster Dictionary* (1995) not only as "sound produced through the mouth by vertebrates and especially by human beings in speaking and shouting" but also as "the power of speaking or the right of expression" (p. 586). It is the latter definition that we speak of in this section. *Having a voice* means feeling confident to speak and be heard. In her seminal work *In a Different Voice*, Gilligan (1982/1993) defines voice as follows:

> I mean something like what people mean when they speak of the core of the self. Voice is natural and also cultural. It is composed of breath and sound, word, rhythm, and language. And voice is a powerful psychological instrument and channel, connecting inner and outer worlds. Speaking and listening are a form of psychic breathing. This ongoing relational exchange among people is mediated through language and culture, diversity and plurality. For these reasons, voice is a new key

for understanding the psychological, social, and cultural order—a litmus test of relationships and a measure of psychological health. (p. xvi)

Gilligan emphasizes the necessity of having a voice for one's psychological health, yet many disempowered people in this society do not believe that they have a voice in the matters of their lives. They do not think that they are heard when they speak, and they do not feel that they have access to the dominant discourse, where their voices might make a difference. Many feel silenced and subsequently power-less and hopeless. Bruneau (1973) refers to this as *sociocultural silence.* Others do not have a voice because of cultural restrictions about speaking and silence (Goldberger, 1996). Without a sensitive recognition of cultural differences, many people's needs go unspoken and unheard.

Within the health care arena, clients often feel disempowered and silenced, especially in institutional settings. Many believe that they have no say in what hap-pens to them. For people of color, members of nondominant cultural or ethnic groups, and individuals who are poor, predominantly White settings raise barriers that prevent adequate communication and the development of rapport with care-givers. Culturally competent occupational therapy practitioners find ways to break down or bypass these barriers so that each client feels supported and understood and thus safe enough to tell practitioners what they need. They must encourage clients to speak and to have a voice in their own health care.

Political Correctness

A chapter on language, power, and multiculturalism would be incomplete without at least a brief description of *political correctness (PC).* PC became popularized on U.S. university campuses around 1990 and is defined as "a set of ideas, concerns, principles, and directives that stresses social nonoppressiveness, inclusiveness, and sensitivity to diverse groups of people" (Herbst, 1997, p. 183). In simple terms, the aims of this political movement were to limit language that was sexist, racist, clas-sist, and homophobic and to find a common way to engage in multicultural dis-course across various groups without resorting to oppressive language. As a result, terms such as *Native American, Asian American,* and *nondominant group* began to be used in place of other labels that might have been considered pejorative. Although using PC language appears to be a worthwhile endeavor—after all, it encouraged people to think about the words they were using and forced them through societal pressure to clean up their act, so to speak—controversy regarding this movement has been intense. The PC controversy is far too complex and convo-luted to be addressed fully in this chapter and book. We do, however, outline some of the prevalent ideas and the conflicting voices of the theorists.

First, the PC movement is political. It addresses power and power relation-ships and attempts to shift power from one side to another through its rhetoric.

Although there are many voices, they fall within two major points of view: the *neo-conservatives* (a term used by Epstein, 1995, and Kristol, 1999; see also Bernal, 1997) and the *liberatory theorists* (term used by Chodorow, 1978/1999; hooks, 1990; Sidorkin, 1999). The neoconservatives typically are described as right-wing conservatives (Bernal, 1997, p. 19) who are White, male, and elitist. The liberatory theorists are seen as feminists, multiculturalists, and critical theorists and include authors such as Giroux (1988), Friere (1992), McLaren (1998), Sleeter (1991), and hooks (1994). The neoconservatives are perceived to hold much of the dominant power in this country, whereas the liberatory theorists are viewed as more societally marginal. The following section identifies some of the major philosophical points of each group.

Neoconservative Voice

Political correctness as seen from the neoconservative point of view holds to the following beliefs:

- Before the 1960s, there was pure and objective (i.e., without political context or bias) scholarship relating to the Great Books and academic literary canon, and this scholarship was polluted by left-wing radicals who brought in feminist and multicultural scholarship, as well as other voices that do not meet the previous standards (Allsup, 1995; Bernal, 1997; Bloom, 1994).
- The Western canon defines intellectual excellence; the one version of truth is liberal thought that is derived from this canon; and multiculturalism, which is equated with anti-intellectualism, opposes truth (Bloom, 1994).
- Being forced to use PC language takes away the right of free speech. Those pushing for PC are "feminazis" (a term identified by talk show host Rush Limbaugh) or radical militants who are thought police and reside in the universities (Limbaugh, 1992).
- Feminists and multiculturalists are degrading the concept of the one, common, binding culture and value system (Kristol, 1999), which has provided the "unique source of those liberating ideas of individual liberty, political democracy, the rule of law, human rights, and cultural freedom that constitute our most precious legacy and to which most of the world today aspires" (Schlesinger, 1991, p. 32).

Liberatory Theorist Voice

Those who argue against the neoconservative criticisms of the PC movement believe that fear is the emotion that drives the rhetoric. Howard (1996) observes that the United States has a history of fear of diversity and that the anti-PC neoconservatives fear "the loss of European and Western cultural supremacy in the school curriculum" (p. 328). In reality, the PC movement was an effort to increase equality, equity, and inclusiveness in the language of the academy and in society. It was an attempt to "introduce the voices and experiences of those who have been excluded from academic curricula and intellectual discourse" (Epstein, 1995, pp. 5–6). The rash of articles and books by neoconservatives who vehemently argued against the PC movement sound to Epstein like "a group of men who are terrified that their world is falling apart, that their worldview is being rejected" (p. 6).

One way that opponents of the PC movement have attacked the movement is to mock, trivialize, and discredit its language and ideas. This attack has deflected the focus away from the real issues, which are efforts to reduce racism, sexism, homophobia, and other kinds of oppression. Lindsley (1998) reports that the media attack PC by trivializing and exaggerating PC language in an effort to pervert the meaning of the words and language and that, as a result,

> An interesting role reversal emerges: Those who are members of traditionally privileged groups are construed as victims of academic liberals who are mandating impositions on individuals' freedom of speech. Thus, tolerance is artfully construed as an attack on basic human rights and, in particular, on the rights of the most powerful members of our society. The actual effects of intolerance on targeted groups are lost in the margins of this media discourse. . . . Thus, mass-mediated constructs juxtapose intolerance as more desirable than tolerance. (p. 196)

Howard (1996) sees the attack against PC as an attack against diversity. In response, he stated,

> It is not multiculturalism that threatens to destroy our unity—as some neoconservative academics would have us believe—but rather our inability to embrace our differences and our unwillingness to honor the very ideals we espouse (equality, freedom, and justice for all people). (p. 328).

In summary, reviewing these two points of view demonstrates that words and language can be political and powerful and may be used to influence others in subtle and covert ways. Culturally competent occupational therapy professionals must become aware of the power they wield (and sometimes yield) every time they speak.

Professional Language, Jargon, Authority, and Power

Although the specialized language occupational therapy practitioners, educators, scientists, and researchers use is not intended to diminish or oppress others or to be biased, it does in fact separate the former from their clients in a hierarchical fashion. An article in a leading health magazine examined the public's understanding of many common terms used in the health arena and found that more than half of those responding to a poll did not know or had only a rough idea of the meanings of the words (Data Watch, 1997). For example, 51% of respondents did not understand the term *universal health care;* 63% did not know what a "PPO" (preferred provider organization) is; 75% did not understand COBRA health insurance, and 84% could not tell researchers the meaning of "POS" (point of sale; Data Watch, 1997, p. 56). If the results of this poll are representative, how well are health care professionals truly communicating with their clients and with each other?

One of the characteristics of a profession is specialized knowledge (Curry, Wergin, & Associates, 1993). Each profession, including occupational therapy, has its own specialized language. This common language defines the technical aspects and uniqueness of each separate profession and allows its members to communicate with and understand one another. For health care professionals, the specialized language is rooted in the medical model, and they use medical terminology to speak to one another across disciplines. Yet each separate health care profession also has its own specialized language; in occupational therapy, this includes the language of occupation. This specialized language helps the members of a profession form a kind of elite society whose language is known only among one another. Specialized language is somewhat like the secret passwords or handshakes used by gangs and other underground groups around the world. Each specialized language provides entry into a community of members that is quite exclusive. Those who do not speak the language, or know the password or special handshake, are excluded.

Occupational therapy practitioners sometimes separate themselves from or exclude their clients through the use of jargon. *Jargon* is defined as "confused unintelligible language," as "the special vocabulary of a particular group," and as "obscure and often pretentious language" (*Merriam-Webster Dictionary,* 1995, p. 281). The specialized language used in occupational therapy, therefore, is jargon. Its use is not necessarily either bad or good. Within a particular group, jargon can be a shorthanded way of communicating more efficiently. When used with others outside the profession, however, especially with clients, jargon has mixed results.

> *Occupational therapy practitioners sometimes separate themselves from or exclude their clients through the use of jargon.*

Some believe that jargon is acceptable to use as long as terms are defined (McGlade, Milot, & Scales, 1996). When professionals use and then define medical or professional terms in lay terms to clients, they educate clients about their health care experience, empowering them to have a clearer understanding and to make more informed decisions. Others, however, believe that jargon and abbreviations not only separate health professionals from their clients but also constitute "an artificial means of defining staff status levels with the profession—from consultant to auxiliary" (Leitch, 1992, p. 50). Hammond (1993) states that the jargon doctors use "transforms common-sense medicine into a cosy, elite world that is impenetrable to all but the ever-so-clever" (p. 26).

Occupational therapists often use jargon as a (perhaps unconscious) way to remind themselves that they are part of a professional group, and the use of jargon may be viewed as part of the developmental process of learning to talk as a professional. In an article about occupational therapy language, Gilfoyle (1979) identifies four developmental stages in communication patterns during the transition from entering to seasoned practitioner: (a) representational language, (b) private language, (c) socialized language, and (d) communicative language. Gilfoyle believes that, to reach the fourth stage, where the speaker communicates well with a person who is not an occupational therapy practitioner, the inexperienced professional must first have learned to speak jargon (representational and private language). Gilfoyle provides the following example of jargon use:

J., diagnosed as MR, with a birth history of Hyelines and RDS, was referred for an OT eval. . . . OT eval included SCSIT, SCPRN, DDST, reflex testing, and ADL. J. has CP, spastic diplegia with hypertonicity. He has severe SID. His PPL is 2 yr. below age. He has positive footing, TLR, ATNR, STNR: primitive righting, poor protective and equilibrium reaction. Recommend OT 3x weekly using SI and NDT techniques. (p. 9)

Although this text may communicate fully with other pediatric occupational therapy practitioners, it should not be presented to the client or family.

Whatever the reasons for speaking in jargon, it rarely allows occupational therapy professionals to communicate well and fully with their clients. Rather, it is a subtle reminder to clients that the professionals are part of the dominant group—the authorities, the ones with the knowledge—whereas clients and families are the *other*—the recipients of services and knowledge, the disempowered ones. Using the private language of occupational therapy with clients and families may intimidate and silence them. Instead of communicating in a way that stimulates dialogue, this kind of language only emphasizes the differences between the health professional and the client. It does not contribute to the conversation but rather strengthens the sense of hierarchy.

Occupational therapists can change this response by communicating with their clients in language that is clear and at the clients' level of understanding. If it is necessary to use medical or professional language, professionals should define the terms until the meaning is clear to the recipient. They should listen well to the client's questions and stories and carefully observe the body language that accompanies the discussion. If the client is from a cultural group that is different from the professional's, the professional cannot assume that he or she understands the meaning behind the client's words. The professional should ask for clarification and, if necessary, communicate through an interpreter. Interactions with clients must be as clear as possible to achieve true client-centered intervention.

Summary

The language occupational therapists and occupational therapy assistants use has the power to separate them from or connect them with colleagues, supervisors, and clients. Occupational therapy professionals must be aware that language has power; the words they use, the linguistic style of their speech, and the way they use their voice all influence the people around them. All of these language characteristics reflect who they are and how others perceive them, just as they influence how professionals perceive their colleagues, clients, and others with whom they interact.

In particular, occupational therapy professionals must use professional language and jargon judiciously in conversation with clients. Considering the effects of the authority of professional language and the sociopolitical privilege afforded most occupational therapy professionals, professionals must acquire and maintain a sensitivity to disenfranchised members of society. Not only must professionals be culturally aware and sensitive to the language they use and the authority it commands, but they also must develop cross-cultural communication skill with those with whom they work and interact.

Reflection

1. In the cafeteria or another public area in your workplace or school, observe some of your peers in conversation with one another.

   a. Notice the words they use, their intonation, and their linguistic style.

   b. Do the language skills they use match the style of the person to whom they are speaking?

   c. Do you notice any differences between the speech of men and women?

   d. Do these people speak the way you do? Identify any differences.

2. Spend one day paying attention to your own communication and language style. If possible, enlist a friend to spend the day observing you as well.

   a. Can you identify any communication patterns that reflect what you have read in this chapter?

   b. Does your language or style change when you are speaking to different groups of people (e.g., clients, friends, faculty, supervisors)?

   c. Are there aspects of your communication style that you would like to change?

   d. What steps will you take to change these aspects?

3. Observe the communication style of health care providers in a therapeutic setting.

   a. What do you notice regarding their words, intonation, and language style?

   b. Do the clients seem to understand what is said to them?

c. Do the providers use professional jargon when interacting with clients?

d. Does their language change when talking with colleagues?

e. If you were evaluating the communication patterns observed, what would you recommend for changes to ensure client-centered and culturally competent care?

References

Allsup, C. (1995). Postmodernism, the politically correct, and liberatory pedagogy. In C. E. Sleeter & P. L. McLaren (Eds.), *Multicultural education, critical pedagogy, and the politics of difference* (pp. 269–290). Albany: State University of New York.

American Psychological Association. (2001). Expressing ideas and reducing bias in language. In *Publication manual of the American Psychological Association* (5th ed., pp. 32–76). Washington, DC: Author.

Bennett, A. T. (1991). Discourses of power, the dialectics of understanding, the power of literacy. In C. Mitchell & K. Weiler (Eds.), *Rewriting literacy: Culture and the discourse of the other* (pp. 13–34). New York: Bergin & Garvey.

Bernal, A. T. (1997). Politically correct: Mythologies of neoconservatism in the American academy. *New Political Science, 38–39*, 17–28.

Bloom, H. (1994). *The Western canon: The books and school of the ages.* Orlando, FL: Harcourt.

Bonvillain, N. (1997). *Language, culture, and communication: The meaning of messages.* Upper Saddle, NJ: Prentice Hall.

Bruneau, T. J. (1973). Communicative silences: Forms and functions. *Journal of Communication, 23*(1), 17–46.

Chodorow, N. (1999). *The reproduction of mothering: Psychoanalysis and the sociology of gender.* Berkeley: University of California. (Original work published 1978)

Curry, L., Wergin, J. G., & Associates. (1993). *Educating professionals.* San Francisco: Jossey-Bass.

Data Watch. (Ed.). (1997, March). *Parlez-vous* health speak? *Business and Health,* p. 56.

Delpit, L. (1995). *Other people's children.* New York: New Press.

Epstein, B. (1995). Political correctness and collective powerlessness. In M. Darnovsky, B. Epstein, & R. Flacks (Eds.), *Cultural politics and social movements* (pp. 3–19). Philadelphia: Temple University.

Freire, P. (1992). *Pedagogy of hope: Reliving pedagogy of the oppressed.* New York: The Contiuum.

Gee, J. (1989). What is literacy? *Journal of Education, 171*(1), 18–25.

Gilfoyle, E. (1979). Occupational therapy language. In *Training: Occupational therapy educational management in schools: A competency-based educational program* (Vol. 4, Modules 6–8, pp. 1–26). Bethesda, MD: American Occupational Therapy Association.

Gilligan, C. (1993). *In a different voice: Psychological theory and women's development.* Cambridge, MA: Harvard University Press. (Original work published 1982)

Giroux, H. A. (1988). *Schooling and the struggle for public life: Critical pedagogy in the modern age.* Minneapolis: University of Minnesota.

Goldberger, N. R. (1996). Cultural imperatives and diversity in ways of knowing. In N. Goldberger, J. Tarule, B. Clinchy, & M. Belenky (Eds.), *Knowledge, difference, and power* (pp. 335–371). New York: Basic Books.

Hammond, P. (1993). Communication breakdown. *Nursing Times, 89*(20), 26.

Herbst, P. H. (1997). *The color of words: An encyclopedic dictionary of ethnic bias in the United States.* Yarmouth, ME: Intercultural Press.

hooks, b. (1990). Postmodern Blackness. *Postmodern Culture, 1*(1). Retrieved July 29, 2007, from http://muse.jhu.edu/journals/postmodern_culture/toc/pmc1.1.html

hooks, b. (1994). *Teaching to transgress: Education as the practice of freedom.* New York: Routledge.

Howard, G. (1996). Whites in multicultural education: Rethinking our role. In J. A. Banks (Ed.), *Multicultural education, transformative knowledge, and action* (pp. 323–334). New York: Teachers College.

Kozol, J. (1992). *Savage inequalities: Children in America's schools.* New York: Harper Perennial.

Kristol, I. (1999). *Neo-conservatism: The autobiography of an idea.* Chicago: Ivan R. Dee.

Labov, W., Cohen, P., Robins, C., & Lewis, J. (1968). *A study of the non-standard English of Negro and Puerto Rican speakers in New York City: Report on Cooperative Research Project 3288.* New York: Columbia University.

Leitch, C. (1992). Understanding sweet nothing. *Nursing Standard, 6*(48), 50–51.

Limbaugh, R. (1992). *The way things ought to be.* New York: Simon & Schuster.

Lindsley, S. (1998). Communicating prejudice in organizations. In M. L. Hecht (Ed.), *Communicating prejudice* (pp. 187–205). Newbury Park, CA: Sage.

McConnell-Ginet, S. (1983). Intonation in a man's world. In B. Thorne, C. Kramarae, & N. Henley, (Eds.), *Language, gender, and society* (pp. 69–88). Rowley, MA: Newbury.

McGlade, L. M., Milot, B. A., & Scales, J. (1996). Eliminating jargon, or medicalese, from scientific writing. *American Journal of Clinical Nutrition, 64,* 256–257.

McIntosh, P. (1985). *Feeling like a fraud* (Work in Progress No. 18). Wellesley, MA: Wellesley College, Stone Center for the Developmental Services and Studies.

McLaren, P. (1998). *Life in schools: An introduction to critical pedagogy in the foundations of education* (3rd ed.). New York: Longman.

Merriam-Webster Dictionary. (1995). Jargon. Springfield, MA: Merriam-Webster.

Merriam-Webster Dictionary. (1995). Voice. Springfield, MA: Merriam-Webster.

Orvando, C. (1997). Language diversity and education. In J. A. Banks & C. A. Banks (Eds.), *Multicultural education: Issues and perspectives* (3rd ed.). Newton, MA: Allyn & Bacon.

Schlesinger, A. (1991, Winter). The disuniting of America: What we stand to lose if multicultural education takes the wrong approach. *American Educator, 15*(4), 14–33.

Sidorkin, A. (1999). The fine art of sitting on two stools: Multicultural education between postmodernism and critical theory. *Studies in Philosophy and Education, 18*(3), 143–156.

Sleeter, C. E. (Ed.). (1991). *Empowerment through multicultural education.* Albany: State University of New York.

Smitherman, G. (1984). Black language as power. In C. Kramarae, M. Schultz, & W. M. O'Barr (Eds.), *Language and power* (pp. 101–115). Thousand Oaks, CA: Sage.

Tanno, D. V. (1997). Ethical implications in the ethnic "text" in multicultural communication studies. In J. M. Makau & R. C. Arnett (Eds.), *Communication ethics in an age of diversity* (pp. 73–88). Urbana: University of Illinois.

Trenholm, S., & Jensen, A. (2004). *Interpersonal communication* (5th ed.). New York: Oxford University Press.

Wolf, E. (1982). *Europe and the people without history.* Berkeley: University of California Press.

16

Developing a Plan to Achieve Cultural Competence

Histories are important 'cause they point the direction of traditions.

—NIKKI GIOVANNI (CITED IN JOHNSON, 1995, P .145)

Key Points

- Becoming culturally competent can occur by chance or by design. Any plan for achieving cultural competence must include performing a self-assessment, acquiring cultural knowledge, and developing cultural skills.

- The development of cultural competence demands a willingness to learn, risk, explore, and change.

- Any plan for achieving cultural competence entails building a support system to help you make the desired changes. Finding and developing resources—books, courses, places, people, Web sites, and other information sources—that will enlighten your knowledge base and help you implement your plan are essential. These resources are the tools with which you will work.

- A plan for cultural competence also requires outcome goals and concrete action steps to keep it realistic and workable.

228

THE OVERALL GOAL OF THE CULTURAL COMPETENCE MODEL is to provide a framework occupational therapy practitioners and students can use to develop skills and acquire knowledge that increases their ability to function effectively in a multicultural environment and to deliver culturally appropriate health care services. The learning tools for this process encompass a wide variety of dimensions and experiences—cognitive, affective, and experiential. Any plan for becoming culturally competent must address three basic components: (a) self-exploration and awareness, (b) knowledge, and (c) skills. Other areas, such as attitude, perceptions, and behavior, also should be integrated into the plan. All of these components are related integrally in actual practice.

Strategic Planning for Change

Change may occur by chance or by design and in large leaps or in incremental steps. Those who assume the task of becoming culturally competent should engage in strategic planning in developing a plan for competence. Table 16.1 provides an outline for developing a strategic plan for achieving cultural competence. Building a support system to help you make the desired changes is imperative to any plan. Colleagues, advocates, role models, and others can help you in this process. The purpose of the support system is to create a safe environment for you to discuss issues, conflicts, and feelings without the fear of being judged. It should be a place that provides opportunities not only to engage in true self-introspection but also to explore and practice new behaviors, perceptions, attitudes, skills, and knowledge.

Resources—books, courses, places, people, Web sites, and other information sources—will increase your knowledge base and aid in the implementation of your plan. These resources are the tools with which you will work. Finally, the development of outcome goals and concrete action steps will keep your plan realistic and workable. The goals of cultural competence development should be to increase your self-awareness and receptivity to diverse client populations, to develop clinical excellence, and to build strong therapeutic alliances with all clients. The development of cultural competence also requires a willingness to learn, to risk, to explore, and to change. It takes a balance of sensitivity, awareness, knowledge, and skill and a base of common experiences and understanding. The following action steps are recommended:

- Develop a personal action plan with specific goals, steps, timelines, and measurements (see Table 16.2 for a sample plan).
- Plan regular and interesting diversity discussions and activities.
- Plan educational activities.
- Develop active listening skills.
- Become a student of different cultures.

Table 16.1. Strategic Plan to Achieve Cultural Competence

Step	Activities to Promote Change
1. Assessing the personal context	Assess the environment by truly looking at yourself—your values, beliefs, behaviors, roles, biases, perceptions, knowledge, work and personal ethics, health beliefs, orientation to time, family roles and relationships, and communication style. Being honest about yourself is necessary for understanding who you are and how you view the world. It is one thing to wish you were bias free and another to truly live by this principle. Admitting to both the negative and positive aspects of your personality is essential for change and acquiring new knowledge.
2. Developing support	Look for allies, colleagues, advocates, and role models to help you through this process. A safe environment is needed to discuss issues and concerns openly, freely, and without fear of being judged. A support system will help you deal with the pain that occurs when your views and beliefs are challenged.
3. Developing resources	Seek out sources of information and tools, including people, that will enlighten your knowledge base. Locating and securing training materials, advisors, courses, consultants, and mentors are vital to developing cultural competence.
4. Establishing goals and taking action	Develop a comprehensive plan for becoming culturally competent, with concrete action steps and a timeline. Activities addressing the three basic components—self-exploration, knowledge, and skill—must be part of the plan.

Components of a Plan to Achieve Cultural Competence

Training for cultural competence should address the developmental needs of the learner and should include a variety of methods, including minilectures, group discussions, interactive exercises, role-playing, case study analysis, selected readings, videos, videotaping of clients and colleagues with follow-up discussion, and simulations. Community tours, discussions with community members, home visits, cultural immersion, service learning, and writing narratives also are activities that should be a part of your plan. Because this topic can be emotional, training is most effective when it occurs over time to allow you to reflect on the emotions elicited and the desired behaviors in response. Performing a self-assessment, gathering knowledge, and developing skills will help occupational therapists and occupational therapy assistants develop an effective plan for achieving cultural competence.

Performing a Self-Assessment

First, carefully assess the personal environment—yourself—in which the change is desired. This assessment will reveal the barriers to and resources for changes. The

Table 16.2. Personal Action Plan

Goal	Action Step	Date	Measures
1. I will broaden my reading.	Purchase books, magazines, newspapers, and other cultural reading material.	December 1, 2007	Minimum of 1 per month
2. I will explore beliefs about others.	Create a list of at least 10 stereotypes you think people hold about other populations/groups.	March 1, 2008	1 list for each diverse population/group
3. I will take a field trip.	Attend different religious ceremonies.	August 1, 2008	At least 3 religious groups

process of looking inward, reviewing, and examining your values, beliefs, behaviors, roles, biases, perceptions, knowledge, work and personal ethics, health beliefs, orientation to time, family, communication style, and so forth answers the question Who am I? It allows you to explore who you are without being judged by others. Admit to both the negative and positive aspects of your personality and beliefs. Select the attributes you wish to change, and analyze the pros and cons of making these changes. The following questions all apply to your cultural makeup:

- When, how, and why did your ancestors come to the United States?
- What ethnic or racial advantages and disadvantages do you have?
- What stereotypes of other ethnicities do you hold?
- How you would like to be treated, or not to be treated, by an occupational therapist?
- How frequently do you bathe?
- How close do you stand to someone with whom you are talking?
- How do you solve problems?
- How do you respond to stress?
- How do you celebrate the holidays?

Harris and Moran (1979) suggest 10 areas that should be included in a self-assessment: (a) sense of self and space, (b) communication and language, (c) dress and appearance, (d) food and eating habits, (e) time and time consciousness, (f) relationships, (g) values and norms, (h) belief and attitudes, (i) mental processes and learning, and (j) work habits and practices.

The identification and recognition of your values, norms, customs, and attitudes and how they shape your interactions are a first step toward accommodating and adapting your practice to respect differences in others. Cultural value differences are not limited to race and ethnicity alone but extend to socioeconomic status, sexual identity, religion, age, and gender.

Infusing a positive view of diversity and other values that promote healthy outcomes for your clients also is important in this process. The beliefs and mindsets of therapists and clients influence direct care encounters, interactions between the client and provider, the provider's delivery of care, and clients' perceptions of care. Self-assessment will develop your capacity to recognize that your own culture and cultural perceptions play a role in the client–provider exchange. This awareness in turn will lead to a better understanding of other cultures and to the rewards of providing culturally competent care.

Gathering Knowledge

Second, gather information to increase your knowledge. Information about health disparities, the clinical decision-making process, diverse health beliefs and practices, and different cultures will be useful. Professional standards developed by the Joint Commission on Healthcare Organizations (2007), the National Standards on Culturally and Linguistically Appropriate Services (CLAS; Office of Minority Health, 2001), the Accreditation Council for Occupational Therapy Education (1998), and the American Occupational Therapy Association *Code of Ethics* (2005) all address cultural competence, and occupational therapy professionals must be familiar with them all.

Knowing the similarities and differences between folk medicine and the Western biomedical health delivery system can help therapists see the benefits and appropriate uses of traditional health beliefs and behaviors in the treatment process. Understanding the sociocultural climate, the socially dominant forces and hierarchies, and the oppression of those who belong to nondominant groups is foundational information. The knowledge and material gathered during the information-gathering process should be personally and professionally relevant so that you can incorporate it into your practice. Culture-specific information should include the effect of the culture on values, beliefs, and behaviors and the effect of cultural expectations its members. You should explore the ways different cultural groups define health and illness and health beliefs that are in contrast with the biomedical model. The underlying assumptions and ethics of these health beliefs are critical to know. Many health care professionals have an ethnocentrism of the system in which they function, leading them to overlook these cultural assumptions and compromising the care they provide.

Structured opportunities to work with other cultures and ethnicities provide valuable, practical, and specific knowledge. Go into a community that you would like to learn more about. Perform a community assessment. Learn about its history, demographics, traditional health and illness beliefs, health resources, neighborhood health centers, home remedies, childbearing and rearing beliefs and practices, and ritual beliefs surrounding death and dying. Walk or drive through the community, and notice its places of worship, grocery stores and pharmacies, parks and recreational facilities, and neighborhood restaurants. Become engaged with culturally or ethnically organized student groups, medical groups, or community groups and ask about specific health or competence issues important to that community or group. Arrange a panel of traditional healers (e.g., *curanderos,* herbalists, shamans, *santiguadoras,* medicine men or women) or practitioners of alternative medicine to discuss their methods and cultural beliefs. Host brown bag lunches, and invite culturally competent speakers. Clients and other individuals from the community can give valuable insight into the experience of being treated by providers who do not understand their culture and their views on health and illness.

Ongoing training is integral to progress toward cultural competence and must be supported by structured opportunities to learn. The training should be broad based and explore the differences not only among ethnic groups but also among various social groupings defined according to gender, generation, lifestyle, and socioeconomic class.

The result of this exploration is cultural knowledge and the development of cultural skills. *Cultural knowledge* means familiarity with the broad differences, similarities, and inequalities in experiences, beliefs, values, and practices among various groupings within society (Health Resources and Services Administration, 2004). To achieve cultural knowledge, the therapist must be able to identify and understand the cultural worldview and theoretical and conceptual frameworks of patients from different cultures. This knowledge forms the base for *cultural skills,* or the skill set needed to evaluate an individual's background and formulate an intervention plan that is culturally relevant.

Developing Cultural Skills

Third, develop your skills to culturally assess a patient, to avoid relying only on written facts, and to explain an issue from another's perspective while reducing resistance and defensiveness and acknowledging interactive mistakes that may hinder the desired communication (American Medical Student Association, 2004). In today's fast-paced health care environment, therapists must constantly prioritize and choose which goals to address and which approaches to use. Most often these choices are based on institutional or insurance priorities. With training, however, a therapist or student can learn the most accurate methods to assess clients and creative ways to incorporate culturally appropriate approaches into their treatment intervention.

Proficiency in cultural communication techniques encompasses a wide range of skills that facilitate the flow and exchange of information among those providing and receiving care. Interpersonal exchanges occur between clients and individual providers and between clients and health care delivery organizations. Cultural communication includes more than just words: It includes the nonverbal aspects of communication as well. To be proficient, health care professionals must know how to effectively use interpreters, how to address medical safety issues related to language differences, and how to communicate effectively with patients with low health literacy.

Clients and providers each have independent styles of communication. Open communication between the provider and the client and his or her family is critical to promoting understanding when there are different communication styles. Therapists' reliance on their own language skills often is not enough. When one is unable to rely on the usual linguistic cues, informed consent and adequate assessment and evaluation may be impossible. Common obstacles to effective intercultural communication include assumptions of similarity, misunderstandings because of differences in nonverbal communication, preconceptions and stereotypes, the tendency to evaluate negatively or positively, and high anxiety (Taylor, 1998).

In making treatment decisions and ensuring appropriate care, language services, including the use of interpreters and translated materials, for clients with limited English proficiency or for whom English is not the primary language are essential. The CLAS standards (see Appendix A) stress the importance of hiring interpreters to facilitate clients' interactions with the health care delivery system. Family members, especially children, and friends are not adequate substitutes for professional interpreters, who have demonstrated bilingual proficiency, training in the skills and ethics of interpreting, and knowledge of the terms and concepts relevant to clinical and nonclinical encounters.

It is important to gauge the literacy rate of the target population. Patients need to understand health information, but they have little face-to-face time with their providers, whether in outpatient settings or during hospitalizations (Osborne, 2005). Clients' health literacy strongly influences their compliance with a therapy program. Clients with low health literacy require interpreter services or illustrated instructions in printed materials. Misunderstanding of nonverbal communication can lead to misinterpretation and confusion for both clients and therapists. Nonverbal conflicts can arise around issues related to the degree of directness, appropriateness of topics, touch, loudness and pitch, and silence (Gardenswartz & Rowe, 1993).

Communication skills include not just the ability to communicate verbally with others, but also the ability to guide discussions; to communicate nonverbal messages that are consistent with the verbal message; and, most importantly, to listen to and appreciate various points of views. In addition, written communication skills are essential for a therapist to function in the institutional context, which expects report generation, written intervention plans, and e-mail communication with diverse people. An important facet of communication skill is understanding who needs to know what and when; the creation and tailoring of information are necessary to an effective and efficient therapy program (Issel, 2004).

A cultural broker understands how to integrate the cultural knowledge he or she has learned into daily patient care. The cultural broker serves as a mediator between the client and the health care system and views himself or herself as an advocate for the client (Jezewski, 1993). These practitioners are conscious of differences in the health beliefs and practices of ethnically and otherwise diverse clients, the barriers they face in the health care system, and the poor health outcomes they experience, and they provide advocacy on behalf of patients. The variety of interventions cultural brokers make on behalf of their patients are limited only by their imaginations. Cultural brokers take medical histories and conduct initial assessments in a way that accounts for cultural, sociological, psychological, and biological factors, including the level of the client's acculturation. They avoid the stereotyping that results from a superficial understanding of culture-specific characteristics and build on evidence-based evaluations of cultural information identified through literature reviews and interactions with clients.

Summary

Becoming culturally competent requires a focus on self-exploration, cultural knowledge, and cultural skills. Examining personal cultural attitudes and knowledge; fostering an open, sensitive approach to health care beliefs; demonstrating comfort with cultural differences; developing cultural communication techniques; using culturally sensitive interviewing tools; and demonstrating respect are all recommended tasks needed to provide culturally competent care (Bazaldu & Sias, 2004). Self-assessment, educational intervention, and hands-on training are all necessary to make cultural competence possible. Your plan must be designed in accord with your learning style, environment, and needs. A support network is critical in becoming and incorporating cultural competence into your day-to-day practice, and a mindset and philosophy of cultural competence and cultural brokering on behalf of your clients will allow you to practice effectively in a multicultural environment. This enriching and transformative experience is not only a challenge to all of us who care but also a worthy journey to take.

Reflection

Self-Exploration

The following activity will facilitate self-exploration and acknowledgment of your cultural heritage and history. Answer each question; there is no right or wrong answer to these questions (Kabagarama, 1993; Ponterotto & Pedersen, 1993; Randall-David, 1989):

1. What ethnic group, socioeconomic level, religion, age group, and community do you belong to?

2. What experiences have you had with people from ethnic populations, socioeconomic levels, religions, age groups, sexual identities, disabilities, or communities different from your own?

3. What were those experiences like? How did you feel about them?

4. When you were growing up, what did your parents and significant others say about people who were different from your family?

5. How has the cultural setting in which you were brought up influenced your outlook on life?

6. What influences in your experiences led to the development of negative feelings, if any, about your cultural heritage or background?

7. What influences in your experiences led to the development of positive feelings, if any, about your cultural heritage or background?

8. What personal qualities do you have that will help you establish interpersonal relationships with people from other cultural groups? What personal qualities may be detrimental?

9. Complete the following sentences:

    - I like to learn about other cultures because _____.

    - I do not like to learn about other cultures because _____.

    - I get along with other people because _____.

    - I do not get along with other people because _____.

10. What changes, if any, would you like to make in your own attitudes or experiences in relation to people of other ethnic or cultural groups?

11. Describe an experience in your life in which you feel you were discriminated against for any reason, not necessarily because of your culture.

12. How do you feel _____ (fill in the blank with the name of an ethnic, racial, or cultural group) should deal with issues of cultural diversity in American life?

Cultural Programming

Analyze your cultural programming in each of the 10 areas listed in the following grid, and then analyze what you think about the programming of members of a group different from your own (modified from Harris & Moran, 1979).

Aspect of Culture	You	Other
1. Sense of self and space		
2. Communication and language		
3. Dress and appearance		
4. Food and eating habits		
5. Time and space consciousness		
6. Relationships, family, and friends		
7. Values and norms		
8. Beliefs and attitudes		
9. Mental processes and learning styles		
10. Work habits and practices		

Note. Adapted from *Managing cultural differences,* P. T. Harris and R. T. Moran, 1979, Houston, TX, Gulf Publishing. Copyright © 1979 by Gulf Publishing. Adapted with permission.

Assessing How You Relate to Various Groups of People

The following are different levels of response you might have toward a person:

- *Greet:* I feel I can greet this person warmly and welcome him or her sincerely.

- *Accept:* I feel I can honestly accept this person as he or she is and be comfortable enough to listen to his or her problems.

- *Help:* I feel I would genuinely try to help this person with his or her problems as they might relate to or arise from the label or stereotype given to him or her.

- *Background:* I feel I have the background of knowledge or experience to be able to help this person.

- *Advocate:* I feel I could honestly be an advocate for this person.

The following is a list of types of individuals. Read the list and place a check mark by anyone you would not greet or would hesitate to greet. Do the same for the other levels of response. Try to respond honestly, not as you think might be socially or professionally desirable. Your answers are only for your personal use in clarifying your initial reactions to different people.

Type of Individual	Greet	Accept	Help	Background	Advocate
1. Haitian					
2. Child abuser					
3. Jew					
4. Person with hemophilia					
5. Neo-Nazi					
6. Mexican American					
7. IV drug user					
8. Catholic					

Type of Individual	Greet	Accept	Help	Background	Advocate
9. Elderly person with senility					
10. Teamsters Union member					
11. Native American					
12. Prostitute					
13. Jehovah's Witness					
14. Person with cerebral palsy					
15. Vietnamese American					
16. Gay man or lesbian					
17. Person with AIDS					
18. African American					
19. Protestant					
20. Ku Klux Klan member					
21. Alcoholic					
22. White American					
23. Amish person					
24. Nuclear armament proponent					
25. Unmarried pregnant teenager					

Note. Adapted from *Strategies for working with culturally diverse communities and clients,* by E. Randall-David, 1989, Washington, DC, Association for the Care of Children's Health. Copyright © 1989 by author. Adapted with permission.

The previous activity may help you anticipate difficulty in working with some clients. If you have a concentration of check marks at specific levels, you may have a conflict that could hinder you from rendering effective professional help.

Cultural Knowledge

The following activities will provide you with a broad base of knowledge about diverse populations.

- Assume that you have been asked to select and describe a diverse population to a class of 5th graders. Prepare a 10-minute presentation that you could use to fulfill the request.

- Identify 10 sources of information (e.g., books, articles, journals, or other media) about diverse populations.

- Develop a list of similarities and differences between diverse populations.

- Select a population of interest to you. Create a multiple-choice test using factual questions about this group.

- Interview a health care provider from a diverse population. Inquire about the professional problems and issues that he or she most frequently encounters in professional activities and professional–client interactions.

- Conduct a community assessment for a diverse population. Identify all of the institutions that the targeted population uses (e.g., schools, churches, hospitals), all of the social services agencies that serve the population, and all community businesses the population patronizes.

- Interview at least 5 people from the diverse population to explore their attitudes about the health care system and medical professionals (Wells, 1994).

The following questions may be useful to explore with health professionals:

- How are traditional healers different from Western-educated health care providers?

- How can I work with traditional healers without compromising my beliefs?

- What are common problem areas in dealing with multicultural populations?

- What are some of the unique problems in serving your specific community?

The following assessment questions may be useful in interacting with clients (Kleinman, Eisenberg, & Good, 1978):

- What do you think caused your problem?

- Why do you think it started when it did?

- What does your sickness do to you? How does it work?

- How severe is your sickness? How long do you expect it to last?

- What problems have your sickness caused you?

- What do you fear about your sickness?
- What kind of treatment do you think you should receive?
- What are the most important results you hope to receive from this treatment?

Cultural Skills

The following activities should help you put into practice all that you have learned about diverse groups (Wells, 1994):

- Have one person role-play the part of a health care provider and another the part of a person from a given group. Have a third person serve as an observer. Role-play an interview session for about 5 minutes, then stop and critique the activity. Change roles in the activity, and repeat 2 or more times. Offer suggestions for improving the interaction.

- Prepare a critique of an audio- or videotape of a treatment session between a health care provider and a person from a particular group.

- Solicit volunteers from various populations. Role-play the part of a health care provider working with them as part of a health care team or as colleagues. Critique the simulation, offering suggestions on how to improve the interaction.

- Practice carrying on a telephone conversation with someone from a different culture. Allow someone to listen to your conversation and give feedback on your performance.

- List the questions that you may want to ask a client from another culture during your first encounter or interview.

How Differently We Say . . .

The meaning of words does not change, but intonation patterns, word order, volume, pauses, facial expression, and gestures can change everything. The word one stresses in any sentence can drastically alter its meaning. Try the following sentence, stressing a different word each time (Gardenswartz & Rowe, 1993):

- *I* am going to do this for you tomorrow.
- I *am* going to do this for you tomorrow.
- I am *going* to do this for you tomorrow.
- I am going to do *this* for you tomorrow.
- I am going to do this for *you* tomorrow.
- I am going to do this for you *tomorrow*.

Case Study

Mrs. Lee is a 49-year-old Cantonese-speaking woman who emigrated several years ago from China to the United States. She lives with her husband and youngest son, a 22-year-old college student. Mrs. Lee recently fell and broke her left hip. Her medical records revealed that she had been diagnosed with osteoporosis, and this was her third bone break in 2 years. She also has lung cancer with metastasis to her lymph nodes. Her son has asked that the therapist not discuss either diagnosis with Mrs. Lee. He did not want his mother to be told any "bad news" that might cause her to lose hope.

- As the therapist, what will you do to obtain Mrs. Lee's consent for you to provide treatment?

- How will this information influence your treatment approach?

- Try to see her son's point of view: What might he be thinking culturally?

- How do cultural differences in the telling of bad news differ between you and the family?

- How do the ethics of informed consent and autonomy fit into the belief system of Mrs. Lee and her family?

References

Accreditation Council for Occupational Therapy Education. (2007). Accreditation Council for Occupational Therapy Education (ACOTE) standards and interpretive guidelines. *American Journal of Occupational Therapy, 61.*

American Medical Student Association. (2004). *Cultural competence in medicine.* Retrieved June 13, 2004, from www.amsa.org/programs/gpit/cultural.cfm

American Occupational Therapy Association. (2005). Occupational therapy code of ethics (2005). *American Journal of Occupational Therapy, 59,* 639–642.

Bazaldu, O. V., & Sias, J. (2004). Cultural competence: A pharmacy perspective. *Journal of Pharmacy Practice, 17,* 160–166.

Gardenswartz, L., & Rowe, A. (1993). *Managing diversity: A complete desk reference and planning guide.* New York: Business One Irwin/Pfeiffer & Company.

Harris, P. T., & Moran, R. T. (1979). *Managing cultural differences.* Houston, TX: Gulf.

Health Resources and Services Administration. (2004). *Health Resources and Services Administration study on measuring competence in health care delivery settings.* Retrieved May 31, 2006, from www.hrsa.gov/culturalcompetence/measures/default.htm

Issel, L. M. (2004). *Health program planning and evaluation: A practical, systematic approach for community health.* Boston: Jones & Bartlett.

Jezewski, M. A. (1993). Cultural brokering as a model for advocacy. *Nursing and Health Care, 14*(2), 78–84.

Joint Commission on Healthcare Organizations. (2007). *Standards revisions.* Retrieved July 2007 from http://www.jointcommission.org/standards/

Johnson, V. (1995). *Heart full of grace: A thousand years of Black wisdom.* New York: Simon & Schuster.

Kabagarama, D. (1993). *Breaking the ice: A guide to understanding people from other cultures.* Boston: Allyn & Bacon.

Kleinman, A., Eisenberg, L., & Good, B. (1978). Culture, illness and care: Clinical lessons from anthropologic and cross-cultural research. *Annals of Internal Medicine, 88,* 251–258.

Office of Minority Health. (2001). *National standards on culturally and linguistically appropriate services.* Retrieved July 27, 2007, from http://www.omhrc.gov/templates/browse. aspx?lvl=2&lvlID=15

Osborne, H. (2005). *Health literacy from A to Z: Practical ways to communicate your health message.* Boston: Jones & Bartlett.

Ponterotto, J. G., & Pedersen, P. B. (1993). *Preventing prejudice: A guide for counselors and educators.* Newbury Park, CA: Sage.

Randall-David, E. (1989). *Strategies for working with culturally diverse communities and clients.* Washington, DC: Association for the Care of Children's Health.

Taylor, R. (1998). Check your cultural competence. *Nursing Management, 29*(8), 30–32.

Wells, S. A. (1994). *A multicultural education and resource guide for occupational therapy educators and practitioners.* Bethesda, MD: American Occupational Therapy Association.

III

Integrating Cultural Competence

It is the responsibility of the educational institutions in the United States to nurture cultural sensitivity . . . by providing students the opportunity to explore and examine other cultures as well as their own.

—ZELLER (1995, P. 8)

Objectives

The information in Part III will help readers

- Apply the concepts of cultural competence in clinical practice,
- Compare and contrast various models and pedagogies used in the education and training of cultural competence,
- Recognize and understand the complexities in community integration programs, and
- Understand and integrate the concepts of cultural competence using an occupational justice framework.

17

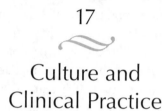

Culture and Clinical Practice

We ain't what we want to be; we ain't what we gonna be; but thank God, we ain't what we was.

—African American folk saying (cited in Johnson, 1995, p. 14)

Key Points

- Every clinical interaction is a cross-cultural interaction with at least three cultures involved: (a) the personal or familial culture of the provider, (b) the culture of the client and his or her family, and (c) the culture of the health care system. There may be a fourth culture—the traditional medical culture of the client.

- Standardized evaluation tools, which are based largely on the sociocultural norms of the White, middle-class population, should be interpreted within the context of the client's culture when used with members of other racial, ethnic, or cultural populations.

- Awareness of the relationships among culture, clinical reasoning, and practice enable a culturally holistic approach to health care. Occupational therapists and occupational therapy assistants must examine their perceptions of culturally diverse clients to understand potential discriminatory practices and promote change.

Understanding the meaning of culture, cultural competence, and health disparities and incorporating these meanings into practice constitute a mission many occupational therapy practitioners and students have embraced. Much has been published in the area of diversity and cultural sensitivity that educates therapists and students about different cultural values and norms and describes the health beliefs and practices of various racial, ethnic, and cultural groups (Blakeney, 1993; Bonder, Martin, & Miracle, 2002; Kirsh, Trentham, & Cole, 2006; Meghani-Wise, 1996). This literature supports the assertion that understanding the influences of health beliefs and behaviors of particular cultural groups can lead to a better understanding of how clients perceive and take action to address illness and will improve clinical judgment (Yuen & Yau, 1999).

In occupational therapy, however, this acknowledgment of cultural diversity has occurred primarily on a theoretical and philosophical level (Krefting & Krefting, 1991). Therapists and students seldom have a clear understanding of how to integrate culture into their daily practice of decision making, assessment, and intervention. It is one of the least developed aspects of occupational therapy knowledge on a practical level.

Poor integration of cultural knowledge into clinical practice can result in a sense of dissatisfaction and disharmony for both client and provider. Providers may feel inadequate in their intervention choices, leading to inappropriate treatment models, and poor integration can impede communication between client and provider (Fitzgerald, 1992; Wells, 1994). Lawlor and Mattingly (1998) found difficulties in bridging cultural boundaries between professionals and between practitioners and families on a practical level in their study of family-centered models of services.

Although the occupational therapy profession espouses the principle of client-centered or person-centered care, the manner and extent to which this principle is implemented with respect to the experiences of culturally diverse groups are largely unknown. Cultural competence is not executed uniformly in occupational therapy practice, and no strategies have been proposed to ascertain what occupational therapy practitioners are currently doing on an individual basis (American Occupational Therapy Association [AOTA], 2005). This issue is key for the profession, because a lack of attention to diversity among and within cultures, as well as a shortage of culturally competent professionals, can create barriers to effective health care (Coridan & O'Connell, 2001).

Using the cultural competence model, this chapter presents practical ways to integrate culture into one's daily clinical reasoning process and practice. It focuses on incorporating culture into assessments and evaluations and using cultural knowledge and skills to design intervention strategies.

Culture and the Clinical Interaction

A plethora of literature focuses on the influence of culture on health and health care, the therapeutic relationship, and treatment outcomes, as well as the need for training and education of providers (Dresser, 1996; Good, 1996; Jang, 1995; Kavanagh & Kennedy, 1992; Kelly, 1995; Kreps & Kunimoto, 1994; Levine, 1984; McCormack, 1987; Pope-Davis, Prietor, Whitaker, & Pope-Davis, 1993). Jackson, Carlson, Mandel, Zemke, and Clark (1998), for example, described cultural clashes among participants in a well-elderly program, an unexpected outcome that led to "an attempt to open new doors of understanding about other cultures within the context of occupations" (p. 331) within the intervention program.

Every clinical encounter or interaction involves multiple cultures. According to Fitzgerald (1992), at least three cultures are involved in clinical interactions: (a) the personal or familial culture of the provider, (b) the personal or familial culture of the client and his or her family, and (c) the culture of the primary medical system (see Figure 17.1). In some cases, especially when the individual is from a non-Western background, a fourth culture—the traditional medical culture—must be taken into account. The first step in establishing a satisfying and productive relationship is acknowledging that multiple cultures are involved in the therapeutic relationship and that every clinical encounter is a cross-cultural interaction. This awareness is fairly easy to maintain when the participants in the interaction come from obviously different cultural backgrounds, but it is more difficult when the participants have similar backgrounds and appearances.

Every person is a product of multiple cultures and interprets reality through his or her cultural filters. According to Barney (1991), because of people's individual cultural filters, "we may be ignorant of the customs, language, social relationship patterns, religion, and other practices of various ethnic and minority groups. In other words, we often do not know what we don't know" (p. 590). And with the tensions surrounding race relationships and political correctness in the United States, many health care providers unsurprisingly are unsure how to approach their clients about cultural beliefs and practices.

In a multicultural health care environment, therapists must engage in *cultural brokering*, which entails helping decrease the degree of disparity among the varieties of cultures by negotiating mutually acceptable solutions to different cultural perspectives. The strength of cultural brokering is in its emphasis on respect, caring, understanding, and patience in health care encounters (Warda, 2000). Therefore, therapists must be comfortable, skilled, and experienced in integrating culture into all aspects and procedures of the health care system. To provide effective guidelines for practice, occupational therapists need more education about evaluation,

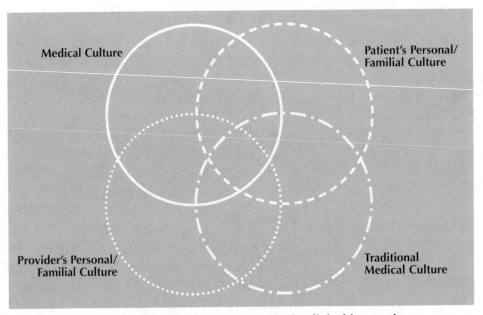

Figure 17.1. The four overlapping cultures present in clinical interactions.

Note. From "Multicultural clinical action," M. H. Fitzgerald, 1992, *Journal of Rehabilitation, 55,* pp. 38–42. Copyright © 1992 by the National Rehabilitation Association. Adapted with permission.

intervention, disease prevention, and wellness as they affect cultural groups confronting a variety of disparities (AOTA, 2005).

Culture in Clinical Reasoning

Occupational therapy practitioners use clinical reasoning and critical thinking to develop interventions that are acceptable, meaningful, and satisfying to clients. Clinical reasoning helps practitioners establish a framework for intervention and care that preserves or maintains the client's cultural perspective, accommodates and negotiates some change to promote the client's health, and repatterns and restructures cultural beliefs and behaviors as necessary (Kavanagh, 1991; Leininger, 1988). Therapists already use clinical reasoning as a guide to organize and articulate thinking in clinical practice (Neistadt, 1998) to individualize treatment, facilitate functional performance, and create positive outcomes for their clients (Fleming, 1991b; Parham, 1987; Rogers, 1983; Slater & Cohn, 1991); thus, it is the perfect process for infusing culture into daily practice.

Thinking Strategies

Clinical reasoning is an umbrella term to include all the complex processes that health care providers use when thinking about their client, the disability, the situation, and the personal and cultural meanings that the client gives to the disability, the situation, and the self (Fleming, 1991a). Practitioners use clinical reasoning to integrate the client's history, assessment information, and cultural context into an individualized intervention plan. Occupational therapists and occupational therapy assistants reconstruct the client's ability to function and perform daily life tasks within his or her cultural context. Therapists and clients together work on rebuilding clients' sense of self, ways of accomplishing tasks and engaging in activities, and ways of viewing themselves and their lives. The practitioner, to accomplish this, uses a variety of thinking strategies.

The occupational therapy literature has identified several types of thinking strategies health care practitioners use to accomplish their outcomes. According to Fleming and Mattingly (1994), for occupational therapists the term *clinical reasoning* refers to "not one, but several forms of thinking. Therapists, in other words, think in more than one way" (p. 9). The types of clinical reasoning therapists use are narrative, interactive, procedural, pragmatic, and conditional:

- *Narrative reasoning* focuses on the client's occupational story, life history, and cultural background and activities and roles that the client values (Clark, 1993; Neistadt, 1996).
- *Interactive reasoning* is used in looking for the meaning of the disease or disability to the client (Crepeau, 1991). It also encompasses the interpersonal interaction between the therapist and the client (Fleming, 1991b; Mattingly & Fleming, 1994).
- *Procedural reasoning* is used in identifying problems and interventions on the basis of the client's disease or impairment. The practitioner's general knowledge and understanding about a specific disease or impairment are called on (Fleming, 1991b; Mattingly & Fleming, 1994).
- *Pragmatic reasoning* is used in considering the treatment environment and possibilities for treatment within the given environment. The therapist's values, knowledge, abilities, and experience, as well as the client's social and financial resources, also are considered (Schell & Cervero, 1993).
- *Conditional reasoning* is used to continuously modify treatment to enable the person to function in the future (Fleming, 1991b; Mattingly & Fleming, 1994).

Culture and Connection

A basic premise of clinical reasoning is that people have reasons for their decisions and behaviors, regardless whether they can articulate those reasons or whether the health care worker recognizes what they are. Culture plays a significant role in the decisions and behaviors of not only clients but also providers. Using a set of behavioral standards developed according to the norms of the therapist or medical system to assess a client from another culture is a cultural imposition based on eth-nocentricity. Neistadt, Wight, and Mulligan (1998) examined the use of case stud-ies to teach clinical reasoning and found that the use of clinical reasoning resulted in intervention plans that placed the client in social as well as cultural contexts: "It allows practitioners to view the client as real human being and integrate the whole-person picture into all aspects of the intervention plan" (p. 129). For exam-ple, the fact that a traditional form of health care is an important part of a client's cultural and social context would be revealed through the use of the clinical reason-ing process.

Occupational therapists and occupational therapy assistants use clinical rea-soning to understand clients from the clients' own point of view—in other words, to see clients as they see themselves. Using narrative and interactive reasoning, prac-titioners attempt to understand the meanings people make of themselves and their lives, families, environment, and culture. Failure to assess cultural considerations in the clinical reasoning process can prevent practitioners from establishing a thera-peutic relationship based on equality and mutual respect and from clearly perceiv-ing the feelings and needs of the client. It may create reluctance in the client to par-ticipate in the treatment program (Wells, 1991). The practitioner's understanding that all people are products of their own culture, have knowledge of other cultures, and have the ability to bridge other cultures can lead only to positive and reward-ing clinical interactions.

Awareness of the relationships among culture, clinical reasoning, and practice enables a culturally holistic approach (Barney, 1991) to health care, which leads to culturally sensitive and appropriate intervention strategies. Gathering explicit details and in-depth information about the client's background and cultural beliefs provides a realistic clinical image of clients and paints a picture of the client as an individual with unique interests, values, goals, abilities, and priorities. Clinical rea-soning helps practitioners center on the particulars of the client rather than on their own general condition or limiting factors (Fleming, 1991a). It moves the clinical intervention from a diagnostic to a more holistic and client-centered approach.

Culture and Evaluations

Many of the evaluation and assessment tools used in health care settings are based largely on the sociocultural norms of the White, middle-class population (Skawski, 1987). These tools have overwhelmingly incorporated Western values, ethics, the-ories, and standards. Such assessment tools are not always appropriate for ethnic and culturally diverse populations (Hinkle, 1994), however, and interpretation of their results may lead to nonoptimal treatment approaches. Standardized tests and evaluation tools intend to assess performance skills, not behaviors, but these tools can produce inaccurate results even regarding performance skills. For example, the

Denver Developmental Test (Frankenburg & Dodds, 1967), which was standardized on a North American sample, may not provide valid results for an East Asian immigrant child, who might be labeled as developmental delayed based on results of this test. Because of differences in child-rearing practices and cultural behaviors, developmental milestones are not necessarily achieved at the same age in all populations.

The behaviors of the evaluator and the person being evaluated may be influenced both by the assessment context and by cultural background. Behaviors such as eye contact, tone of voice, and greetings are culturally dependent and varied. Evaluators run the risk of making an incorrect assessment if they interpret clients' behaviors by what they mean in the mainstream culture (Cross, Bazron, Dennis, & Isaacs, 1989; Gaw, 1993). For example, clients evaluated in an unfamiliar system or by a provider who is culturally different often exhibit adjustment behavior: They are likely to be more reserved than usual, they may be apprehensive or fearful that the evaluator will judge them negatively, or they may try to fit in by displaying behaviors commonly associated with the mainstream culture. If the therapist judges these individuals on the basis of these behaviors, language usage, or emotional expressiveness, he or she may mislabel or misdiagnose the client, which in turn may lead to inappropriate intervention strategies and an unsatisfactory therapeutic relationship.

> *Evaluators run the risk of making an incorrect assessment if they interpret clients' behaviors by what they mean in the mainstream culture.*

Tests should be used as an aid to understanding the client: "Providers choosing to use a standard evaluation tool on a different population need to take an individual's sociocultural background into consideration in interpreting its score" (Paul, 1995, p. 158). Standardized tests and assessments, therefore, need to be interpreted in the context of the client's culture and other forms of assessment also should be used with ethnic and diverse populations.

Accurate evaluation is the first step in effective and culturally appropriate treatment provision. Lack of knowledge about other cultures, as well as lack of awareness of one's own biases and values, can lead to possible misinterpretation of evaluation results. Because there are few culturally specific tests and evaluations, therapists should continue to use standardized assessments with culturally different clients but should carefully consider their sociocultural background and cultural foundation (Cross et al., 1989; Paul, 1995).

General Cultural Information

The need for general knowledge about other cultures is as necessary to the reasoning process as general medical knowledge. Cultural knowledge promotes understanding, sensitivity, and empathy. Information about the general characteristics and life experiences of different racial, ethnic, and cultural groups enables practitioners to recognize individual differences and similarities, affirm the culture of the client, and open avenues to learning and growth. Such information, however, should never be used as part of a cookbook approach to treatment or clients. Rather, general cultural knowledge provides a starting point for gathering information, asking questions, and establishing rapport with the client.

Table 17.1 provides a general overview of basic cultural values, family roles and structures, religious practices, perceptions of time, communication styles, support networks, health practices and utilization, and beliefs. This overview can help practitioners

- Interpret assessments and evaluation tools,
- Determine whether standardized treatment methods and approaches need to be modified, and
- Determine whether the use of Western standards, ethics, and ideas may negatively affect clients and their families.

Table 17.1. Comparison of Cultural Foundations

"Mainstream" America	Ethnocultural Groups
Mastery over nature	Harmony with nature
Personal control over the environment	Fate
Doing—active	Being/being-in-becoming
Time dominates	Personal interaction dominates
Human equality	Hierarchy/rank/status
Individualism/privacy	Group welfare
Youth	Elders
Self-help	Birthright inheritance
Competition	Cooperation
Future orientation	Past or present orientation
Informality	Formality
Directness/openness/honesty	Indirectness/ritual/"face"
Practicality/efficiency	Idealism
Materialism	Spiritualism
Nature of man is good and bad	Nature of man is good

Note. Data from *Family therapy with ethnic minorities*, M. K. Ho, 1987, Thousand Oaks, CA: Sage; *Strategies for working with culturally diverse communities and clients*, E. Randall-David, 1989, Washington, DC: Association for the Care of Children's Health.

Cultural Clinical Reasoning Process

Practitioners can easily incorporate cultural queries into the clinical reasoning process for clinical decision making (Opacich, 1991). Exhibit 17.1 provides a summary of the steps in the cultural clinical reasoning process.

Phase 1: Problem Setting

The initial assessment phase is the "process by which data are gathered, hypotheses formulated, and decisions are made for further action" (Opacich, 1991, p. 356). The information gathered during this phase guides the establishment of treatment goals and interventions. A general knowledge of the client's culture, including basic beliefs, values, and behaviors, can help the practitioner determine at the outset whether standard treatment approaches should be modified. Examples of general cultural knowledge include the following:

- In most ethnic cultures, older people are addressed more formally than younger individuals.
- African Americans tend to look at someone when talking and to look away while listening.
- Practitioners should avoid a highly casual manner with Asian American clients.
- The interaction should be conducted in the preferred language of the client, if possible.

How the practitioner approaches the individual sets the stage for all therapeutic interactions and influences the client's ability to trust the provider and health system. A basic knowledge of specific cultural and ethnic groups and an awareness of one's own values and biases will enable practitioners to create a wide range of appropriate responses to the needs of the client. Culturally skilled and competent providers are aware of and comfortable with differences between themselves and their clients and are sensitive to circumstances that may prompt them to refer clients to others for provision of services. For example, a practitioner has been asked to provide occupational therapy services to someone who is gay. The practitioner feels uncomfortable interacting with this person because of religious beliefs; therefore, to ensure that the client receives quality care, the practitioner refers him to another therapist.

Phase 2: Framing and Delineating the Problem

During the second phase of the cultural clinical reasoning process, the practitioner explores clients' problems using assessment tools and instruments as well as his or her general cultural knowledge and professional and technical knowledge. For

Exhibit 17.1. Culture and the Clinical Reasoning Process

Phase 1: Problem Setting

Client's Referral Information + General Cultural Knowledge = Initial Response

Initiate information about the client:

- Racial/ethnic identifier
- Age
- Gender
- Diagnosis/disability
- Medical history
- Family/social history (limited)

Provide clues to (narrative reasoning)

- What culturally sensitive approaches to take;
- What additional information is needed regarding the client's occupational history; cultural background, life history, and values; and
- What potential cultural and performance problem(s) might arise.

Phase 2: Framing and Delineating the Problem

General Cultural Knowledge + Professional Knowledge = Preliminary Assessment

Gather additional information about the client:

- Performance level
- Goals and concerns
- More family/social history
- Life experiences
- Present-life situation
- Health beliefs
- Values

Provide clues to (interactive and procedural reasoning)

- The meaning of disease or disability to the client,
- The interaction between the client and provider, and
- The provider's professional knowledge and understanding about the disease or disability.

Phase 3: Forming Hypotheses and Developing Intervention Plans

Client's Information + General Cultural Knowledge + Professional Knowledge = Cultural Intervention Strategies

Provide clues to (pragmatic reasoning)

- The health care provider's values, knowledge, abilities, and experiences;
- The client's social functioning and financial resources; and
- The treatment environment and possibilities of treatment within a given environment.

Phase 4: Implementing the Intervention Plan

Client's Information + General Cultural Knowledge + Professional Knowledge + Cultural Intervention Strategies = Beneficial Outcome

Gather information about the client:

- Performance changes
- Personal cultural and lifestyle situation.

Provide clues to (conditioning reasoning)

- The continuation or modification of treatment and
- The future functioning of the client.

example, some Hispanic clients do not differentiate between physical and emotional illness. They may present with physical complaints, when in fact the cause is an emotional problem. Thus, culturally sensitive practice with Hispanics might involve not only looking for physical causes of complaints but also encouraging clients to talk about why they are ill.

When selecting an assessment strategy, the provider should be aware of the validity, reliability, and test construction process of any instruments or tools he or she is considering. Many test instruments have not been standardized for ethnic populations. Therefore, caution should be used in the interpretation of the test results, because unless cultural differences are accounted for, inappropriate treatment strategies may be selected. For example, a 6-year-old child raised on a Native American reservation is labeled a slow learner because he is shy and quiet in class, responds only when called on or when spoken to, avoids eye contact and looks down at the floor, does not engage in conversations with the other children, and has trouble writing his name on a piece of paper. Within the Native American culture, children are taught to respect and honor their elders; a bowed head is a sign of respect. Also, looking at people directly in the eye is considered a sign of hostility or impoliteness, while children are expected to be seen but not heard (Champagne, 1994; Wells, 1994). Providers also should inquire about the use of traditional healing practices and healers, which can alter the results of some standard tests and assessments.

Constructing a narrative and life history of the client, whether formally or informally, allows the provider to frame the problems and limitations in a cultural context. This process also gives the provider a way to share with colleagues his or her ideas about what is going on with a particular client; to discuss with the family specific client-centered issues; and to plan with the client, treatment team members, and other professionals culturally appropriate strategies. A working knowledge of sociocultural questions to ask is an essential tool for health care providers. One mechanism for learning about a client's life history, cultural beliefs, and attitudes toward illness and health is to use an opening statement and series of questions, examples of which are provided in Exhibit 17.2.

Phase 3: Forming Hypotheses and Developing Intervention Plans

During Phase 3, the provider articulates and applies theoretical reasoning and his or her understanding of clients' problems from a contextual and cultural perspective. The provider examines the facts he or she knows about clients, general cultural information, and professional and technical data and develops goals and intervention strategies. This process ensures that treatment matches clients' expectations, which are grounded in cultural values and behaviors, and the health care provider's responsibilities, which are grounded in his or her professional orientation. This type

Exhibit 17.2. Eliciting Cultural Information in Clinical Interactions

Proposed opening statement:

"Mr./Mrs./Ms. _____, sometimes clients and health care providers have different ideas about health and illness as well as outcome expectations. To design and provide individualized care, it is important for me to have a clear picture and understanding of your thoughts and concerns about this illness. I would like to ask you some questions about your culture, values, and beliefs. This way we can work together to improve your health/function and address your concerns."

Questions regarding current illness:

- What is your general understanding about your illness?
- What do you think caused your problem?
- Why do you think it started?
- How severe is your illness? How long do you think it will last?
- What are the main problems your illness has caused for you?
- Have you tried any home remedies, medicines, folk/traditional treatment for your illness? Did it help? Are you still using it/them?
- What type of treatment do you think you should receive?
- What results do you hope to receive from the treatment?
- Is there any other information that would be helpful in designing a workable treatment plan?

Questions regarding health beliefs and practices:

- Do you adhere to a religious healing system (e.g., Seventh Day Adventist, West African voodoo, Fundamentalist, Pentecostal)?
- Do you adhere to a cultural healing system (e.g., Asian healing system, Raza/Latina *curanderismo*)?
- How is illness explained in your culture (e.g., germ theory, presence of evil spirits, imbalance between "hot" and "cold," yin and yang, disequilibrium between nature and man)?
- Do you rely on cultural healers (medicine men, shamen, *curanderos*, Chinese herbalists, spiritualists, ministers, *hougans* [voodoo priests])?
- What types of cultural healing practices and remedies do you or your family practice (e.g., massage to cure *empacho*, coining, wearing of talismans or charms for protection against illness)?
- How would you describe a state of "wellness" or "good health"? A state of "poor health" or "illness"?

Questions regarding cultural beliefs and values:

- Are there any taboos or restrictions on who can see a woman's or man's body?
- Are there any taboos or other beliefs connected with mental illness?
- Describe your spirituality or religious practice and beliefs.
- With what culture/racial/ethnic group do you identify?
- How would you describe your family structure?
- What type of support system or network is available to you?
- Who is the primary decision maker in your family?

of integration increases the likelihood that therapeutic goals will be accomplished, treatment requests complied with, and satisfaction with the treatment outcome achieved for both clients and providers.

Phase 4: Implementing the Intervention Plan

During the implementation phase, the provider implements, monitors, reassesses, and modifies the intervention strategies. The provider continually and systematically collects specific information not only about performance changes but also about cultural values, beliefs, and behaviors. If the intervention is not beneficial or in line with clients' cultural expectations, the provider can alter or terminate the therapy.

Case Example

Phase 1: Problem Setting

Client's Referral Information

- The client is a single, 29-year-old man.
- His health problems are the result of a traumatic brain injury and right hemiparesis.
- He is Asian American.
- Before the accident, he lived alone and worked as a laborer.

General Cultural Knowledge: Asian American and Pacific Islander Culture

- The family system is extremely important. Members may have varying levels of acculturation, depending on generation.
- Regarding communication style, touching strangers is inappropriate, eye-to-eye contact with a stranger is considered shameful, and high value is placed on emotional restraint. This group tends to be nonconfrontational and noncommunicative of personal feelings.
- Members of this cultural group may hold the belief that time is flexible, so there is no need to hurry.
- Health practices may involve the concept of yin and yang, meditation, traditional healers, hot–cold theory, and partial acceptance of Western medicine. A typical health belief is that illness may result from bad conduct of an individual or family member.

Initial Response

- Avoid a highly casual manner, and be cautious about touching the client.
- Small talk at the beginning of a session is considered good manners and keeps you from appearing too rushed.

- The client may be hesitant to admit he has health problems. Encourage him to share his feelings about the injury and disability.
- The client may feel personally responsible for the injury. Be prepared to provide a careful explanation of the etiology of his health problems.
- Formulate additional questions to explore. For example, What specific group of Asian Americans is the client a member of (e.g., Korean, Japanese, Vietnamese)?

Phase 2: Framing and Delineating the Problem

Client's Presenting Information

- The client sustained injury in a motorcycle accident; he was not wearing a helmet.
- The client is a second-generation Cambodian American and demonstrates assimilative patterns.
- Before the accident, he contributed much of his time to working in the family store.
- The client completed high school, but he has expressed little interest in higher education.

Specific Cultural Knowledge

- Khmer is the official language of Cambodia, and many Cambodian Americans speak this language at home. Children usually are fluent in speaking and writing English. When interpreters are required for communication, most prefer same-sex interpreters.
- When Cambodians greet each other, they hold their palms together near their faces and often state the greeting *chum reap sur*. They appreciate hearing this greeting from individuals other than Cambodians as well.
- Cambodian Americans value interdependency among family members, and members of an extended family are expected to share or pool resources to meet the needs of the family and its members. The family takes basic responsibility for the care of its members.
- The role of the sick person is viewed as being dependent and passive, and family members may even discourage the sick person from doing physical self-help. They may believe that the member is ill because of the sins committed by family members. The family is jointly responsible for all decisions. The senior man is the head of the household. The relationships between the father and his sons are especially emphasized. This relationship can be both a strength and source of conflict.
- Most Cambodians are Buddhist and attend temple regularly.

- Rice typically is the base of each meal and is accompanied by a clear or vegetable soup, fish, or meat and vegetables (fresh and dried). Most families eat all three meals together.
- It is very insulting to touch an individual's head, which is considered the most important part of the body and the place where the spirit is found. Feet are considered the lowest in value of the body parts, and it is insulting to point them at someone. When the client is lying down, it is impolite to step over his or her feet and legs. It is impolite to walk in front of someone, except children. It also is impolite to have eye contact with someone who is older or someone who is considered a superior.
- Cambodians traditionally have dealt with illness through self-care and self-medication. The assistance of a health practitioner is sought if one's own remedies don't work. Traditional healers (a *Khru Khmer*) or spiritual healers may be sought for illness thought to be caused by spirits. Spirit possession or sickness may be the result of evil spells cast by another, mistakes made in various rituals through the life cycle, or neglect of rituals. Cupping, pinching, and rubbing are the most commonly used treatments and are thought to restore balance by releasing excessive air. Western medicine is generally considered hot, and herbal remedies have cooling properties.
- Western health care is confusing and overwhelming for many Cambodians. Language and cultural barriers, crowded waiting rooms, multiple interviews, mysterious procedures, and the abrupt behavior of personnel make obtaining health care an unpleasant experience. Cambodians expect to receive medications for every illness, which makes them feel that something is being done to alleviate their discomfort. Many Cambodians are hesitant to share the fact that they are using other forms of health care, because they believe Western medical providers will think it is wrong to use alternatives.
- Some principle stressors in everyday life for Cambodians are language barriers, limited education, fear of children becoming involved in gangs, and economic difficulties. (The information in this section is found in Wetzel, 1995).

Professional Knowledge

- Two months have elapsed since the injury; the client has impaired gross and fine motor coordination.
- The client is unable to perform some self-care activities and has problems with memory, organization, and judgment.
- The standard treatment approach emphasizes the individual's independence and self-help.

Preliminary Delineation of Problems

- Impaired motor functioning
- Impaired self-care skills
- Cognitive impairments
- Intra- and interpersonal difficulties
- Productivity and return-to-work issues
- Cultural and ethical conflicts.

Phase 3: Forming Hypotheses and Developing Intervention Plans

Forming Hypotheses

- The client will demonstrate upper extremity dressing with minimum assist of family members within 3 weeks.
- The client will engage with family members during at least one family meal daily.
- The client will participate in one traditional healing practice to restore spiritual balance.

Developing Cultural Intervention Strategies

- Involve the family in the treatment process. Use them as aides.
- Teach family members why independence in function is important and good for the client and family.
- Ascertain the family's perception of the causes of the illness.
- Ascertain the family's cultural traditional medicine practices. Work with traditional healers or diviners.
- Use a directive rather than a nondirective approach.

Phase 4: Implementing the Intervention Plan

Re-evaluate and modify treatment as needed to reflect the client's performance, lifestyle, and culture.

Cultural Approach to Healthy Service Delivery

According to Leininger (1991), in creating a multicultural approach to the delivery of care, three strategies should guide the practitioner's actions:

1. *Cultural preservation and maintenance.* The client's beliefs, values, and practices should be preserved and incorporated into the intervention process as much as possible. This strategy allows the client to be a partner in his or her health care and facilitates the selection of intervention methods that work within his or her cultural context.
2. *Cultural negotiation and accommodation.* Negotiation and accommodation should be used when there is a conflict between Western medical practice

and the client's traditional health practices. The practitioner should work with the client to develop a plan that incorporates both approaches, modifying when necessary what is perceived as best or optimal treatment.

3. *Cultural repatterning and restructuring.* Repatterning and restructuring are used when a shift or change in cultural beliefs is needed for the client's overall health or safety. The practitioner must explain why and how a certain cultural practice is detrimental to the client's health and safety in terms that the client understands. In addition, the practitioner should discuss with the client how potential treatment outcomes may alter typical cultural roles and practices and let the client decide when and to what extent he or she wishes to engage in the new behavior (Wells, 1991).

When a cultural issue interrupts the therapeutic interaction, practitioners can try the LEARN (*L*isten, *E*valuate, *A*cknowledge, *R*ecommend, and *N*egotiate) approach (Berlin & Fowkes, 1983; Carballeira, 1997).

- *Listen:* Listen with sympathy and understanding to the client and family about their perception of the illness and problem. Concentrate on actively listening rather than on preparing your response. When you respond, respond to both what is being said and how it is being said. Listen for both facts and feelings.

- *Evaluate:* In clear and everyday terms, evaluate your perceptions, as a health care provider, of the problem. Openly discuss your personal views and the sources of those views. Evaluate both the cultural context and the cultural effects of your advice and intervention. This type of discussion helps clients better understand their options and resolve any ethical conflicts.

- *Acknowledge:* Acknowledge and discuss the similarities and differences in perceptions between you and the client. Acknowledge that some health beliefs and practices are derived from basic human needs and may have little basis in science. Even practices you consider primitive serve a purpose for the person within the culture and must be respected.

- *Recommend:* Offer options or alternative treatment interventions. Suggest several ways the client might view a given treatment approach from your, as well as his or her own, cultural point of view.

- *Negotiate:* Collaborate with the client in determining intervention options and agreements. Allow the client to choose, as long as the choice avoids harm. Go as far as your health care system will allow in accommodating the client's needs. If necessary, advocate for change within the health care system to make it more accommodating for cultural variation.

Bazaldua and Sias (2004) describe the interaction between a provider and a client as a cross-cultural exchange of attitudes that require RESPECT:

- *R*apport is vital. Develop it by understanding the client's point of view and avoiding assumptions.

- *Empathy* also is important. Remember that clients are seeking advice.
- *Support* clients by understanding their social context and involving their family.
- *Partner* with clients regarding the intervention plan and negotiate if necessary.
- *Explain* or teach concepts and verify that clients understand them.
- *Cultural* competence is your responsibility, and you must respect the client's beliefs.
- *Trust* is essential and requires patience.

Exhibits 17.3 to 17.5 provide additional intervention strategies.

Summary

Because cultural differences are present in many health care encounters, occupational therapy practitioners must serve as cultural brokers among the many cultures with whom they interact. Integrating culture into the daily clinical reasoning process and activities allows the therapist to not only bridge cultures but also use a culturally holistic approach to care and see each client as an individual with his or her own identity, culture, experiences, background, and lifestyle. Interacting in this manner moves the clinical intervention from a diagnostic approach to a client- and family-centered approach.

Accurate assessment of the client is the first step in culturally appropriate treatment intervention. Practitioners should review the cultural validity of the standard assessment tools they use and interpret the results of assessments within the context of the client's culture. Any bias present in the tool should be acknowledged in the documentation. Equally important to consider are the environment in which the client functions, which directly influences the client's ability to adhere to an intervention program (Dyck, 1992), and differences in communication styles and expressions of emotions, which are directly influenced by culture, age, geography, ethnicity, race, gender, generational conditioning, and acculturation.

Occupational therapy practitioners should not be afraid to ask culturally specific questions. General cultural information and knowledge provide only a starting place for communication and interaction. Exploring an individual's values, beliefs, environment, and life history promotes practitioner–client collaboration and builds a relationship based on mutual respect and equality. Potential cultural issues, concerns, and conflicts must be addressed beginning with the initial interaction to ensure that the clinical interaction is beneficial to all parties involved: client, health care provider, and health system. Occupational therapists and occupational therapy assistants must make every effort to develop critical analytical skills that address cross-cultural interaction and shift occupational therapy into enactments of client centeredness and holism that incorporate diversity (Kirsh et al., 2006).

Exhibit 17.3. Creating a Multicultural Approach: Treatment Implications

African Americans/Blacks
- Involve the extended family in the treatment process.
- Identify the significant decision maker and involve him or her in the treatment process.
- Address older adults by their title and last name.
- Work within the religious belief system of the client. Involve the minister in the treatment process.
- Help the client identify the causes of illness and the specific actions he or she can take.
- Focus on the immediate situation rather than future plans.
- Be aware that guilt may influence the client's perception of the illness.
- Give the client permission to have problems.
- Focus on survival issues.
- Use action- and task-oriented activities.
- Remember that some clients may be reluctant to discuss family problems and personal relationships with outsiders.

Hispanic/Latino Americans
- Allow the client to define body space parameters.
- Address older adults more formally than younger clients.
- Focus on immediate solution rather than long-term goals.
- Be aware of the roles each family member plays.
- Encourage the client to talk about why he or she feels ill or depressed.
- Probe for the causes of physical complaints.
- Conduct the session in the preferred language of the client.
- Use an interpreter.

Asian Americans/Pacific Islanders
- Remember that the family system is extremely important.
- Involve the family members in the treatment process. Use them as aides.
- Teach the family members why independence in function is important and good for the client and family.
- Avoid a highly casual manner. Be cautious about touching.
- Encourage the client to express feelings and see him- or herself as an equal partner with the practitioner.
- Use small talk at the beginning of a session, which will be considered good manners and keeps the provider from appearing too rushed.
- Realize women may experience conflict between traditional roles and mainstream America female roles.
- Ascertain the client's perception of the causes of his or her illness.
- Take a directive rather than a nondirective approach.
- Encourage the client to begin to take initiative in making changes.

Native Americans/Alaska Natives
- Involve the extended family in the treatment process.
- Address older adults in a formal way.
- Acknowledge and work with traditional "healers."
- Focus on the immediate situation rather than future plans.

Exhibit 17.4. General Guidelines for Creating a Multicultural Approach and Environment

- Expect every client, family, colleague, or person to be different. (A "patient" is not "just a patient.") Each individual has his or her own identity, culture, ethnicity, background, experiences, and lifestyle.

- The culture and lifestyle of people do matter. Being "aware of" or "respecting" differences is not enough. Knowledge about the effects of these differences must be integrated into all your interactions.

- Take into account the client's culture and how it affects and shapes the individual.

- Acknowledge that some health beliefs and practices are derived from basic needs and may have little basis in reality. Also be aware that some practices that you may consider to be "primitive" do serve a purpose for the person within the culture and must be respected.

- Be cognizant of gender and age. These characteristics do affect the clinical approach used as well as the perceptions held by the client, family, or caregiver about the practitioner.

- Use good basic health care practices, such as completing a thorough assessment with the client and the family, checking diet restrictions before planning or initiating a cooking activity, involving the client and the family in the program, and doing an assessment of the home environment.

- Look for cues, both verbal and nonverbal, that will help you involve the client in the treatment session.

- Be flexible and adaptable in your treatment of the client and, by all means, avoid a "cookbook" approach.

- Be aware of your personal biases and how they may affect the therapeutic relationship.

- Don't misjudge people because of their accent or grammar.

- Avoid being patronizing or condescending. Use language that fosters trust and alliance.

- Use an interpreter if you are not fluent in the client's preferred language. If an interpreter is unavailable, learn basic words, phrases, or sentences in that language. This will show that you are making an effort to identify with the client.

- Be aware of discriminatory *intent* versus discriminatory *effect*.

- Be an agent of change.

- *Listening* to the client and being responsive to his or her needs is a demonstration of cultural competency. It is important to understand the view of the world from the perspective of the client, family, and caregiver.

Note. From American Occupational Therapy Association. (1996). *Creating a multicultural approach and environment.* [Video]. Bethesda, MD: Author. Copyright © 1996 by the American Occupational Therapy Association.

Exhibit 17.5. Culturally Sensitive Intervention Strategies

- Become aware of the diverse group's inclinations on issues of privacy, self-disclosure, familial power and distribution, discussion of intimate matters with persons outside the family, use of formally organized helping institutions, and the context in which help is or should be offered.
- During the assessment, consider the social–environmental effects as well as psycho–individual reactions.
- Become familiar with local medical beliefs and practices.
- Take advantage of opportunities to learn about people and their cultures. Listening and showing a willingness to learn and share experiences can be invaluable.
- During discharge or termination planning, make an effort to connect clients to positive elements of support in their community.
- Avoid recommending and training in use of equipment that may be financially impractical, culturally inappropriate, or culturally unacceptable to the client and his or her family.
- Avoid patronizing or condescending approaches.
- Understand the communication style of the group. Observe for clues—verbal or nonverbal—that may indicate preferences.
- Develop a wide variety of verbal and nonverbal responses that will facilitate involvement of the client.
- Become familiar with special terminology used by the client.
- Use an interpreter if you are not fluent or effective in the preferred language of the client. Learn basic words, phrases, and sentences in the target language.
- If an interpreter is used, meet with him or her on a regular basis to discuss information to be given and received from the client, the interpreter style and approach to the client, and cultural practices and beliefs of the client.
- Involve the client and family members in goal setting.
- Discuss with the client or family how potential treatment goals and outcomes may alter typical cultural roles and practices. Let the client or family decide how and to what extent they wish to engage in the new behavior.
- Be flexible and adaptable in your approach. Take into account the client's culture, environment, age, gender, religion, life history, principle stressors, geographic location, sexual identity, educational level, appearance, nationality, ethnicity, communication style, and abilities.

Note. Adapted from "Clinical considerations in treating minority women who are disabled," by S. A. Wells, 1991, *Occupational Therapy Practice, 2,* 13–22. Copyright © 1991 by the author.

Reflection

- Using the clinical reasoning process, outline how you would solicit and integrate cultural information in the assessment and treatment planning for a client from a different culture. If you do not have such a client, create a case study.

- Select an occupational therapy assessment or evaluation tool, and evaluate its usefulness with culturally diverse clients. Has it been standardized on a variety of racial and ethnic populations? How would you interpret its results for members of culturally diverse groups?

References

American Occupational Therapy Association. (1996). *Creating a multicultural approach and environment* [Video]. Bethesda, MD: Author.

American Occupational Therapy Association. (2005). *Task Force on Health Disparities.* Bethesda, MD: Author.

Barney, K. (1991). From Ellis Island to assisted living: Meeting the needs of older adults from diverse cultures. *American Journal of Occupational Therapy, 45,* 586–593.

Bazaldua, O. V., & Sias, J. (2004). Cultural competence: A pharmacy perspective. *Journal of Pharmacy Practice, 17,* 160–166.

Berlin, E. A., & Fowkes, W. C. (1983). A teaching framework for cross-cultural health care: Application in family practice. *Western Journal of Medicine, 12*(139), 93–98.

Blakeney, A. B. (1993). Cultural diversity: Teaching cultural skills to health providers in Appalachia. *OT Week, 7*(30), 18–19.

Bonder, B., Martin, L., & Miracle, A. (2002). *Culture in clinical care.* Thorofare, NJ: Slack.

Carballeira, N. (1997, January–February). The LIVE and LEARN model for cultural competent family services. *Continuum,* pp. 7–12.

Champagne, D. (1994). *Native America: Portrait of the peoples.* Detroit: Visible Ink.

Clark, F. (1993). Eleanor Clarke Slagle Lecture—Occupational embedded in a real-life: Interweaving occupational science and occupational therapy. *American Journal of Occupational Therapy, 47,* 1067–1078.

Coridan, C., & O'Connell, C. (2001). *Meeting the challenge: Ending treatment disparities for women of color.* Alexandria, VA: National Mental Health Association.

Crepeau, E. B. (1991). Achieving intersubjective understanding: Examples from an occupational therapy treatment session. *American Journal of Occupational Therapy, 45,* 1016–1025.

Cross, T. L., Bazron, B. J., Dennis, K. W., & Isaacs, M. R. (1989). *Towards a culturally competent system of care* (Vol. 1). Washington, DC: CASSP Technical Assistance Center.

Dresser, N. (1996). *Multicultural manners: New rules of etiquette for a changing society.* New York: Wiley.

Dyck, I. (1992). Managing chronic illness: An immigrant woman's acquisition and use of health care knowledge. *American Journal of Occupational Therapy, 46,* 696–704.

Fitzgerald, M. H. (1992). Multicultural clinical interaction. *Journal of Rehabilitation, 58,* 38–42.

Fleming, M. H. (1991a). Clinical reasoning in medicine compared to clinical reasoning in occupational therapy. *American Journal of Occupational Therapy, 45,* 988–996.

Fleming, M. H. (1991b). The therapist with the three-track mind. *American Journal of Occupational Therapy, 45,* 1107–1114.

Fleming, M. H. & Mattingly, C., (1994). Giving language to practice. In: C. Mattingly & M. H. Fleming (Eds.). *Clinical reasoning: Forms of inquiry in therapeutic practice.* (pp. 3–21). Philadelphia: F.A. Davis.

Frankenburg, W. K., & Dodds, J. B. (1967). The Denver Developmental Screening Test. *Journal of Pediatrics, 71,* 181–191.

Gaw, A. (1993). *Culture, ethnicity, and mental illness.* Washington, DC: American Psychiatric Press.

Good, D. (1996). Cultural sensitivity: Integrating cultural concepts into clinical practice. *Work: A Journal of Prevention, Assessment, and Rehabilitation, 6,* 61–65.

Hinkle, J. (1994). Practitioners and cross-cultural assessment: A practical guide to information and training. *Measurement and Evaluation in Counseling and Development, 27,* 103–115.

Ho, M. K. (1987). *Family therapy with ethnic minorities.* Thousand Oaks, CA: Sage.

Jackson, J., Carlson, M., Mandel, D., Zemke, R., & Clark, F. (1998). Occupation in lifestyle redesign: The Well Elderly Study occupational therapy program. *American Journal of Occupational Therapy, 52,* 326–336.

Jang, Y. (1995). Chinese culture and occupational therapy. *British Journal of Occupational Therapy, 58*(3), 103–106.

Johnson, V. (1995). *Heart full of grace: A thousand years of Black wisdom.* New York: Simon & Schuster.

Kavanagh, K. H. (1991). Social and cultural influences: Values and beliefs. In J. L. Creasia & B. Parker (Eds.), *Conceptual foundations of professional nursing practice* (pp. 167–210). St. Louis, MO: Mosby.

Kavanagh, K. H., & Kennedy, P. H. (1992). *Promoting cultural diversity: Strategies for health care professionals.* Thousand Oaks, CA: Sage.

Kelly, L. (1995). What occupational therapists can learn from traditional healers. *British Journal of Occupational Therapy, 58*(3), 111–114.

Kirsh, B., Trentham, B., & Cole, S. (2006). Diversity in occupational therapy: Experiences of consumers who identify themselves as minority group members. *Australian Occupational Therapy Journal, 53,* 302–313.

Krefting, L. H., & Krefting, D. V. (1991). Cultural influences on performance. In C. Christiansen & C. Baum (Eds.), *Occupational therapy: Overcoming human performance deficits* (pp. 101–124). Thorofare, NJ: Slack.

Kreps, G. L., & Kunimoto, E. N. (1994). *Effective communication in multicultural health care settings.* Thousand Oaks, CA: Sage.

Lawlor, M. C., & Mattingly, C. F. (1998). The complexities embedded in family-centered care. *American Journal of Occupational Therapy, 52,* 259–267.

Leininger, M. M. (1988). Leininger's theory of nursing: Cultural care diversity and universality. *Nursing Science Quarterly, 1*(4), 152–160.

Leininger, M. M. (1991). *Culture, care, diversity, and universality: A theory of nursing.* New York: National League of Nursing.

Levine, R. (1984). The cultural aspects of home care delivery. *American Journal of Occupational Therapy, 38,* 734–738.

Mattingly, C., & Fleming, M. H. (1994). *Clinical reasoning: Forms of inquiry in a therapeutic practice.* Philadelphia: F. A. Davis.

McCormack, G. L. (1987). Culture and communication in the treatment planning for occupational therapy with minority patients. *Occupational Therapy in Health Care, 4,* 17–36.

Meghani-Wise, Z. (1996). Why this interest in minority ethnic groups? *British Journal of Occupational Therapy, 59,* 485–489.

Neistadt, M. E. (1996). Teaching strategies for the development of clinical reasoning. *American Journal of Occupational Therapy, 50,* 676–684.

Neistadt, M. E. (1998). Teaching clinical reasoning as a thinking frame. *American Journal of Occupational Therapy, 52,* 221–233.

Neistadt, M. E., Wight, J., & Mulligan, S. E. (1998). Clinical reasoning case studies as teaching tools. *American Journal of Occupational Therapy, 52,* 125–132.

Opacich, K. J. (1991). Assessment and informed decision-making. In C. Christiansen & C. Baum (Eds.), *Occupational therapy: Overcoming human performance deficits* (pp. 62–89). Thorofare, NJ: Slack.

Parham, D. (1987). Nationally Speaking—Toward professionalism: The reflective therapist. *American Journal of Occupational Therapy, 41,* 555–561.

Paul, S. (1995). Culture and its influence on occupational therapy evaluation. *Canadian Journal of Occupational Therapy, 62*(3), 154–161.

Pope-Davis, D. B., Prietor, L. R., Whitaker, C. M., & Pope-Davis, S. A. (1993). Exploring multicultural competencies of occupational therapists: Implications for education and training. *American Journal of Occupational Therapy, 47,* 838–844.

Randall-Davis, E. (1989). *Strategies for working with culturally diverse communities and clients.* Washington, DC: Association for the Care of Children's Health.

Rogers, J. C. (1983). Eleanor Clarke Slagle Lecture—Clinical reasoning: The ethics, science, and art. *American Journal of Occupational Therapy, 37,* 601–616.

Schell, B. A., & Cervero, R. M. (1993). Clinical reasoning in occupational therapy: An integrative review. *American Journal of Occupational Therapy, 47,* 1033–1037.

Skawski, K. A. (1987). Ethnic/racial considerations in occupational therapy: A survey of attitudes. *Occupational Therapy in Health Care, 4,* 37–46.

Slater, D. Y., & Cohn, E. S. (1991). Staff development through analysis of practice. *American Journal of Occupational Therapy, 45,* 1038–1044.

Warda, M. R. (2000). Mexican Americans' perceptions of culturally competent care. *Western Journal of Nursing Research, 22,* 203–224.

Wells, S. A. (1991). Clinical considerations in treating minority women who are disabled. *Occupational Therapy Practice, 2,* 13–22.

Wells, S. A. (1994). *A multicultural education and resource guide for occupational therapy educators and practitioners.* Bethesda, MD: American Occupational Therapy Association.

Wetzel, L. (1995). *Cambodian Cultural Profile.* Ethnomed Organization, Harborview Medical Center, University of Washington. Retrieved January 20, 1999, from www.ethnomed.org/ethnomed/cultures/cambodian/cambodian.html

Yuen, H. K., & Yau, M. K. (1999). Cross-cultural awareness and occupational therapy education. *Occupational Therapy International, 6,* 24–34.

Zeller, C. (1995). Cultural vignettes: A multi-cultural educational teaching strategy. Nurse Educator, 20(2), 8–9.

18

Educating for
Cultural Competence

*H*ope *is something shared between teachers and students. The hope that
we can learn together, teach together, be curiously impatient together,
produce something together, and resist together the obstacles that prevent the
flowering of our joy.*

—FREIRE (1998, P. 69)

Key Points

- Teaching about diversity enhances student learning and increases critical thinking.

- Multicultural education provides learners with the ability and skills to cross ethnic and cultural boundaries and to participate and interact with other cultures and groups.

- There are multiple approaches to multicultural education and numerous pedagogical strategies.

- Educators must consider the classroom climate, pedagogical assumptions, and curricular fit as they plan the diversity curriculum.

- The model of multicultural education chosen must fit the existing curriculum or program.

- Careful planning and intentional learning strategies to develop cultural competence are the hallmarks of a transformational curriculum.

THE EDUCATIONAL LITERATURE INCLUDES compelling evidence that teaching about diversity enhances student learning and increases critical thinking (Gay, 1994; Merryfield, 2003; O'Grady, 2000). Educating for cultural competence can produce the same skills. Cultural competence can be facilitated through various educational methods: by total immersion in a group or culture different from the learner's own; by interacting with people culturally different from oneself; by reading, researching, and learning about others through self-education; or through more formal means of education, such as courses, workshops, or academic programs. The accreditation agencies of most, if not all, health professions have mandated that their educational programs include multicultural content. This mandate reflects the compelling arguments made in this book for the need for multicultural content in health professions education. However, questions remain. How does one educate learners for cultural competence? What models does one use? What kinds of exercises and teaching or learning strategies should one use? How does one recognize one's own blind spots? Are videos or speakers available that will support what is taught? What are one's goals in providing multicultural education?

The answers to these questions depend somewhat on the context of the teaching situation. One must consider the educational model of the health professional program, the curricular fit of the multicultural content, the interest and knowledge of the faculty, and the demographics of the student population when determining which approach to take to multicultural education. This chapter discusses issues that arise in multicultural education in responding to these questions.

Definitions of *Multicultural Education*

The multicultural literature provides many definitions of multicultural education. Diaz (1992) states that the only commonality among these definitions is the "view that *multicultural education* is a reform movement designed to improve schooling for students of color" (p. 24, italics added). This view seems far too simplistic, however, given the plethora of definitions now available in the literature.

Parekh (1986) sets the overall tone for multicultural education by stating that it is good education for all children. He defines multicultural education as "an education for freedom" (quoted in Banks, 1994, p. 1). Hernandez (1989) also asserts that multicultural education is important for all students and observes that it is synonymous with effective teaching. Banks (1994) clarifies this concept: "Multicultural education should help students to develop the knowledge, attitudes and skills to participate in a democratic and free society.... [It] promotes freedom, ability and skills to cross ethnic and cultural boundaries to participate in other cultures and groups" (p. 81). Bennett (1995) is more thorough when she states, "A comprehensive definition includes the following four dimensions of multicultural education: the movement toward equity, the multicultural curriculum approach, the process of becoming multicultural, and the commitment to combat prejudice and discrimination" (p. 14).

Multicultural education is not a narrow concept but rather is broadly conceptualized and comprehensive. It is an interdisciplinary process that fosters understanding, acceptance, empathy, and constructive and harmonious relations among people of diverse cultures. It encourages learners of all ages to view different cultures as a source of learning and enrichment. It also is a transformative educational movement that produces critically thinking members of society who are active in areas of social justice. Although much of the multicultural education literature examines elementary and secondary education, these ideals hold true for occupational therapy education as well and are important for culturally competent practice.

Goals of Multicultural Education

As health professionals, occupational therapists and occupational therapy assistants are aware of and embrace the importance of writing goals to direct their actions. Intervention goals direct practice, whereas educational goals frame teaching and learning. Similarly, when considering where multicultural content fits within occupational therapy curricula, educators must explicitly define the reasons and goals for its inclusion.

The goals or aims of multicultural education are many and varied. Banks (1994) believes that one important goal is "to increase educational equality for both gender groups, for students of diverse ethnic and cultural groups, and for exceptional students" (p. 6). Although this goal has merit, educators must consider the demographics of health professions' classrooms. The occupational therapy professional membership is 90.1% White and 92.4% female, and only 5.6% have disabilities (American Occupational Therapy Association, 1998). Occupational therapy classrooms reflect these numbers. Although most educators would agree that there is a need for increased student diversity, and although the profession is working diligently to attract diverse people to the profession, the reality is that there is little diversity in the classroom at the beginning of the 21st century. Therefore, Banks's goal may not address the focus of multicultural content in an occupational therapy curriculum. Other, more appropriate goals found in the literature include the following:

- Helping all students, including White mainstream students, develop the knowledge, skills, and attitudes needed to survive and function effectively in the society of the future (Banks, 1994)
- Helping students develop empathy and caring toward diverse groups of people (Banks, 1994)
- Eliminating stereotypes (Bennett, 1995)

- Fostering the intellectual, social, and personal development of students to their highest potential and providing each student with an equal opportunity to learn (Bennett, 1995)
- Promoting the strength and value of cultural diversity (Gollnick & Chinn, 1990)
- Promoting social justice and equality for all people (Gollnick & Chinn, 1990).

These goals are representative of those found throughout the literature on multicultural education. To these we would add the vitally important goal, one not identified in the literature, of recognizing one's own beliefs and biases as they relate to groups other than one's own. We believe that culturally competent professionals must begin with the awareness of themselves as cultural beings and then gain knowledge of how their own culture influences their beliefs, attitudes, and behaviors. This goal, we believe, should be incorporated into any approach to multicultural education, even those in which self-awareness is not a focus.

Approaches to Multicultural Education

As with many educational reform movements, multicultural education has changed and developed over the years. Initially, it was designed to examine only ethnic and racial diversity, but now it encompasses other issues involving oppression and injustice, including gender, sexual identity, class, ability, and age. The real-world practice of multicultural education varies, however. Although several authors have described various approaches, Sleeter and Grant (1987) developed the most comprehensive taxonomy on the basis of a review of the literature at that time, and this taxonomy continues to be used. Sleeter and Grant found five distinct approaches used in multicultural education: (a) teaching people who are culturally different, (b) the human relations approach, (c) single group studies, (d) multicultural education, and (e) education that is multicultural and social reconstructionist.

Teaching People Who Are Culturally Different

The first approach Sleeter and Grant (1987) described is assimilating students of color in the cultural mainstream by offering transitional bridges in existing school programs. One goal of this approach is to help nonmajority students develop cultural and social competence in the dominant group. This approach also emphasizes maintaining one's own cultural heritage, often by trying to establish a positive group identity, but tries to find areas in which to build bridges between the home and the dominant cultures. The focus is on the nondominant group; no attempt is made to have members of the majority group examine themselves or do any self-reflection. Most authors using this approach discuss race and ethnicity without mentioning other forms of human diversity, and examining issues of power and privilege is not a goal. Bilingual education and English as a second language programs fit within this structure.

Human Relations Approach

The human relations approach is used to help students of different backgrounds get along better and appreciate one another. Advocates of this approach emphasize improving communication between people of different cultural backgrounds with the hope that it will lead to increased cooperation between different ethnic groups and White Americans. Although positive in its ideals, a critique of this approach is that it "has produced almost no literature that links practical application theoretically and conceptually with social psychology and theory on intergroup conflict and prejudice formation. . . . Nor is there conceptual linkage with research on cross-cultural differences" (Sleeter & Grant, 1987, p. 427). Although this approach may result in immediate and short-term benefits, most scholars of multicultural education do not subscribe to its methods as the sole approach to teaching multicultural content because of the lack of a theoretical base and of development of long-term goals and outcomes.

Single Group Studies

The single group studies approach fosters cultural pluralism by teaching lessons, units, or courses about the experiences, contributions, and concerns of distinct ethnic, gender, and social class groups. The emphasis is on specific groups in an attempt to foster appreciation of cultural and linguistic diversity. This approach seems to focus more on prescription and application rather than on goals or theory. Although single group studies usually discuss the victimization and accomplishments of each group, they often do not stress social change as a goal. However, if a faculty member in Minnesota, for instance, incorporated a single group study of a local Native American tribe to apply the principles of the Cultural Competency Model described in Chapter 4, this approach might prove effective.

Multicultural Education

Although advocates of other approaches use the label *multicultural education* as well, Sleeter and Grant (1987) select it for this approach because it truly "promotes cultural pluralism and social equality by reforming the school program for all students to make it reflect diversity" (p. 429). The five major goals of this approach are

1. Human rights and respect for cultural diversity,
2. Strengths and value of cultural diversity,
3. Alternative life choices for people,
4. Social justice and equal opportunity for all, and
5. Equity distribution of power among members of all groups.

This approach addresses institutional racism in society and schools, unequal power relationships among groups, and economic stratification and social class.

The multicultural education approach differs from the first three in that it requires a shift in thought and pedagogy, resulting in a critical analysis of the dominant paradigm and curriculum reform. This approach involves more than just adding a little multicultural content into the curriculum and stirring; it requires making a conscious effort to critically analyze the current power structure of various groups within society.

Although Sleeter and Grant (1987) identify many positive aspects of this popular approach to multicultural education, they suggest that "the literature should grapple more with the relationship of social stratification to culture, as well as consider the integration of race, class, and gender factors when examining oppression" (p. 434). They suggest that "authors should also endeavor to connect the approach more directly with established bodies of inquiry on educational history and social policy, curriculum theory, the hidden curriculum, and the sorting function of schools" (p. 434).

Education That Is Multicultural and Social Reconstructionist

The final multicultural education approach Sleeter and Grant (1987) identify prepares students to challenge social structural inequality and promote cultural diversity. The emphasis on social action is what differentiates this approach from that of multicultural education. Suzuki (1984, quoted in Sleeter & Grant, 1987) suggests that, with this approach, more emphasis is placed on helping students "gain a better understanding of the causes of oppression and inequality and ways in which these social problems might be eliminated" (p. 435). The categories of gender and social class or stratification receive more attention than in any other approach.

Of the five approaches, however, this one is the least developed and the most controversial in many ways. There also is less agreement as to what to name this approach. It has been called *emancipatory education* by Gordon, Miller, and Rollock (1990); *transformative education* by Giroux (1988); and *critical teaching* by Shor (1992). Sleeter and Grant (1987) warn that "particularly lacking is material on achieving the goals in schools; without this material the approach runs the risk of being passed off as a good, but impractical and unrealistic idea" (p. 436). Shor, however, approaches these issues in a more pragmatic manner than many of his colleagues, providing concrete examples of good and effective pedagogical practice.

In summary, multicultural education means different things to different people and is practiced in the classroom in many ways. It is a curriculum model that is here to stay given the changing demographics in the United States and the increasing awareness of educators. However, continued study and research are needed for this model to continue to progress. Because the Accreditation Council for Occupational Therapy Education (ACOTE, 2007) has mandated multicultural content in occupational therapy education programs, occupational therapy educators must choose an approach to theory and pedagogy that complements their own style, beliefs, values, and goals.

Pedagogy and Multicultural Education

Pedagogy is not limited to the teaching methods a teacher selects; it also includes educational philosophy, specific curriculum content and design, classroom strategies and techniques, and methods and evaluation. All of these aspects of educational practice influence what happens in classrooms:

> Together, they organize a view of how teachers work within an institutional context which specifies a particular version of what knowledge is of most worth, what it means to know something, and how we might construct representations of ourselves, others, and our physical and social environment. (Simon, 1987, p. 370)

We support and promote a model of multicultural education that promotes empowerment and transformation. A transformative curriculum that supports the development of cultural competence cannot be constructed merely by adding content about ethnic groups and women to the existing Eurocentric curriculum or by integrating or infusing ethnic content or content about women and other groups into the mainstream curriculum (Banks, 1991). Such an additive approach does not challenge or substantively change the basic assumptions, perspectives, and values of the dominant culture or curricula. Transformational education is thoughtfully constructed, intentionally delivered, and comprehensive in scope, addressing all aspects of the thinking–teaching–learning process. Examples of transformational education are included in the following discussion of classroom climate, pedagogical assumptions, and teaching strategies.

Classroom Climate

The tone or climate of the classroom is an important consideration when teaching about diversity. Because issues of diversity often elicit strong emotions, a climate of emotional safety is vital. Students must be told, and must believe, that their ideas, beliefs, and comments will be heard and respected, even if they do not match the prevailing attitude of the rest of the class. Teachers should encourage students to challenge and discuss ideas but also make it clear that personal attacks, humiliating remarks, name calling, accusations, and ridicule are never appropriate and will not be allowed in the classroom.

An aspect of classroom safety is confidentiality. Students must believe that whatever is said or disclosed will not be revealed outside the classroom. If the teacher assigns reaction papers in response to classroom discussions, he or she must remind students not to share the contents of their papers with friends or leave them lying around so that others can read them. To further ensure confidentiality in written work, classmates' full names should never be used; initials are better. It is important to discuss climate and confidentiality issues at the beginning of the course and to elicit consensual agreement about classroom safety from each class member.

Classroom climate is strongly influenced by the teacher's attitude. The teacher must model and create an open and accepting atmosphere that encourages a willingness to share ideas and beliefs, to explore values, and to confront and grapple with concepts that may be new, uncomfortable, and possibly frightening (see Figure 18.1). When a student is compelled to examine ideas that conflict with lifelong family and personal values, he or she may experience anxiety and discomfort. Teachers must present information and respond to each student in a way that provides a model of behavior for all students to emulate. Educators establish this open and accepting climate by treating each student and his or her ideas and beliefs with respect. Foss (1991) defines a *safe classroom* as a place where everyone experiences equality in terms of personal value, where students and the professor have equal respect for each other as people, and where this respect affects all aspects of the interaction and learning in the class.

Pedagogical Assumptions

The professor's assumptions about diversity play an important role in multicultural education. For the educational process to be empowering or transformative, the teacher must hold the following four pedagogical assumptions:
1. Each student has a unique and equal capacity to learn.
2. Students must be active participants in the learning process.
3. Effective teaching and learning is dialogic.
4. Learning is facilitated in an affective classroom.

Fostering Students' Unique and Equal Capacity to Learn

Faculty expectations influence a student's academic performance. Nieto (1996) summarizes some of the numerous research studies illustrating that teachers' low expectations of students on the basis of gender, race, or class result in lower academic performance. This phenomenon exemplifies the self-fulfilling prophecy concept Merton identified in 1948. If a professor believes a student does not have the capacity to learn because of some inherent quality, he or she will not expect that student to perform at the same level as other students. The teacher then (often unconsciously) treats the student differently than other students, which causes the student to believe that he or she cannot learn as well as others (a reaction called "internalized oppression"), resulting in loss of self-esteem and diminished academic performance. The student's less-than-stellar performance affirms to the teacher that his or

Photo by Roxie M. Black

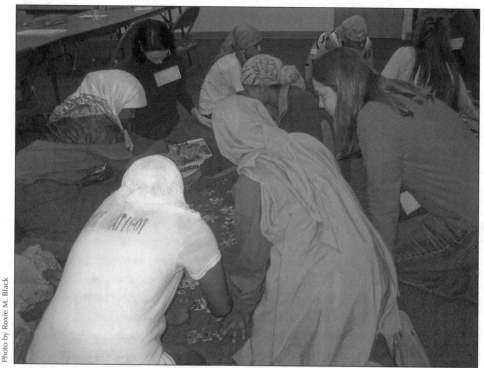

Figure 18.1. An occupational therapy student works with Somali schoolgirls in a service–learning project where she applies the knowledge of teen development and participation with an immigrant population in the process of developing cultural competence.

her initial assumption of the student's abilities was correct and justifies the lowered expectations. And the cycle continues.

High teacher expectations for all students regardless of personal characteristics contribute to an attitude of positive potential, resulting in increased academic performance, increased success, and a perceived and real sense of empowerment for students. Open, accepting, and positive teacher attitudes, coupled with a commitment to facilitating success for all students, are necessary for a climate of learning. According to LaBelle and Ward (1994), "Attention to increasing student achievement, including enhancement of basic skills, is a vital component of an empowerment curriculum model" (p. 170).

Promoting Active Participation in the Learning Process

The traditional approach to teaching almost exclusively uses the lecture method, where the all-knowing professor fills the minds of students with knowledge as if they were empty vessels. Students are passive recipients of this wisdom, taking in information and regurgitating it on an exam in a process that Shor (1992, p. 20) labels *endullment*—the dulling of students' minds as a result of nonparticipation. Brazilian educator Paulo Freire (1970/1986) calls this process the *banking method* of education, where instead of "communicating the teacher issues communiqués and makes deposits that the students patiently receive, memorize and repeat. . . . The scope of action allowed to the students extends only as far as receiving, filing, and storing the deposits" (p. 58). Freire sees this approach as oppressive to students, establishing the teacher as the knowledgeable authority and keeper of wisdom and the student as knowing nothing except what the teacher chooses to impart to them.

A more empowering approach to education is a student-centered classroom, where students are active participants in the learning process. Participation is vitally important, because action is essential in gaining knowledge and developing intelligence (Shor, 1992). Educational theorists Jean Piaget and John Dewey both support the importance of action for learning. According to Piaget (1969/1979), "Knowledge is derived from action. . . . To know an object is to act upon it and to transform it" (p. 28). Dewey (1938/1963) argues that participation in school is crucial to learning; he often is credited with the notion that learning is doing.

Experiential education is an important aspect of an occupational therapy educational curriculum. Learning labs where specific skills are taught and practiced are a standard and expected part of the learning process. In addition to participating in lab situations, students engage in discussion groups, role play experiences, case study applications, problem-based learning experiences, simulated and real client–practitioner interactions within the classroom, research and presentations, and field-based internships. Many of these approaches and strategies can be used when learning about diversity and engaging in cross-cultural experiences. All of these activities allow and encourage active student participation from which students can construct meaning.

Having a student-centered philosophy and participatory classroom does not mean that lecture is never used, however. A fact of occupational therapy curricula is that there often are courses (particularly in the sciences) that lend themselves more to the lecture method because of the extent of factual content needing to be taught. In a human anatomy course, for example, students must memorize the origins and insertions of each muscle to know their location and function. Learning facts and data does not lend itself to more active approaches to inquiry such as discussion groups or reflection papers. Shor (1992) suggests, however, that even facts-based courses can be taught in an empowering manner if the information is offered in a context that is functional to the students' lives and work and that reveals critical problems in society. For example, an assignment to analyze a work site for stress on the human musculoskeletal system provides an effective, experiential method of applying the knowledge gained in an anatomy course. Because it personalizes the information by bringing it into the context of the students' lives, their interest in the topic is increased, new meaning is constructed and remembered, and improved quality of learning occurs.

Encouraging Dialogue

Students learn best when teachers talk *with* them rather than *at* them. Mutual discussion is the heart of the dialogic classroom. *Dialogue* is a conversation among two or more people. A conversation implies that two or more voices will be heard. A dialogic classroom, therefore, is one where students are encouraged to have a voice, a say, and an opinion. Within the context of a climate of safety, students who often are silent and silenced in traditional classrooms gain the courage and feel empowered to present their ideas and questions, actively entering the conversation in a dialogic classroom. For very shy and introverted students, small group discussions or conversations in dyads provide forums for their voices to be heard and included. A dialogic classroom, therefore, results in an increased sharing of diverse ideas and facilitates learning.

Shared interaction between students and teachers results in mutual learning, in which all reflect together on the meaning of their experience and knowledge (Shor, 1992). For dialogue to be effective, each person must enter the conversation with an attitude of openness and a willingness to learn. In his last book, published shortly after his death, Freire (1998) discusses the condition of openness in this way:

> To live in openness toward others and to have an open-ended curiosity
> toward life and its challenges is essential to educational practice. To live
> this openness toward others respectfully and, from time to time, when
> opportune, critically reflect on this openness, ought to be an essential
> part of the adventure of teaching. (p. 121)

Some may see this openness and willingness to learn from students as diminishing the authority of the educator, placing him or her in a more horizontal rather than hierarchical position *via-à-vis* the student (Freire, 1970/1986). Dialogue transforms teachers' unilateral authority to a shared authority; it calls on them to relinquish some authority and requires students to codevelop a joint learning process.

Developing an Affective Classroom

Many authors believe that cognitive learning should be integrated with affective learning to ensure the engagement of the students in the learning process (hooks, 1994; Shor, 1992). Shor (1992) discriminates between empowering and traditional pedagogies by the emotions they elicit:

> In traditional classrooms, negative emotions are provoked in students
> by teacher-centered politics. Unilateral teacher authority in a passive

curriculum arouses in many students a variety of negative emotions: self-doubt, hostility, resentment, boredom, indignation, cynicism, disrespect, frustration, [and] the desire to escape. (p. 23)

Shor believes that these negative emotions interfere with learning. In contrast, he believes that, in a participatory class, "some of the positive affects which support student learning include cooperativeness, curiosity, humor, hope, responsibility, respect, attentiveness, openness, and concern about society" (p. 24).

Learning should be fun! There can and should be joy in the discovery and mutual construction of knowledge. Freire (1998) discusses the importance of joy in the classroom and its relationship with hope: "Hope is something shared between teachers and students. The hope that we can learn together, teach together, be curiously impatient together, produce something together, and resist together the obstacles that prevent the flowering of our joy" (p. 69).

In classrooms where emotions are expressed and accepted, the passion of learning is patently evident. hooks (1994) strongly supports the notion of a passionate and emotional learning environment, but she believes that little of this kind of teaching and learning takes place in contemporary classrooms: "Even when students are desperately yearning to be touched by knowledge, professors still fear the challenge, [and] allow their worries about losing control to override their desires to teach" (p. 199).

Teaching for cultural competence evokes strong emotions because it often challenges students' (and faculty members') personal values and beliefs. It is important to allow the expression of feelings, even though passionately debating the issues may be uncomfortable for students and teachers alike; most of us have been taught that a dispassionate, objective stance is the appropriate and rational way to examine ideas. Multicultural education strongly refutes that philosophy. Multicultural content is inherently emotive, personal, conflictual, and involving. Consequently, students must be given ample opportunities to express their beliefs and emotions, to interact with their classmates, and "to express rage or pride when multicultural issues are discussed" (Banks, 1994, p. 96).

Affective learning, or using the emotions in the process of constructing knowledge, involves engaging the self in learning. One cannot remain aloof and objective when emotions are involved. By engaging themselves in learning, students become the subjects rather than the objects of the learning experience. The focus of the teaching–learning experience is on the student rather than the teacher, and the student has more control and agency in his or her own learning and construction of knowledge.

Teachers of diversity must therefore "take the experiences and voices of students themselves as a starting point [of the curriculum]. We must confirm and legitimatize the knowledges and experiences through which students give meaning to their everyday lives" (McLaren, 1998, p. 225). Knowledge must be meaningful to students before they can critically analyze it. By starting with the students' experiences framed within the context of their lives, educators help them first comprehend the information from their own personal and subjective point of view and then add new information to construct new knowledge. In this way, learning becomes personal, meaningful, critical, and often useful.

Within an occupational therapy curriculum, for example, students can receive facts about how sensory processing changes as a person ages. They can be taught the theories of social disengagement and the isolation of older adults. And they can be taught the resultant diminishing of purposeful and productive activities. Students even can be examined on how well they have learned these facts. Yet many will soon forget this information if they have little or no experience with older adults. But if, in addition to imparting theoretical and factual information, the teacher requires students to visit the nursing home where their neighbor or great aunt resides and lead activities for people with sensory deficiencies and diminished social interaction skills, the theories and facts will take on new meaning. Personal experiences, imbued with the feelings and emotions that accompany any action and interaction, brighten and highlight the interpretation of knowledge and make meaning in a way that often is remembered and available for future use. Whereas a traditional curriculum often disempowers students by not considering the context of the students' lives or allowing them to have a voice in the classroom,

> *Knowledge must be meaningful to students before they can critically analyze it.*

> A curriculum designed to empower students must be transformative in nature and help students to develop the knowledge, skills, and values needed to become social critics who can make reflective decisions and implement their decisions in effective personal, social, political, and economic action. (Banks, 1991, p. 131)

Teaching Strategies

Once the classroom climate has been established and the pedagogical assumptions identified, teachers must determine which model or models of multicultural education they will use, how the models will fit within the curriculum, and which learning strategies will be the most effective.

For example, a teacher who chooses Sleeter and Grant's (1987) conceptual model of multicultural education may transform the curriculum so that students view concepts, events, issues, and problems from the perspective of a particular cultural group. Far from merely adding specific content, the teacher would reconceptualize the curriculum and make this group's content an integral part (Banks, 1994).

If a teacher were to choose to examine the history of African American leaders in the profession of occupational therapy, identifying and listing African American occupational therapy practitioners would just be adding ethnic content. If students, however, interviewed contemporary African American occupational therapy leaders and subsequently gave their interpretation of these leaders' achievements from their own perspectives, or if students researched the thoughts and ideas of deceased African American occupational therapy leaders as described in these leaders' publications, journals, or letters, students would benefit from a transformed and more balanced curriculum.

Beyond the theoretical approach and model chosen, curricular fit and integration of multicultural content are determined by the philosophy of the institution in which the occupational therapy educational program is housed, the requirements of the accrediting agency, the model and structure of the program's curriculum, the interests and desires of the program director and the teacher, and the demographics of the student body. Curricular fit (developing teaching strategies and approaches that support the curricular goals and student outcomes) determines whether one chooses to teach a separate course focusing on diversity or multicultural content; to include a multicultural module within a course; to provide an individual class, lecture, or short workshop devoted to diversity issues; to integrate or infuse multicultural content throughout the curriculum; or to do a combination of approaches.

Separate Course

In a separate course covering social issues and ethics, critical multicultural theory can be presented, discussed, grappled with, and applied in the context of an analysis of the ethical issues involved. An examination of poverty might be part of this course; readings could include current government statistics on the subject, chapters from Sidel's (1998) book *Keeping Women and Children Last,* and a journalist's interview with a homeless man. As part of this course, the instructor also might provide an opportunity for class discussion with a woman on welfare and a short field experience in a homeless shelter for destitute families.

Analyses of these experiences might include an examination and comparison of the students' perceptions of poverty, a discussion of the ethnic and cultural characteristics of the impoverished groups the students observe, identification of access and barriers to health care for this population, and a discussion of the ethical principles of beneficence, malfeasance, and occupational and distributive justice. Institutionalized oppression could be examined, especially at the intersection of gender, race or ethnicity, and class, and evaluated for its effect on people whose incomes are below the poverty line. Students could relate and reflect on their own experiences with poverty and class issues in both professional and personal settings and how these experiences influenced or were influenced by their personal values. A comprehensive examination of poverty in a course such as this would reflect a transformative curriculum.

The positive aspects of teaching a course with a multicultural focus include the following:

- An opportunity to examine multicultural issues in depth
- More time to allow a wider breadth of information about the issues
- Time and opportunity for community and field-based application and experiences
- A semester- or quarter-long opportunity for personal reflection on a topic that may result in personal growth, increased knowledge about and sensitivity to socioeconomic issues and people caught within the class power struggle, and positive movement toward cultural competence.

The negative implications of this approach include the following:

- Additional time needed, perhaps more than is available in an already packed curriculum
- Possible "ghettoization," or marginalization, of the course and its content if multicultural and diversity issues are not included elsewhere in the curriculum
- Student view of the course as "too liberal" or not technical enough to warrant the same attention as other professional courses
- Need for a faculty member with enough interest and knowledge in a transformative multicultural approach to coordinate, plan, and deliver the course
- Need for fairly extensive faculty development.

Multicultural Module Within a Course

Including a focused module within an existing course is another way to present multicultural content. In a course on clinical conditions or etiology of disease, a professor might choose to examine one ethnic group in the community—for example, a Great Plains Native American tribe. To engage in a transformational examination of this group, students would not only look at the experiences, contributions, and concerns of this population but also study their view of health and wellness by reading resources such as Spector's (2004) *Cultural Diversity in Health and Illness* or Silko's (1986) *Ceremony* or by bringing a native healer to class to present his or her concept of health through ritual. The module might include an assignment requiring students to examine the power structure of the Bureau of Indian Affairs within the context of the delivery of and access to adequate health services both on and off reservations. Students could examine the incidence of medical conditions such as coronary heart disease, diabetes, and alcoholism within this tribe and others and the sociocultural factors that contribute to these conditions.

The benefits of including a multicultural module within a course include the following:

- A cost-effective, resource-saving way to present multicultural content in a focused manner
- An opportunity for some depth in a single topic
- An administratively easier approach to covering the content by hiring an adjunct teacher who can teach a limited portion of the curriculum
- Provision of an opportunity for a beginning understanding of and increased sensitivity to the group that is examined, which may spark student interest that might result in independent research on this topic or in other courses and assignments where appropriate
- An affirmation and opportunity to share his or her culture for any local Native American student in the class.

Negative implications of this approach include the following:

- Less opportunity for depth of study because of limited time
- View of the information as only theoretical, lessening its value and meaning to any student who is not Native American or has had no interaction with Native people (experiential application of the material can compensate for this disadvantage)
- Risk of confirming stereotypes and prejudice rather than increasing awareness and cultural competence if the information is presented in a superficial way.

Individual Class, Lecture, or Short Workshop

Providing multicultural content in an individual class, lecture, or short workshop is another way that occupational therapy programs can address diversity issues. An African American man could talk about his experiences with racism and discrimination in the small, rural, White community in which he lives. Or a class discussion might feature a lesbian couple who has experienced discrimination by medical insurers. Other examples include a 3-hour workshop on prejudice reduction strategies and a lecture on bilingualism or English as a second language in a course on communications for the health professions.

Many education programs favor this approach for the following reasons:

- It provides an introduction to a variety of diversity issues that may spark an interest in students.
- It can be included in the curriculum without much course revision or additional planning.

- Because a guest speaker can present these lessons, program faculty do not need special knowledge about diversity or multicultural theory.
- It allows for numerous effective and informational "spots" in a variety of classes throughout the curriculum.
- It meets most accreditation and institutional requirements for diversity content without great expense.

Negative effects of this approach include the following:

- A lack of breadth and depth on any topic
- A lack of opportunity for extended personal reflection about the topic
- Possible disregard and devaluation by students of the information presented because of the lack of opportunity to apply the concepts in a meaningful way
- Limited ability to promote cultural competence.

Integration or Infusion of Multicultural Content Throughout the Curriculum

Integration of multicultural content has proved to be an effective pedagogical approach (Bailey, 2000). Consciously including culture as a factor of analysis in multiple curricular areas lessens the marginalization of the content, increases the visibility and awareness of diversity, and facilitates ongoing critical awareness and analysis by students. The following are strategies for infusing multicultural content throughout the curriculum:

- Teachers can provide experiences and opportunities for students to examine their own values and belief systems and to recognize how their values and belief systems flow from their culture and social location. Increasing cultural self-knowledge is the first step in developing cultural competence.
- Educators can model inclusive language for students by teaching them to use accepted terms for all groups, to use the word *partner* rather than *spouse* when speaking of committed relationships, to use person-first language with people with disabilities, and to use *White* as an identifying racial and cultural designation.
- A variety of cultural groups can be used when developing case studies, which should be realistic rather than contrived. Teachers should learn in detail about a cultural group before developing a culture-specific case and should be aware and careful not to promote stereotypes in these cases.
- When evaluating clients, students should know how to include questions about the client's culture and cultural perspectives on health, wellness, illness, independence, family relationships, and other important concepts.
- Educators can help students be sensitive to subtle cultural cues when providing intervention. These cues often are expressed in body language, such

as the distance required for personal space, the use of eye contact, comfort
with touch, the response to someone of the opposite gender, tone of voice,
and the practice of smiling or using silence rather than saying no to the
practitioner.

- Students must learn not to make assumptions based on White American,
middle-class, heterosexual standards; not to assume that all partnered people are married or that all families reflect the traditional structure; not to
expect that all White Americans have attended college or that others are less
educated; and not to assume that all people hold the same values they do
regarding health and hygiene, work and play, or education and money.

- Teachers can model and teach students how to take cultural risks. Learners
must be made aware that they have much to learn about and from people
who are different from themselves. To be culturally competent, they must
be willing to make mistakes, to admit that they do not know or are unsure,
and to ask questions. Humility is an important characteristic to maintain
when engaged in this process.

- Students can learn to be critical sociopolitical analysts. When studying
third-party payers and health maintenance organizations, students can
examine the power of those groups over access to health care of groups who
vary by class, race, sexuality, gender, age, and ability. Classroom interactions
can be used as opportunities to examine power differentials among students and between students and faculty. The teacher can encourage students to ask why social standards exclude and oppress certain groups. A
transformative curriculum teaches students to think and reflect critically
on the materials they read and the voices they hear (Banks, 1991).

- Educators must model respect for each person in the classroom and their
ideas and feelings, openness to and acceptance of differences in opinion and
perspective, and good listening skills. They must encourage the development
of each student's voice and of a sense of power in the learning community.

Although this list is by no means exhaustive, it does present some considerations for facilitating and empowering classrooms and students. The inclusive
approach to multicultural education

- Makes sociocultural and sociopolitical issues more apparent by removing
the shroud of invisibility and increases the awareness and possibly sensitivity of students to these issues;

- Recognizes White privilege as an important issue in the examination of
sociopolitical power, making all students more aware of their own place
within this society's power structure;

- Sensitizes students to the oppression of people who are members of nondominant groups;

- Encourages critical analysis and underscores the need for social justice; and
- Does not require the addition of extra courses within an already packed curriculum.

The negative effects of this approach may include the following:

- All faculty need to be knowledgeable about critical multicultural issues and skilled enough to present these issues in the classroom through both planned and spontaneous activities and lessons. Supporting faculty in acquiring this knowledge and skill may require increased faculty development, which requires time, money, and personal commitment.
- There is less opportunity for formal presentation of the theoretical constructs that support analysis of multicultural issues.
- There is a lack of structured, sequential, and formal approaches to gaining knowledge of this content in any depth, perhaps resulting in superficial and fragmented learning of the information.

In our experience, we find that a combination of these approaches is most effective for providing multicultural content and developing cultural competence. Achieving cultural competence is a process that cannot be mastered by a one-shot approach. Students will not move toward cultural competence by taking only one class or one workshop, by reading one book or article on the subject, or by engaging in only one or two learning activities.

Applying the Cultural Competence Model in an Academic Setting

This chapter has suggested multiple ways to incorporate diversity and multicultural issues into an academic curriculum. Multicultural education is most effective when one goal of the occupational therapy program is the development of cultural competence in students. Using the information in this chapter, combined with the Cultural Competency Model outlined in Chapter 4, the educator can begin to plan an effective curriculum. Educators must intentionally incorporate the three main characteristics of cultural competency—self-exploration and self-awareness, knowledge, and cultural skills—into the content of the course through their teaching and learning strategies.

Self-Exploration and Self-Awareness

A first step in diversity work should be to encourage self-exploration and self-awareness in learners. There are multiple ways to encourage students to examine themselves and their sociocultural standing within their environments. Some educators encourage students to reflect on their own values and beliefs in a private manner—for example, by requiring the examination of inclusive texts, provocative articles, and videos or assigning reflective journaling or diversity games. Others, within the context of a safe classroom, engage students in critical dialogue that examines particular beliefs (including biases and prejudices) and their etiology and the ways these values might affect client–practitioner interactions. Whatever strategies are used, this area of concentration should occur early in the curriculum so that the skills learned provide the foundation for the next steps in the development of cultural competence.

Knowledge

Students must attain multiple areas of knowledge to become culturally competent. Knowledge of self, knowledge of groups different from oneself, knowledge of the historical and current sociopolitical systems that sustain privilege and nonprivileged status, knowledge of language and behavior that oppress and discriminate, and knowledge of the many strategies to eliminate discriminatory patterns are only a sample of what they must learn. Any of the curricular approaches discussed in this chapter can help educators present and explore these areas of knowledge. Multiple teaching and learning strategies can be used, including discussion of selected articles, books, documentaries, and videos; guest speakers and panel discussions; independent reading and research; and other favored approaches to learning. In many ways, this is the easiest part of applying the model, because it involves a more traditional educational approach.

Cultural Skills

Learning the skills of cultural competence often is missing from diversity education. Developing an attitude of open respectfulness takes work. Necessary skills in communication include the ability

- To constantly self-monitor one's language, feelings, attitudes, and behavior when interacting with others who are different from oneself;
- To empathize with others, develop rapport through honest and open dialogue, and be willing to risk exposing one's own lack of or developing knowledge and sensitivity;
- To use inclusive language and to ask appropriate and culturally sensitive questions during interviews and assessments; and
- To be culturally inquisitive in an inoffensive manner.

Other skills that are necessary in diversity work include the ability to recover quickly when one makes a mistake and to avoid blaming oneself or others when there is discomfort in interactions.

Although some of this material can be introduced in the classroom with simulations, role plays, and games, much of the skills will be learned in the workplace, in the homes of clients, and during other field-based experiences (MacDonald, 1998), including service learning experiences. Therefore, academic and fieldwork programs must work together in developing culturally competent practitioners.

Summary

There are multiple models of multicultural education, and numerous pedagogical approaches and strategies can be used to effectively teach and present these models. The most effective way to incorporate multicultural content within occupational therapy curricula is to simultaneously use all of the approaches delineated in this chapter. Each model and strategy complements, supports, and enhances the knowledge gained from any other method. A curricular model that aims to facilitate the development of cultural competence in students and faculty will be most successful in meeting this goal if there are resources to support multiple learning strategies and approaches.

The reality in institutions of higher learning, however, is that resources, including money, faculty, and time, are inadequate. In the face of limited resources, occupational therapy educational programs must present multicultural content in the best way possible that meets the needs of both the students and the program. What is important is that educators continue to educate students not only to actively and effectively participate in the health care and community arenas of tomorrow but also to be culturally competent practitioners who are active agents in the fight for equality and social justice.

Reflection

- Analyze your academic program or practice arena. What resources are available to add more diversity content to your curriculum?

- Consider issues of personnel (their interest and commitment), financial support (for consultants, guest speakers, faculty and staff development, materials, and resources), and time. Which educational models will fit well with your workplace? What teaching and learning strategies will you use?

- Determine what else you need to know to begin. Develop a 1-year strategic plan that outlines the steps you will take to add more diversity content to your curriculum. How will you assess the results?

References

American Occupational Therapy Association. (1998, March). Demographic information [of] occupational therapists and occupational therapy assistants [Unpublished raw data]. Bethesda, MD: Author.

Bailey, D. (2000). Introducing an awareness of cultural diversity into an established curriculum. In P. A. Crist (Ed.), *Innovations in occupational therapy education* (pp. 134–145). Bethesda, MD: American Occupational Therapy Association.

Banks, J. A. (1994). *An introduction to multicultural education.* Newton, MA: Allyn & Bacon.

Bennett, C. I. (1995). *Comprehensive multicultural education: Theory and practice* (3rd ed.). Newton, MA: Allyn & Bacon.

Dewey, J. (1963). *Experience and education.* New York: Collier. (Original work published 1938)

Diaz, C. (Ed.). (1992). *Multicultural education for the 21st century.* Washington, DC: National Education Association.

Foss, S. K. (1991, November). *What is feminist pedagogy?* Paper presented at the annual meeting of the Organization for Research in Gender and Communication, San Antonio, TX.

Freire, P. (1986). *Pedagogy of the oppressed.* New York: Continuum. (Original work published 1970)

Freire, P. (1998). *Pedagogy of freedom: Ethics, democracy, and civic courage.* New York: Rowman & Littlefield.

Gay, G. (1994). *A synthesis of scholarship in multicultural education.* NCRL's Urban Education Program. Retrieved January 14, 2007, from www.ncrel.org.sdrs/areas/issues/educatrs/leadrshp/le0gay.htm

Giroux, H. A. (1988). *Teachers as intellectuals.* Westport, CT: Bergin & Garvey.

Gollnick, D. M., & Chinn, P. C. (1990). *Multicultural education in a pluralistic society* (3rd ed.). New York: Macmillan.

Gordon, E. W., Miller, F., & Rollock, D. (1990). Coping with communicentric bias in knowledge production in the social sciences. *Educational Researcher, 19,* 14–19.

Hernandez, H. (1989). *Multicultural education: A teacher's guide to content and process.* Columbia, OH: Merrill.

hooks, b. (1994). *Teaching to transgress.* New York: Routledge & Kegan Paul.

LaBelle, T. J., & Ward, C. R. (1994). *Multiculturalism and education: Diversity and its impact on schools and society.* Albany: State University of New York.

MacDonald, R. (1998). What is cultural competency? *British Journal of Occupational Therapy, 61,* 325–328.

McLaren, P. (1998). *Life in schools: An introduction to critical pedagogy in the foundations of education* (3rd ed.). New York: Longman.

Merryfield, M. (2003). Like a veil: Cross-cultural experiential learning online. *Contemporary Issues in Technology and Teacher Education, 3,* 146–171.

Merton, R. (1948). The self-fulfilling prophecy. *Antioch Review, 8,* 193–210.

Nieto, S. (1996). *Affirming diversity: The sociopolitical context of multicultural education* (2nd ed.). White Plains, NY: Longman.

O'Grady, C. R. (Ed.). (2000). *Integrating service learning and multicultural education in colleges and universities.* Mahwah, NJ: Erlbaum.

Parekh, B. (1986). The concept of multicultural education. In S. Modgil, G. K. Verma, K. Mallick, & C. Modgil (Eds.), *Multicultural education: The interminable debate* (pp. 19–31). Philadelphia: Farmer.

Piaget, J. (1979). *Science of education and the psychology of the child.* New York: Penguin. (Original work published 1969)

Shor, I. (1992). *Empowering education: Critical teaching for social change.* Chicago: University of Chicago Press.

Sidel, R. (1998). *Keeping women and children last: America's war on the poor.* New York: Penguin.

Silko, L. M. (1986). *Ceremony.* New York: Penguin.

Simon, R. (1987). Empowerment as a pedagogy of possibility. *Language Arts, 64,* 370.

Sleeter, C. E., & Grant, C. A. (1987, November). An analysis of multicultural education in the United States. *Harvard Educational Review, 57,* 421–444.

Spector, R. E. (2004). *Cultural diversity in health and illness* (6th ed.). Upper Saddle River, NJ: Prentice Hall.

19

Assessment Methods in Culturally
Competent Community Practice

*D*estroy the culture and you destroy the people.

—FRANZ FANON (CITED IN JOHNSON, 1995, P. 57)

Key Points

- *Community* means different things to different people. A community consists of people with a shared belief, shared geography, shared interests, shared values, shared experiences, shared traditions, shared culture, or shared kinship, whether virtual or in person.

- *Community practice* is an interchange in which each person is altered through coming together. It involves learning to engage with one another with respect and trust and developing partnerships. It may require that one confront racism, sexism, classism, ableism, professionalism, and homophobia in oneself, in others, and in institutions as one struggles to incorporate diversity.

- An array of assessment methods is used to determine the health of communities.

- An appreciation of people, problems, goals, and places—of past history, current conditions, and future dreams—is the critical basis for working with culturally diverse communities. When practitioners fail to recognize and take into account the many ways in which issues of oppression and racism affect the community, they can perpetuate the objectification and exploitation of groups who are at risk.

- To build a community practice that is successful in improving conditions and resolving problems, practitioners need to understand and appreciate many cultures, establish relationships with people from cultures other than their own, and build strong alliances with different groups.

- Community interventions are actions done intentionally to have a direct effect on the health of a community. Interventions are the heart of all health programs or services and should be presented in culturally competent ways.

COMMUNITIES ARE THE ARENAS in which health disparities are identified and public health challenges addressed. Community practice is grounded in the notion that more doctors, more clinics, and more sophisticated diagnostic and treatment advances will not reduce the major health problems facing culturally diverse populations; instead, the greatest gains will come from what people do or do not do for themselves collectively.

Community participation and empowerment have been central components of the design of social and health programs in the United States. Yet the extent of involvement of the individuals affected by these initiatives has not been fully realized or explored in practice. In the practice environment of the community, health professionals often have imposed "necessary" interventions on targeted communities or populations without soliciting or taking into account the needs and wants of the affected groups and individuals (Israel, Schultz, Parker, & Becker, 1998). One of the many challenges facing community practice is to establish a structure by which community members and health care professionals can work together to identify and implement actions to improve health. Practitioners must be willing to find ways to work together with partners who may be different from themselves to see justice happen.

Communication directed toward a mutual understanding between affected parties best establishes the foundations of trust and collaboration in the presence of different points of view (Aday, Begley, Lairson, & Balkrishman, 2004). Ideally, establishing trust and collaboration is facilitated by combining the knowledge base and skills of practitioners with residents' in-depth understanding of their communities and the resources within them. By using their skills in community building, practitioners can enhance the quality, relevance, and application of interventions to more effectively address community-identified needs (Schulz et al., 2003). This chapter examines the form and quality of community participation by both occupational therapy practitioners and residents of culturally diverse backgrounds and describes opportunities to design consumer-oriented health and neighborhood services.

What Is a *Community*?

Although *community* ultimately is an indefinable concept, generally communities can be thought of as aggregates of individuals who share common characteristics or other bonds (Turnock, 2004). They encompass people, some form of proximity or place that enables interaction (both virtual and in person), and shared values or culture (Bell & Newby, 1971; Issel, 2004). They can consist of an associated group of people, including families, groups of colleagues, and neighbors. They can be affixed to a locale in combination with a spirit of sharing, membership, and commitment (Fazio, 2001). A community also may be characterized by a sense of identification with and emotional connection to other members, common symbol systems, mutual influence, common interests, and commitment to meeting shared needs (Israel et al., 1998).

Thus, a community is a group of people who have common characteristics that can be defined by location, race, ethnicity, age, occupation, interest in particular problems or outcomes, or other common bonds. Communities also allocate available assets and resources through collective discussion, decision making, and action (Turnock, 2004).

Community Practice

Communities and their associated emotional and cultural components are the settings for health programs and evaluation. *Community practice* involves engaging communities to work collectively on their own behalf. According to Issel (2004), when the program planners of a health program target a community, they must define which community members are the intended recipients and delineate the community's boundaries. They must view the community in terms of the sociopolitical and economic factors that can influence the program. In addition, they must identify influential individuals from the community and solicit their participation in program development and evaluation. Community members involved in the planning process become part of the immediate, intimate context of the program intervention.

Several terms related to community practice merit defining. *Community based* indicates that the program or service is physically located in the community. Community-based programs or services are delivered at a variety of locations within the community, such as churches, schools, recreation centers, clinics, or libraries rather than at a centralized location outside community boundaries. Alternatively, health programs or services that are designed to affect the community as a whole unit are *community focused*. Community-focused programs seek to change health-related norms or behaviors of community members.

If a health program or service is the result of the involvement of community members and is driven by their expressed preferences, it is referred to as *community driven*. The design and implementation of community-driven programs are driven by the passion and persistence of key representatives from the community (Issel, 2004).

Using these terms correctly can be important in describing the types of community practice and the nature of the program or service offered, especially when working with culturally diverse communities. The terms indicate the strategy used to address the health disparities of the community, the cultural tailoring of the services, and the involvement of the culturally diverse community in defining the issues to be addressed (Issel, 2004). The type of community practice implies the framework that will be used to educate and empower members of a culturally diverse community to take leadership roles. It denotes a sharing of power and control of the program and services, and it symbolizes the tenet of "diversity is strength" (Gutierrez & Lewis, 2002).

Successful community development efforts are driven not only by the commitment of those investing themselves but also by the resources devoted to the effort. Higher rates of morbidity and mortality exist in communities with few economic and social resources and communities of color (Israel et al., 1998), and addressing these disparities in health status is a major challenge for researchers, practitioners, community leaders, is the affected communities. Community health improvement seldom occurs as a result of the actions of outside interests alone, and many community interventions have not been successful in improving the health and well-being of the target population. Racially and ethnically diverse communities have a long history of outsiders coming into their community to "rescue" their members from some inherent danger. Community members often resent it when outsiders receive funds to work in the community while the community itself experiences economic stressors, and many believe that community members are in the best position to provide culturally appropriate interventions because they best know the community network and culture (Minkler, Blackwell, Thompson, & Tamir, 2003).

Community Assessment Methods

A positive approach to understanding the sociocultural aspects of a community and identifying needs and assets is through the performance of a community assessment. An array of assessment methods can be used to determine the health of communities. These methods cover many areas of potential need. A thorough community health assessment, however, requires an appraisal not only of needs but also of the various structures and resources available to a community that can have a positive effect on its health, as well as processes such as educating children, reducing crimes, decreasing unemployment, and improving water quality taking place and the outcomes of those processes.

According to Turnock (2004), the primary building blocks of a community include both individual and organizational assets. Individual assets include the skills, talents, and experiences of residents, individual businesses, and home-based enterprises as well as personal income. Organizational assets include business, citizens, cultural, communications, and religious organizations. Secondary assets are the private, public, and physical assets that are under the control of the community and can be used for community improvement. These assets include higher education institutions, hospitals, social services agencies, public schools, police departments, libraries, fire departments, parks, vacant land, commercial and industrial structures, housing, energy, and waste disposal resources. Table 19.1 summarizes the community assessment methods discussed in this section.

Medical Community Health Assessment

The medical community health assessment, used in primary care, is a method that is individual focused and based because the health of the community is determined

Table 19.1. Comparison of Community Assessment Methods

Assessment Method	Strengths	Limitations	Data Sources
Medical community health assessment	Individual focused Focus on tertiary and secondary disease prevention Health education	No community involvement or input	Physical examination and laboratory testing Health care providers' opinions regarding needs and deficits
Selective community health assessment	Population focused Primary prevention Health education Measurable outcomes	Little to no community involvement or input	Screening and surveillance Immunizations
Community needs assessment	Community focused Problem oriented	Limited community involvement	Health statistics Health indicators
Community health assessment	Community based Community health profile	Community involvement limited to leadership	Vital statistics Health statistics Demographics
Healthy community (or comprehensive community health) assessment	Community driven and owned Community profile Community capacity building and empowerment Advocacy for social and system changes Harm-minimization approach	Outcomes hard to measure Difficult to establish timelines for achievement	Community asset mapping Demographic data Socioeconomic data Opinion data, key informant interviews, focus groups, participant observation Geographic data Health data, mortality and morbidity data Program evaluations, service data Behavioral risk data

by the health status of its members. Drawn from a biomedical model, a *medical community health assessment* is a plan of care that identifies the specific needs of the individual and how the facility or community can address those needs. It focuses on the individual's specific illnesses or disease conditions with the expectation that they can be eradicated or lessened. Medical community health assessments concentrate on early diagnosis, timely and effective treatment, and case management. The individual is targeted for change rather than the social or environmental conditions that underlie the disease or condition.

This type of assessment generally includes a medication and immunization review; assessment of blood pressure, pulse rate and rhythm, physical functioning, activities of daily living, cognitive functioning and mental status, hearing and vision, nutrition screening, and routine screenings; and a review of social support and lifestyle. The outcome tends to depend on the physical examination and laboratory testing. These measurements are quantitative rather than qualitative and static rather than dynamic (Rifkin, Muller, & Bichmann, 1988). They rely on health care providers' professional opinions, which are based on detailed comprehensive clinical assessments of needs and deficits (Carr, Szapiro, Heisler, & Krasner, 1989).

This traditional approach to community assessment requires individual community members to enter the health system if they need active assistance. It demands a single or intermittent assessment and management of the person's specific illness or condition with an expectation of client–provider interaction. The outcome of this interaction is geared toward disease prevention at the primary level, early treatment to minimize complications at the secondary level, and rehabilitation at the tertiary level. Because this assessment method is concerned with health risks, it includes some form of health education to encourage the individual to take measures that will improve his or her health (Keleher, 2001). This form of education is commonly conducted in the client–provider interaction, thereby limiting community interaction and assessment to activities such as consultations with consumer groups about health needs or perceptions of health services.

Although the medical community assessment method can help health professionals identify improvements in perceived health status, decreases in hospital admissions and length of stay, and decreases in age-specific mortality, it cannot help them identify individuals' perceptions of change in their quality of life. It cannot help them identify specific correlations, such as the relationship between increased educational level or improved income and individual health status. And it cannot be used to measure the influence of increased health services on improved health status (Rifkin et al., 1988). In addition, a medical community health assessment does not provide a measurement of participation in health programs or indicate whether the desired community outcomes have been achieved.

Selective Community Assessment

Health systems and governments frequently provide funding for selective programs aimed at improving population health, such as immunizations and screenings. A selective community assessment is conducted to evaluate the prevalence of and changes in targeted illnesses or conditions. This assessment method is used in efforts to improve the health of the greatest number of people by providing primary intervention and health education using the most recent technology and medical interventions. Such efforts tend to focus on a minimum number of severe health problems that affect many people and for which interventions of established efficacy can be provided at low cost.

Using a selective community assessment method, health professionals identify health problems on the basis of morbidity, prevalence, mortality, and feasibility of control and establish measurable outcome objectives and goals (Magnussen, Ehirl, & Jolly, 2004). By targeting specific conditions, such programs can be proved to improve health statistics.

The selective community assessment method requires limited community input and involvement, especially in the planning phases. Evaluators do not consider the needs of the local people, society, organizations, or cultures. They do not directly assess the concerns of community members. Technology and medical intervention programs are considered sufficient for improving and sustaining targeted health outcomes, regardless of the society or community. Evaluators do not recognize or solicit the help of nonprofessionals in defining or making decisions about the health problems of the community, nor do they promote social equity and social justice for the recipients of technologically driven medical interventions. Health initiatives tend to maintain the status quo of vertical objectives (a top-down approach to addressing and intervening with problems), allowing only a modest level of service coordination (Magnussen et al., 2004). This method may be population focused but centers the assessment on medical interventions and the cost-effectiveness of those interventions (Rifkin & Walt, 1986).

Community Needs Assessment

A community needs assessment is used in determining the gaps, lacks, and wants relative to a defined population and a specific health problem. This type of assessment often addresses the question, What health problems exist in the community, and to what extent?

Program planners use the community needs assessment to analyze health status (risk factors, problems, protective factors, and assets) within a population; establish priorities; and then plan, implement, and evaluate public health interventions.

This assessment method provides the data necessary for program development, specifically what health interventions are needed, where, and with what target group. It helps make program decisions more defendable and acceptable to stakeholders, ensuring that money and effort are channeled to meet the needs of the community (Issel, 2004).

The community needs assessment is problem oriented. It begins with a stated health problem about which additional information is wanted and required. Data from vital records, national registries, surveys and databases (e.g., Behavior Risk Factor Surveillance Survey [Centers for Disease Control and Prevention, 2007a], U.S. Census Bureau [2007], National Health Interview Survey [CDC, 2007b]), and state and local records (e.g., health care data reported by hospitals) are used to identify which health problems or conditions should be addressed and which interventions developed. A community needs assessment also includes data that describe the strengths pertaining to a specific group, community, or problem. The written report provides detailed information about the expressed (in words or behavior), normative (viewed through the eyes of an observer), relative (comparative), and perceived (wanted and preferred) needs of a community. The report also includes data that describe the socioeconomic and political context affecting the health of individuals, as well as the assets, strengths, abilities, and resources that are available to the community or group (Issel, 2004).

The community needs assessment can serve political purposes ranging from system maintenance and control to promotion of social change and consciousness raising. It can be narrowly conceived, defined, and designed. When conducted by outside experts to justify and provide raw data for a predetermined community health need, this method may be effective in achieving its objectives, but it may fail to involve community members in determining the goals of the assessment process; outside experts may focus solely on addressing needs rather than on identifying and building on the community's strengths and empowering the people.

Community Health Assessment

The community health assessment is a systematic examination of the health status indicators for a given population to identify the key health problems in a community. The data used to describe the health status of a community at a given time include vital statistics, health statistics such as mortality (death rate) and morbidity (incidence and prevalence of disease), and demographics such as socioeconomic factors, housing, education, and income. A community health assessment is used to establish the magnitude of the health problem relative to the strengths and resources within the community and to determine the priority the community should give to addressing the problem. A community health assessment takes into account the tangible and intangible characteristics of the community; its formal and informal networks and support systems; its norms and cultural nuances; and its institutions, politics, and belief systems. It encompasses the entire community (Issel, 2004).

One important reason to conduct a community health assessment is to engage the community's leaders in identifying and resolving health problems. It is an effective tool for developing consensus about the most important problems to be managed and obtaining the commitment of community members to work together on the problems. As with other forms of community assessment, consideration of lay opinions is essential if a community health plan is to be meaningful to the community and obtain its support. An effective community health assessment reflects the fact that communities are not simply collections of needs or problems but entities possessing many strengths and assets.

> *An effective community health assessment reflects the fact that communities are not simply collections of needs or problems but entities possessing many strengths and assets.*

A community health assessment takes into account the broad determinants of health, such as income and social status, housing, nutrition, employment and working conditions, social support networks, education, neighborhood safety and violence issues, physical environment, personal health practices and coping skills, cultural customs and values, and the community's capacity to support family and economic growth. The assessment examines the entire range of factors that promote or prevent health rather than just personal health risks or disease. Evaluators collect, organize, analyze, prioritize, and report data on health and social indicators, including health care data reported by hospitals and by local, state, and federal health agencies and national health care groups. Evaluators also obtain input from community members and public health experts. The assessment report identifies a comprehensive list of health problems, risk factors, and protective factors and provides an inventory of community resources and assets.

A community health assessment provides information, and information is needed for change and for empowerment. But an initial assessment alone will not provide information about the process of change or of action. It provides the baseline information that will enable program planners to assess the impact of the intervention on community health. Regular repetitions of measures via surveys and other methods must be conducted to assess change (Hancock & Minkler, 2002).

Healthy Community Assessment

A healthy community assessment, also called a *comprehensive community health assessment,* evaluates the development of all segments of the community—social climate, economy, access to care, prevention, sanitation, nutrition, education, immunization, and family planning. It is "concerned with a development process by which people improve both their lives and life-styles" (Rifkin & Walt, 1986, p. 560). A healthy community assessment is a process rather than a status. This method takes into account resources, processes, and outcomes. It assesses the whole range of social and environmental factors that both cause ill health and sustain and create good health, including economic, human, and social capital; emotional and mental health and well-being; material and physical health and well-being; productivity; safety; and community involvement.

A community health assessment is one component of a healthy community assessment. A variety of outcome indicators are used to scan communities and draw attention to changing conditions or circumstances that have particular needs. The geography and environment of the community reveal factors likely to affect health, such as climate, natural resources, air and water quality, and natural hazards. The community's history provides important information on the major economic, political, and social forces that shaped the community's evolution and may explain many of the present circumstances that influence the health of the community. The community's present demography, including age and gender distribution and racial or ethnic and socioeconomic characteristics, provides further information that can be used to anticipate some of the health-related issues the community faces (Hancock & Minkler, 2002).

A healthy community assessment also looks at the processes under way in the community that are believed to be related to health and the extent to which health is taken into account or is a focus for action. It takes the time to identify not only the formal leadership of the community at the local level but also its informal leaders. By appraising the processes of community action and change on multiple levels and uncovering multiple players in these processes, the healthy community assessment broadens the program's potential to involve a diversity of stakeholders in building a healthier community. For this approach to work, every component of the community, as well as outside agencies, must make not only an emotional but also a financial commitment to improving the health of the community.

There is no one specific way to conduct a healthy community assessment. There are, however, basic assessment guides in current use (Issel, 2004). The first steps are to establish a coalition of community leaders and organizations to define what a good state of health means for the community, design the assessment, oversee the conduct of the assessment, interpret its findings, prioritize the health problems to be managed, and design a health plan for the community. Program planners then identify the health indicators to be measured, including indexes of community strengths and resources available to resolve the health problems, indexes of illness and causes of death, and risk factors representing behaviors and conditions that lead to poor health and that may be modified.

The next step is the collection and interpretation of the health indicators data. Numerous types of data are used in a healthy community assessment, including archival data (e.g., medical records and other types of agency records, public data), national surveys, vital statistics, census social indicators, primary data (those specifically collected around a need of interest), provider data, proprietary data sources, case studies, community stories, community mapping, and published literature. The last step is to prepare a summary report of the findings and present them to interested parties (Issel, 2004).

Program planners using the healthy community assessment method accept the fact that radical health improvement outcomes will be a long time coming, because changes must occur on all levels from the individual to the community. Timelines for achievement and measurable outcomes and objectives are hard to define as well. Planners must overcome barriers to community involvement such as time constraints on busy individuals, competing interests for available time and resources, and community members' insecurity about being involved or lack of awareness of the opportunity for community involvement. A healthy community assessment requires a considerable commitment of time, leadership, and financial resources by individuals and lead agencies. Overall, the healthy community model emphasizes prevention of community problems and the development and empowerment of communities and people.

The health of individuals, of families, and of populations is a state in which physical, mental, social, and spiritual well-being is integrated so that optimal functioning is possible. It is not a commodity or product. It is a blending of the elements and resources needed to master the developmental tasks necessary to enjoy a satisfying and productive life. Health is achieved and maintained not merely through the absence of illness but also through the synthesis of complex, elaborate, and intricate events. It has many dimensions and is largely culturally defined. Health cannot be valued just by looking at the physical needs and functions of individuals. It must be assessed and measured through the relationship between wellness and key components of the living and working environments, including housing, education, religion, employment, nutrition, leisure and recreation, health and medical care, and a clean environment.

Assessing Culturally Diverse Communities

An understanding of cultural beliefs and practices can aid community efforts to improve health. Enhancing cultural competence helps build cross-cultural relationships and create more inclusive and culturally appropriate interventions. To be successful, community efforts must mobilize and engage all individuals who can benefit and contribute, especially those of diverse cultures and experiences. The more specific components of the intervention should reflect an analysis of contributing factors and available assets.

It is vital to establish an inclusive definition of the community from diverse perspectives, to share the decision-making power, and to develop effective collaboration. To understand what community members view as strengths and weaknesses, one must listen to the voices of a diverse group of community leaders, residents, and professionals. It also is crucial to distinguish between problems (what outsiders identify as "something wrong") and issues (what the community identifies and is willing to work on to bring about change). *Community capacity* represents the capabilities that exist within communities and the networks of individuals, communities, and institutions that strengthen the individual; this capacity also involves the community members' ability to define their own values and priorities and competence to act on them.

The key to successful intervention is translating community needs and issues into language that makes sense to all participants. This translation process entails starting where the people are, emphasizing and building on community strengths and assets, and using the power of dialogue to help people examine the whys of their lives and the sources and implications of their own knowledge. How this information is collected, the purposes for which it is sought, and whether the findings then are returned to the community play a critical role in determining the empowering potential of the assessment process.

A host of tools, methods, and approaches can be used to help communities identify their strengths and assets as well as the problems or issues they wish to address. Program planners should begin by asking questions, starting conservations, and holding dialogues with various community individuals and groups, always engaging in active listening. Planners may set up meetings, enlist community participation in assessing needs and resources, and facilitate the process of developing goals and priorities. Program development must start from within the community.

Numerous techniques and approaches can be used to obtain the types of information needed. According to Hancock and Minkler (2002), methods vary in terms of their degree of contact with the community (see the following sections). Because contact with and high-level involvement of the community residents in the assessment process are vital to community building and developing culturally appropriate approaches to health, methods that promote contact should be paramount. However, lower contact methods that produce hard data also should be included in any community assessment.

No-Contact Methods

An epidemiological assessment often is the first type of data collection. Demographic and social indicators such as mortality, morbidity, and life expectancy statistics and behavior and environmental factors are reviewed. No-contact statistical methods using multivariate analysis can document such factors as the effect of race, ethnicity, and class on mortality rates. These methods can provide information that is vital in demonstrating health disparities in a format that legislators and advocacy groups can use to obtain resources. In addition to statistical studies, this method can include data from newspapers, health departments, agencies, and community bulletin boards (Hancock & Minkler, 2002).

Minimal Contact Observation Methods

Minimal contact observation methods include the "windshield tour" or walk-through. Program planners walk or drive through the community looking for potential indicators of community health and well-being. This activity provides social, cultural, and economic information about residents and their health issues. This method can be modified to enable more contact in the form of community involvement. Community residents can conduct a needs survey or capacity inventory of community assets and capacities. Assets identified include those located inside the community and under the control of the community, those located in the community and outside community control, and those located outside community and outside community control (Hancock & Minkler, 2002).

Interactive Contact Methods

Interactive contact methods include qualitative techniques such as key informant interviews, door-to-door surveys, and focus groups to elicit data and stories about the community. Interviews should be conducted with both formal and informal leaders; the latter are natural helpers people go to for advice or help and who often are key behind-the-scenes players (Hancock & Minkler, 2002). Interviews with community members and long-time residents also are key to identifying a core group of participants and leaders. Program planners should ask a variety of questions, including the following: What do you like about living in this community? What would you most like to see changed? What are some of the things people are proud of in the community? Program planners also should conduct interviews and focus groups with professionals who serve or work with the priority population. The nominal group process method is a good way to encourage the participation of marginal group members in small group meetings (Debecq, Van de Van, & Gustafson, 1975).

Program planners also can conduct a social assessment, or "the process of determining people's perceptions of their own needs or quality of life" (Gielen & McDonald, 2002, p. 412) Engaging community members in dialogue or guided discussions about their community is another means of community assessment and issue selection. The Delphi survey is one method of collecting information and opinions from a large group of people (Alder & Ziglio, 1996).

Asset Mapping

In community asset mapping, program planners and community representatives identify local resources, abilities, and other building blocks for community growth and change and lay them out in a visual format. The result is a map of the physical assets of the community—for example, library, playgrounds, schools, parks, houses of worship—that may constitute important physical and social support structures for achieving community goals. Risk mapping, which involves the identification of threats to safety in the community (e.g., poorly lit areas), also can be a part of this process and can be a potent method for issue selection.

After collecting all of this information, program planners should hold a visioning process with a group of the community members. Participants collectively define a shared dream of what the community can become and the types of intervention that are needed to help them achieve their goals. The visioning process could be a day-long retreat or a year-long process under the leadership of trained facilitators. Common themes recognized as being fundamental to the health of the community are identified and become the basis for issue development.

These approaches will provide a wealth of data and stories about the community and its resources, strengths, perceived problems or needs, and dreams for the future. In this process, health practitioners ask questions that can help community members build the competence needed for decision making. Health practitioners help community members look at the pros and cons of an issue and intervention approach. Because the ultimate goal is to bring about social change that will promote the health and well-being of the priority population, the process of intervention selection should involve dialogue about whether and how the intervention can improve the health of the community. Communities need to consider many factors as they decide on issues and interventions. By fostering dialogue, asking questions, and guiding considerations, practitioners can enhance the capacity of the community members to select the best course of action.

Approaching the Community

An appreciation of people, problems, goals, and places and of past history, current conditions, and future dreams is a critical foundation when working with culturally diverse communities. By failing to recognize the many ways in which issues of oppression and racism affect the community, practitioners can perpetuate the objectification and exploitation of groups who are at risk. Practitioners whose own racial or ethnic stereotypes distort their view of culturally diverse communities will be ineffective in working in partnership (Rivera & Erlich, 1995). Therefore, practitioners are encouraged to take the role of learner in approaching a community and discovering its problems and strengths.

Effective community-organizing efforts should build on the traditions of the community. The role of the practitioner should vary according to his or her relationship to the community or the issue being addressed. Rivera and Erlich (1995) identified three levels in approaching culturally diverse communities. If the practitioner is a member of the community, then primary contact is appropriate. Primary contact involves immediate and personal grassroots work with the community. If the practitioner is of a similar cultural background but is not a member of the community, he or she should be involved on a secondary level by participating as a liaison between the community and the larger society. The tertiary level of contact is most appropriate for those who do not have backgrounds similar to those of the population. At this level, the practitioner can provide valuable contributions to the community through consultation and the sharing of technological knowledge. The principal activity of the practitioner is to learn the strengths of the community as they are exemplified in daily activities within the community. In time, community members will recognize the practitioner's willingness to use the culturally competent approach of noninterference, and more opportunities to work with the community might be presented (Lewis, 1993).

Gutierrez and Lewis (2002) recommended the use of an empowerment framework that stresses the core concepts of education, participation, and capacity building as a way to develop sensitive and effective methods for community practice. The education component includes the following activities:

- Learning about, understanding, and participating in the community
- Recognizing and building on ways in which diverse community members have worked effectively within their own communities
- Building on existing structures
- Serving as a facilitator and viewing situations through the lens or vision of the diverse members.

The participation component includes the following:

- Using the process of praxis to understand the historical, political, and social context of the organizing effort
- Forming small groups
- Recognizing and embracing the conflict that characterizes cross-cultural work.

The capacity-building component includes the following:

- Involving diverse members in leadership roles
- Understanding and supporting the need that diverse members may have for their own separate programs and organizations.

This empowerment framework emphasizes several critical principles in working effectively with culturally diverse communities, including being an active learner and facilitator, viewing a given situation through the lens of diverse members, accepting the conflict inherent in cross-cultural work, and involving diverse members in leadership roles.

Israel and colleagues (1998) state that working with culturally diverse communities requires the development of a common language, trust, and mutual respect; understanding of the cultural context; recognition that participants may have different goals, agendas, experiences, and degrees of commitment; conflicting loyalties; multiple demands on their time; and varying levels of ability to contribute to the effort. Practitioners also should consider how structural inequities contribute to the cultural differences that exist within and across communities and partnerships.

Cultural competence is particularly germane for practitioners working in community settings. Chavez, Duran, Baker, Avila, and Wallerstein (2003) observe that working with culturally diverse communities is like dancing. It has the potential to make practitioners feel "exhilarated, awkward, controlled, and free" (p. 81). Understanding the roots of oppression and its relationship to trust and community building is part of the dance. To engage in effective community practice, practitioners must do all of the following:

- Acknowledge the diversity within racial and ethnic groups.
- Acknowledge that race is a social construct and not a biological determinant.
- Address the present-day existence and impact of racism.
- Examine the role of racism in diminishing the health of a population.
- Use the intervention process and outcomes to mobilize and advocate for change to reduce disparities and enhance race relations.
- Listen, listen, listen.
- Recognize that privilege, especially White privilege, is continually operating to some degree and creating power imbalances.
- Accept that outsiders cannot fully understand community and interpersonal dynamics.
- Build true multicultural working relationships.

Siegel, Howard, Adams, and Wasongarz (2003) found in their review of several community-based programs to address health disparities that these programs achieved positive results in many communities, but their efforts could not completely solve the greater social issues of poverty, racism, and lack of health insurance for millions of Americans. The features that fostered successful programs in culturally diverse communities included the following:

- Mobilizing and managing a continuum of resources
- Engaging in one-to-one outreach
- Practicing cultural competence
- Improving physical access to care
- Building bridges to the provider community
- Formally seeking community input.

In these programs, cultural competence took the forms of linguistic competence; understanding of the client population's barriers to care; and knowledge of the client population's predominant diet, lifestyle, culture, and beliefs. At some sites, it meant including minority representation on governing boards and among upper-level management. Some sites placed a strong emphasis on understanding the belief systems and everyday lives of their clients. They hired and trained workers and volunteers from the culture they were serving. Clearly, practicing cultural competence means more than just speaking the language. It also means deliberately infusing the client's culture in the programs and interventions.

Community Intervention

The cultural and ethnic background of the recipients of services affects both program development and the interpretation of outcomes. The intervention or action used in community practice must be tailored to the target audience if the program is to be successful in achieving the desired health effects. The choice of intervention and manner of delivery ought to be based on both the sociocultural diversity of the target audience and the biological diversity within the target audience. In addition, the diversity and cultural competence of the health professionals play a role in the effectiveness of program intervention (Issel, 2004).

Community interventions are actions done intentionally to have a direct effect on the health of a community. In community practice, interventions can include a broad range of actions, such as medical treatment, pharmacological treatment, education, psychological strategies, and policy formation. They can encompass strategies that typically are not considered to be treatment, such as transportation or community development. Community interventions may follow a social model of intervention rather than a medical model. Interventions are the heart of all health programs or services and should be presented in culturally competent ways.

Getting Started

What kind of cultural community practice or action do you envision? Which approaches and strategies will prove the most promising in building a caring community practice? To build a community practice that is successful in improving conditions and resolving problems, practitioners need to understand and appreciate many cultures, establish relationships with people from cultures other than their own, and build strong alliances with different groups. As you envision the kind of diverse community practice you want to engage in, consider these questions (Community Tool Box, 2006):

- Who lives in your community right now?
- What kind of diversity already exists?
- What kinds of relationships already are established between cultural groups?

- Are the different cultural groups well organized?
- What kinds of struggles between cultures exist?
- What kinds of struggles within cultural groups exist?
- Are these struggles openly recognized and talked about?
- Are there efforts to build alliances and coalitions between groups?
- What issues do different cultural groups have in common?

Each person in your target area must feel welcome regardless of background. Each needs to know that his or her culture is important to others, but treating everyone the same unintentionally may be oppressive. Often people are afraid that recognizing differences will divide people. Learning about cultural differences, however, actually can bring people together. You should seek to create an environment that is inclusive.

Cultural differences can either enrich or impede the success of your community practice. Creating multicultural coalitions will challenge you to deal with differences and use them to strengthen your work. Awareness of sensitive issues can help you detect potential obstacles and develop approaches to address them either before or after they arise. According to Wolff and Kaye (1995), building effective multicultural coalitions involves articulating a vision, conducting strategic outreach and membership development, setting ground rules that maintain a safe and nurturing atmosphere, establishing a structure and operating procedures that reinforce equity, practicing new modes of communication, creating leadership opportunities for everyone (especially people of color and women), and engaging in activities that are culturally sensitive or that directly fight oppression.

Practitioners and communities concerned with social change are increasingly using computer networks to organize online surveys and chat rooms in which community members jointly identify community problems and resources, engage in dialogue, and actively participate in solutions. New community groups can evolve around common interests, such as a specific disease or health condition. This technology can be used to share strategies with colleagues across town or around the world that may be effective in addressing health and social problems (Cart, 2002). Program components, of course, then must be tailored to individual behaviors and the community agencies addressing the health issue.

Media advocacy is another way to facilitate change and advance social or public initiatives. A range of mass media and advocacy strategies can be used to define the problem and stimulate broad-based coverage in an effort to change public policies. Media advocacy is used to reframe and shape public discourse to increase support for and advance healthy public policies. According to Wallack (2002), the fundamental steps in media advocacy are

(1) Establish what your group's policy goal is—what do you want to happen? (2) Decide who your target is—to whom do you want to speak?

Do they have the power to effect the change you want to see happen? (3) Frame your issue and construct your message, (4) Construct an overall media advocacy plan for delivering your message and creating pressure for change, and finally (5) Evaluate how well you have done what you set out to do. (p. 342)

The process and success of media advocacy are linked to how well the advocacy is rooted in the community. The more support and participation at the local level for media initiatives, the more likely journalists will be to define the issue as relevant and newsworthy.

Issel (2004) notes that the final choice of a community action or package of interventions should be evaluated against six criteria for usefulness: A good intervention must be (a) technologically feasible (changeable using available knowledge); (b) clearly linked to health gains; (c) politically feasible (acceptable to the target audience); (d) linked to societal priorities (important in the big picture); (e) manipulable (able to adjust to specific needs of the participants); and (f) reasonable, rather than prohibitive, in cost.

Summary

Members of culturally diverse communities must be involved as much as possible throughout the process of developing a community practice, their concerns must be heard and responded to, and collaboration must be achieved in assessing the situation. It is important to focus not only on the needs but also on the strengths or assets of the community. Community practice must be of the community, by the community, and for the community if it is to be truly empowering and health promoting. Community health assessment methods address the relationship between wellness and components of the living and working environments. They are used to assess not only the needs and deficiencies of the individual and community but also the capacity of the community to design and solve problems. They help practitioners understand the kinds of information that will enable a community to decide what a health problem is, how to solve it, and then how to act to carry out the solution. They provide a context in which health can be expressed in multiple ways and used to magnify the power of citizens. These assessment methods are not the source of analysis or solutions; rather, they are the source of information not easily discovered by local citizens.

Systematic assessments are needed to enable the development of purposeful and culturally appropriate health policies, to change lifestyles, and to improve community and individual health. It is equally important to evaluate the effect of the community program on the population it serves. The approach selected to improve the health of a community often is based on the types of measurements done and the desired outcomes. Unless people are empowered to take charge of their own lives and health, no sustainable achievement in improving health is possible. Regardless of the community assessment method chosen, it will be most effective if it combines multiple methods of data collection and community measurements and involves community members in assessing the effects of change, the realities of the community, and the empowerment of the people.

When working within culturally diverse communities, building formal or informal bridges is important. One-on-one outreach and ongoing contact are essential for success. Practicing cultural competence, fostering volunteerism, and formally seeking community input are vital. Community input can be integrated with a conscious attempt to change the environment through advocacy by way of linkages or grassroots appeal. Local observations, organizational sponsorship and mission, and the identities of willing community partners are important in determining what community programs are needed and what these programs may accomplish. These factors will drive the model, intervention, and community action.

By engaging in community practice in partnership with members of culturally diverse communities, health professionals can reduce health disparities at the local level. Detecting breast cancer early in a community member or keeping members with diabetes healthy is an invaluable service. Creating networks of services, assisting diverse clients in gaining access to these services in a coordinated fashion, and providing culturally competent care may be the best way to promote physical, mental, social, and spiritual well-being not only for individuals but also for communities as a whole.

Reflection

- Design a community outreach program for a specific group of clients, such as young Hispanic women, that provides AIDS education and prevention.

- Start by conducting a community assessment. Make a list of agencies and organizations that serve the target population, places where community members gather, businesses the target population patronizes, key community leaders, and sources of materials.

- Review methods of gathering information about this population.

- Conduct interviews with professionals or agency staff, community leaders, and members of the target group. Talk with as many people as possible.

References

Aday, L. A., Begley, C. E., Lairson, D. R., & Balkrishman, R. (2004). *Evaluating the healthcare system: Effectiveness, efficiency, and equity* (3rd ed.). Chicago: Health Administration.

Adler, M., & Ziglio, E. (Eds.). (1996). *Gazing into the oracle: The Delphi Method and its application to social policy and public health.* London: Jessica Kingsley.

Bell, C., & Newby, H. (1971). *Community studies: An introduction to the sociology of the local community.* London: Allen & Unwin.

Carr, W., Szapiro, N., Heisler, T., & Krasner, M. (1989). Sentinel health events as indicators of unmet needs. *Social Sciences and Medicine, 29,* 705–714.

Cart, C. U. (2002). Online computer networks: Potential and challenges for community organizing and community building now and in the future. In M. Minkler (Ed.), *Community organizing and community building for health* (pp. 325–338). New Brunswick, NJ: Rutgers University.

Centers for Disease Control and Prevention. (2007a). *Behavioral Risk Factor Surveillance System (BFRSS).* Retrieved August 1, 2007, from www.cdc.gov/brfss

Centers for Disease Control and Prevention. (2007b). *National Health Interview Survey (NHIS).* Retrieved August 1, 2007, from www.cdc.gov/nchs/nhis.htm

Chavez, V., Duran, B., Baker, Q., Avila, M. M., & Wallerstein, N. (2003). The dance of race and privilege in community-based participatory research. In M. Minkler & N. Wallerstein (Eds.), *Community-based participatory research for health* (pp. 81–97). San Francisco: Jossey-Bass.

Community Tool Box. (2006). *Community building tools.* Retrieved August 17, 2006, from http://ctb.ku.edu/tools

Delbecq, A., Van de Van, A. H., & Gustafson, D. H. (1975). *Group techniques for program planning: A guide to nominal group and Delphi processes.* Glenview, IL: Scott Foresman.

Fazio, L. S. (2001). *Developing occupation-centered programs for the community: A workbook for students and professionals.* Englewood Cliffs, NJ: Prentice Hall.

Gielen, A. C., & McDonald, E. M. (2002). Using the Precede–Proceed planning model to apply health behavior theories. In K. Glanz, B. K. Rimer, & F. M. Lewis (Eds.), *Health behavior and health education: Theory, research, and practice* (pp. 405–436). San Francisco: Jossey-Bass.

Gutierrez, L. M., & Lewis, E. A. (2002). Education, participation, and capacity building in community organizing with women of color. In M. Minkler (Ed.), *Community organizing and community building for health* (pp. 216 – 229). New Brunswick, NJ: Rutgers University.

Hancock, T., & Minkler, M. (2002). Community health assessment or healthy community assessment. In M. Minkler (Ed.), *Community organizing and community building for health* (pp. 139–156). New Brunswick, NJ: Rutgers University.

Israel, B. A., Schulz, A. J., Parker, E. A., & Becker, A. B. (1998). Review of community-based research: Assessing partnership approaches to improve public health. *Annual Review of Public Health, 19,* 173–202.

Issel, L. M. (2004). *Health program planning and evaluation: A practical, systematic approach for community health.* Boston: Jones & Bartlett.

Johnson, V. (1995). *Heart full of grace: A thousand years of Black wisdom.* New York: Simon & Schuster.

Keleher, H. (2001). Why primary health care offers a more comprehensive approach for tackling inequities than primary care. *Australian Journal of Primary Health, 7*(2), 57–61.

Lewis, E. (1993). Continuing the legacy: On the importance of praxis in the education of social work students and teachers. In D. Schoem, L. Frankel, X. Zuniga, & E. Lewis (Eds.), *Multicultural teaching in the university* (pp. 279–292). New York: Praeger.

Magnussen, L., Ehirl, J., & Jolly, P. (2004). Comprehensive versus selective primary health care: Lessons for a global health policy. *Health Affairs, 23,* 167–176.

Minkler, M., Blackwell, A. G., Thompson, M., & Tamir, H. (2003). Public Health Advocacy Forum—Community-based participatory research: Implications for public health funding. *American Journal of Public Health, 93,* 1210–1213.

Rifkin, S. B., Muller, F., & Bichmann, W. (1988). Primary health care: On measuring participation. *Social Sciences and Medicine, 26,* 931–940.

Rifkin, S. B., & Walt, G. (1986). Why health improves: Defining the issues concerning "comprehensive primary health care" and "selective primary health care." *Social Science Medicine, 23,* 559–566.

Rivera, F., & Erlich, J. (1995). *Community organizing in a diverse society* (2nd ed.). Boston: Allyn & Bacon.

Schulz, A. J., Israel, B. A., Parker, E. A., Lockett, M., Hill, Y., & Wills, R. (2003). Engaging women in community-based participatory research in health: The East Side Village Health Worker Partnership. In M. Minkler & N. Wallerstein (Eds.), *Community-based participatory research for health* (pp. 293–315). San Francisco: Jossey-Bass.

Siegel, B., Howard, B., Adams, A., & Wasongarz, D. (2003). *Addressing health disparities in community settings: Final report to the Robert Wood Johnson Foundation.* New York: New Schools University.

Turnock, B. J. (2004). *Public health: What it is and how it works* (3rd ed.). Boston: Jones & Bartlett.

U.S. Census Bureau. (2007). *Data tools.* Retrieved August 1, 2007, from www.census.gov/main/www/access.html

Wallack, L. (2002). Media advocacy: A strategy for empowering people and communities. In M. Minkler (Ed.), *Community organizing and community building for health* (pp. 339–352). New Brunswick, NJ: Rutgers University.

Wolff, T., & Kaye, G. (1995). *From the ground up: A workbook on coalition building and community development.* Amherst, MA: AHEC/Community Partners.

20

Cultural Competence and Occupational Justice

If we lose [our principles, values, and beliefs], those we aspire to serve, who really legitimize our existence and our means to power, have more to lose. So whatever choices we make as occupational therapists, individually and collectively, they are political and so are their implications and consequences.

—KRONENBERG & POLLARD (2005, P. 83)

Key Points

- *Occupational justice* involves the right of people and populations to have access and opportunity to engage in activities that have meaning to them.

- *Occupational injustice* occurs when occupational participation is barred, confined, segregated, prohibited, undeveloped, disrupted, alienated, marginalized, exploited, or otherwise devalued.

- Occupational injustice takes the forms of occupational deprivation, occupational alienation, occupational imbalance, and occupational apartheid.

- Occupational justice interventions often occur under a social model of health that requires social action to modify the environmental, social, and political context.

- Occupational injustice can occur globally or locally.

- To provide interventions that focus on occupational justice, practitioners must be culturally competent.

317

DURING THE PAST DECADE, the concept of occupational justice has developed and proliferated in the occupational therapy literature, but most of this work has been published outside the United States. Gradually, however, the literature and the ideas have found their way to this country and have begun to take root. Practitioners have been slower to seek out and embrace these ideas, perhaps because dealing with issues of oppression has been seen as "too political." Perhaps because the U.S. health care system keeps a tight rein on the process of providing care by requiring specific kinds of interventions and by reimbursing selected interventions for a specific number of days, few practitioners have learned, or have had the courage, to think outside the box of traditional health services provision. Or perhaps because occupational therapy is still governed by the dominant and privileged White culture, many practitioners are blind to the health disparities and social inequities that affect so many vulnerable populations in the United States. Whatever the reasons for the delay, occupational justice is becoming more prevalent in the U.S. occupational therapy literature, academic programs, and the vernacular of U.S. occupational therapy practitioners.

Within the literature of occupational justice, an entire new vocabulary has arisen. This chapter introduces and clarifies terms such as *occupational injustice, occupational deprivation, occupational alienation, occupational imbalance,* and *occupational apartheid* and challenges occupational therapists and occupational therapy assistants to address these concepts in their practice.

What Is *Occupational Justice?*

Simplified, *occupational justice* is the right of people and communities to have access and opportunity to engage in activities that have meaning to them. Ann Wilcock, an Australian occupational therapist and her Canadian colleague Elizabeth Townsend (2000), have collaboratively and individually developed and explored this concept, and state that "occupational justice is about recognizing and providing for the occupational needs of individuals and communities as part of a fair and empowering society" (p. 84).

As might be expected, the notion of occupational justice has arisen from the social justice arena, and although the terms are not synonymous, they are complementary. Instead of focusing on the social relations and conditions of life, as does social justice, "occupational justice addresses what people *do* in their relationships and conditions for living" (Wilcock & Townsend, 2000, p. 84). *Social justice* concerns itself with fairness, equity, empowerment, and the right of each person to equal access to goods and services. It addresses social conditions and discrimination that places individuals and groups at a disadvantage on the basis of race, ethnicity, class, religion, gender, age, or sexual orientation (Wilcock & Townsend, 2000). Occupational justice focuses on the inequality, unfairness, discrimination, and other injustices that prevent people from participating in meaningful occupations: "Occupational injustices exist when, for example, participation is barred, confined, segregated, prohibited, undeveloped, disrupted, alienated, marginalized, exploited, or otherwise devalued" (Townsend & Whiteford, 2005, p. 112). The distinction between social justice and occupational justice is somewhat subtle; in effect, occupational therapy professionals are called on to examine issues of social justice using their unique occupational perspective.

Providing occupational therapy using an occupational justice framework involves addressing not only the needs of the person, community, or population with whom one is working but also the social systems that help maintain the injustices. Occupational therapy practitioners are required to work beyond the confines of the health care arena in larger contextual settings, in which resource allocation may involve government, corporate, or philanthropic sources (Townsend & Whiteford, 2005). To understand and work for occupational justice, occupational therapists and occupational therapy assistants must become knowledgeable about the laws and regulations that support or inhibit occupational justice for people and populations and use advocacy and educational strategies for change to enable the people with whom they work. Occupational therapy practitioners also must become cognizant of the social systems that maintain bias, discrimination, and health disparities in vulnerable groups. In other words, occupational therapists and occupational therapy assistants working for occupational justice must become politically savvy. This approach focuses on relevant and effective practice and public accountability (Townsend & Whiteford, 2005). It requires occupational therapy practitioners to work within a social model as well as a medical model.

Social Models and Occupational Therapy

International Classification of Functioning, Disability, and Health

Moving to a social model brings the occupational therapy profession in close alignment with the framework of the World Health Organization (WHO, 2001), the *International Classification of Functioning, Disability, and Health (ICF)*. The purpose of this classification is to provide a scientific basis for the consequences of health conditions; to establish a common language to improve communications; to permit comparison of data across countries, health care disciplines, services, and time; and to provide a systematic coding scheme for health information systems (WHO, 2002). It facilitates global communication, understanding, and research.

In recognition that health and health care are broader than described by medical frameworks, the WHO developed this model with a health (not illness) orientation that is socially based. It is an integrative, universal model that examines human functioning and participation rather than disabilities. "Moving clients toward participation in occupation" is language used both in this model and in occupational therapy.

The medical model views the disablement phenomenon as a personal problem that is directly caused by disease, trauma, or health conditions and that requires medical care in the form of individual treatment by professionals (see Table 20.1). Management of disablement is aimed at promoting the person's adjustment and behavior change. Health care is viewed as the main issue, and at the political level it is health care policy that needs to be modified. The social model of disablement, on the other hand, sees the issue mainly as a societal problem; the goal is to integrate people with disabilities into society. Disablement is an attribute not of a person but of a complex collection of conditions, many of which are created by the social environment. Hence, management of the problem requires social action, and it is the collective responsibility of society to make the environmental modifications necessary for the full participation of people with disabilities in all areas of social life. The issue, therefore, is attitudinal or ideological and requires social change, while at political level it is a question of human rights. Thus, the issue is highly political for all intents and purposes (WHO, 2002). As is evident, viewing health conditions from a social perspective requires a much broader perspective of care delivery.

Community-Based Rehabilitation

In the spring of 2006, the World Federation of Occupational Therapists (WFOT) voted to support the concept of community-based rehabilitation (CBR) as a viable context for occupational therapy practice. This idea was developed and brought to WFOT in a position paper conceptualized by the WFOT–CBR Project Team and

Table 20.1. Comparison of Medical and Social Models of Care

Aspect of Model	Medical Model of Care	Social Model of Care
Locus of problem	Personal problem	Social problem
Means of addressing problem	Medical care	Social integration
Intervention focus	Individual treatment	Social action
Addressee of problem	Professional help	Individual and collective responsibility
Results of intervention	Personal adjustment	Environmental adjustment and manipulation
Characteristic of change	Behavior	Attitude
Philosophy of intervention	Care	Human rights
Influencing regulators	Health care policy	Politics
Outcomes	Individual adaptation	Social change

mainly authored by team member Frank Kronenberg (2003). The team defined *CBR* as

A strategy within general community development for rehabilitation, equalization of opportunities and social inclusion of all children and adults with disabilities. CBR is implemented through the combined efforts of people with disabilities themselves, their families and communities, and the appropriate health, education, vocational, and social services. (p. 4)

The major characteristics of programs that use CBR are as follows:

- *They are community based.* Programs work with people who have disabilities within their own natural environment and community and collaborate with families and community members. By involving the community in the rehabilitation process, the community, as well as the person with disabilities, benefits.
- *They are rehabilitative.* Rehabilitation takes on a broader meaning in this model, one that incorporates the concepts of social inclusion, human rights, and community participation. Considering rehabilitation in this light closely aligns it with occupational justice.
- *They are culturally competent.* The program's occupational therapy practitioners are culturally competent and build on "existing community traditions, structure, networks, and activities" (Kronenberg, 2003, p. 6). Practitioners may work with people of numerous cultures, interacting competently and safely. This work involves "a socio-political overview of practice; a critical awareness of the structures and processes that systematically marginalize people within society" (Kronenberg, 2003, p. 6).
- *They use local resources.* Programs use a skill that most occupational therapy practitioners already have in finding or working with local community members to make low-cost equipment and materials for projects and to involve people with disabilities and their families with the larger community.

Kronenberg (2003) summarizes CBR as benefiting the entire community rather than just individuals; encouraging people with disabilities to actively participate in all aspects, including decision making, of the rehabilitation process; and developing programs that are cross-disciplinary. In community-based rehabilitation, all practitioners involved work beyond the boundaries of traditional institutional-based practice and seek to become active community and world citizens. (Chapter 19 describes community-based occupational therapy in more detail.)

CBR has been used in working with blind children in Tibet (Tenberken & Kronenberg, 2005), with community integration for people in Lebanon (Thibeault, 2005), with child survivors of war (Algado & Burgman, 2005), and with street children in Mexico and Guatemala (Kronenberg, 2005). This work is described in *Occupational Therapy Without Borders: Learning From the Spirit of Survivors* (Kronenberg, Algado, & Pollard, 2005), a book that educates occupational therapy practitioners and others about the possibilities for using CBR within an occupational justice framework.

Occupational Justice Concepts and Terminology

Townsend and Wilcock (2004) state that there are at least three outcomes of occupational injustice and possibly more to be discovered. The three they emphasize are occupational deprivation, occupational alienation, and occupational imbalance. Steinberg (1991) identified another outcome of occupational injustice, *occupational apartheid*.

Occupational Deprivation

One outcome of occupational injustice is occupational deprivation. As defined by Whiteford (2000), *occupational deprivation* is

> A state in which a person or group of people are unable to do what is necessary and meaningful in their lives due to external restrictions. It is a state in which the opportunity to perform those occupations that have social, cultural, and personal relevance is rendered difficult if not impossible. (p. 200)

Multiple factors produce occupational deprivation, including those that are "social, economic, environmental, geographic, historic, cultural, or political in nature" (Whiteford, 2004, p. 222), and these factors are external to the individual. Whiteford (2004) offers five illustrations of occupational deprivation in cases of (a) geographic isolation, (b) extreme conditions of employment, (c) incarceration, (d) sex role stereotyping, and (e) refugeeism. Much of the literature on occupational deprivation examines what people do within the confines of jail or prison (Molineux & Whiteford, 1999; Whiteford, 1995, 1997, 2000). One study examined occupational deprivation with refugees from Kosovo (Whiteford, 2005).

Within the New Zealand prison system, Whiteford (1997) found that the inmates she interviewed experienced "sustained occupational deprivation" (p. 129), and an absence of tools limited their opportunities for the engagement in occupation. Another finding was that time use was impaired; few activities, with the exception of mealtimes, helped inmates mark time. The lack of orientation to time also disrupted typical activity, and many inmates slept throughout large portions of the day. The New Zealand minister of correction stated that "unless they [inmates] learn the value of an honest day's work, they will find it hard to get a job upon release and may reoffend" and that "the government wants inmates to ... work hard towards self improvement" (quoted in Whiteford, 1997, p. 130). Whiteford concludes, however, that her observations of the lack of access to meaningful and productive occupations indicated "a substantive gap between rhetoric and practice" (p. 130). People cannot understand what "an honest day's work" means if they have no opportunity to engage in an honest day's daily activities, including productive work.

A more recent examination of occupational deprivation involved a case study of a man who was a refugee from Kosovo (Whiteford, 2005). *Refugees* are people who are forced out of their native countries for "fear of being persecuted for reasons of race, religion, nationality" (from the definition in the 1951 United Nations High Convention on Refugees, quoted in Whiteford, 2005, p. 79). Refugees often leave their homes with few belongings and often spend time in refugee camps in other countries until they can travel to a host country to begin a new life. Listening to and analyzing "Florim's" story, Whiteford (2005) identified three key issues:

1. Refugees' overt exclusion from occupational participation occurs over time.
2. Trauma and geographic dislocation have a profound effect on refugees' ability to engage in even the most basic occupations.
3. Community and social interaction become the context for occupational participation.

It is yet to be seen if these findings can be generalized to all experiences of occupational deprivation.

Examining the lives of prisoners and refugees has contributed to an understanding of the concept of occupational deprivation. Although most occupational therapy practitioners do not work with these populations, they should recognize the concept and consider whether external structures contribute to occupational deprivation for the people and populations with whom they presently work. There may be laws, regulations, or social systems based on bias and discrimination that prevent people from engaging in meaningful and productive occupation. Because vulnerable groups such as members of ethnic or cultural minorities, poor people, people with mental health disorders, refugees and immigrants, prisoners, older adults, and others often have limited access to social privileges, goods, and services in the United States, it is important that occupational therapy practitioners examine whether members of these groups also are experiencing occupational deprivation.

Occupational deprivation is sustained over time, whereas *occupational disruption* is a temporary or transient phenomenon that, given supportive conditions, resolves itself. Whiteford (2000) describes the experience of occupational disruption as

> When a person's normal pattern of occupational engagement is disrupted due to significant life events (such as having a baby), environmental changes (such as moving house or location), becoming ill or sustaining an injury from which full recovery is expected. (p. 201)

Occupational disruption results from issues internal to the individual rather than the external factors seen in occupational deprivation. For example, an occupational therapy student would experience occupational disruption following a bicycle fall that resulted in a broken wrist on her dominant hand. Her hand would be casted, and she would have little, if any, functional use of the fingers. While her wrist was healing, her ability to perform daily occupations, including writing and using a computer, would be seriously impaired, causing significant disruption of her typical day and activities. However, once the wrist had healed, she would be able to resume all previous activities and occupations. Occupational disruption is not usually considered to be occupational injustice, but we describe the term here to distinguish it from occupational deprivation, which by definition involves occupational injustice.

An interesting article examining occupational disruption for farmers with disabilities clearly described this phenomenon (Molyneaux-Smith, Townsend, & Guernsey, 2003). The authors studied 47 Canadian farmers who had experienced disabling injuries. Of these, 83% returned to farming following their injuries. Using the model of human occupation framework to analyze their findings, Molyneaux-Smith and colleagues found that the farmers felt their habituation (i.e., habits, routines, and roles) had been altered and their performance impaired but that their drive and will (volition) were key in their recovery.

Many occupational therapy professionals work with people who have experienced occupational disruption but will recover much of their ability to continue to engage in beloved occupations, even if in an altered manner. Occupational therapy practitioners' role is to facilitate and engage the internal motivation of the people they work with and help them problem solve ways to successfully participate in their preferred occupations.

Occupational Alienation

Occupational therapy practitioners cannot facilitate motivation or engagement if their clients feel alienated from the activities practitioners present to them. One intervention strategy still used in some clinics is that of stacking cones (see Figure 20.1). For many clients this activity has no meaning or interest. Townsend and Wilcock (2004) define *occupational alienation* as the absence of meaning or purpose in the occupations of daily life. Chronic illness, poverty, and economic and social forces, as well as paid work that does not enrich the worker and is meaningless and boring, may result in occupational alienation. Westwood (1985, cited in Townsend & Wilcock, 2004) describes paid work that may result in occupational alienation as "occupations that are highly standardized, rigidly repetitive, and without opportunities for individual choice, control, decision making, or creativity" (p. 253).

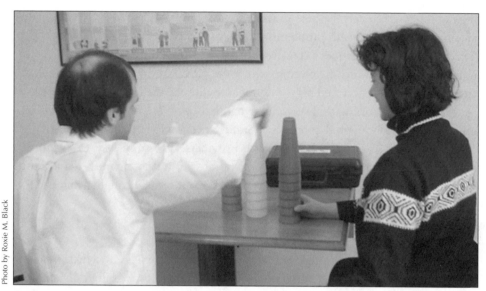

Photo by Roxie M. Black

Figure 20.1. Occupational alienation occurs when activities, such as stacking cones, have no meaning for the client.

Occupational alienation is an emerging concept, and literature on the topic is limited at this time. One study of clients in a mental health day service program in London (Bryant, Craik, & McKay, 2004) found that the study participants felt uncomfortable and estranged when "having to engage in occupations defined and controlled by others" (p. 285). The authors also discovered a sense of internal alienation associated with ongoing mental health issues, which then prevented people from engaging in occupations. As one client said, "I won't move from my bed. . . . Sometimes even in the house you can't do housework and things because you are so down" (p. 285). A third aspect of occupational alienation found in this study was alienation from the wider community. Attendance at the mental health day center in itself separated people there from people who did not have mental illness. Although attending the sessions had unique meaning for each client, the role of day center attendee and the occupation of engaging in therapeutic sessions while there alienated them from the well community.

This study sheds light on the complexity of the injustice of occupational alienation, particularly for those with mental health impairments (Bryant et al., 2004). Often the illness itself caused a person to be unwilling to engage in (i.e., to be alienated from) daily occupations. To engage the person, a practitioner or sometimes a family member or friend coerced (often in subtle ways and with loving intentions) the person into participating in activities that had no meaning for him or her. And finally, the act of entering an institution to receive services for mental illness alienated the person from a community and society that stigmatize anyone with mental health problems.

Bryant and colleagues (2004) conclude that the study results highlight the importance of a sense of belonging, which they felt "can be achieved through the sustained provision of a safe place and meaningful occupation in a social context" (p. 288). As they work with clients, it is vital that occupational therapy practitioners provide client-centered care incorporating occupations that have meaning to clients rather than exclusively to service providers. The only way to ensure the meaningfulness of interventions is to collaborate with each client in determining meaningful activities that will help that person avoid occupational alienation during treatment.

Occupational Imbalance

Another aspect of occupational injustice is *occupational imbalance,* which "refers to situations in which sufficient variations in daily occupations needed to sustain well-being are rendered impossible due to personal or societal circumstances" (Wood, Hooper, & Womack, 2005, p. 380). Occupational imbalance is a temporal issue implying that insufficient time is available for individuals to engage in paid and unpaid work, leisure, and self-care activities (Townsend & Wilcock, 2004). A balance of occupations is important for health. Imbalance occurs in individuals who, for instance, spend too much time in paid labor to the detriment of other aspects of their lives or, conversely, who spend so much time caring for a child or aging parent with a disability that they are unable to work outside the home, resulting in poverty and economic deprivation.

Within societies, occupational imbalance occurs when some groups are "over-occupied while others are underoccupied" (Townsend & Wilcock, 2004, p. 253). In the United States, for example, a huge difference exists in occupational engagement between older adults and adults with disabilities and 30- to 50-year-olds without disabilities. The principal factor in this imbalance is the fact that disabled and older adult groups have limited access to meaningful employment. The societal image of and bias against these populations result in stigma, which lowers access. Occupational imbalance is unjust when societal and "hierarchical classification of occupations drives a labor market in which those with particular skills and knowledge are paid well and have lots of work, while others are unable to find paid work at all" (p. 253).

Refugees are another population that frequently experience occupational imbalance. In Lewiston, Maine, Somali residents who seek paid employment experience many barriers because of cultural and language differences, causing an occupational imbalance for that population.

Occupational Apartheid

The term *occupational apartheid* was first noted by sociologist Stephen Steinberg (1991) who describes it as "a system of occupational segregation that relegates most Blacks to the least desirable jobs or that excludes them altogether from legitimate job markets" (p. 744). Steinberg, the author of *The Ethnic Myth: Race, Ethnicity, and Class in America* (2001) is not an occupational therapist, and he limited his ideas to the occupation of paid labor. His thesis is that the legacy and current reality of racism in the United States maintain the myth that African American people are "inefficient and unproductive workers, deficient in the work habits and moral qualities that have delivered other groups from poverty" (p. 745).

Steinberg's 2001 work provided the foundation for the notion that external social forces affect a group's access to meaningful occupations. The current working definition of *occupational apartheid* by Kronenberg and Pollard (2005) is as follows:

> Occupational apartheid refers to the segregation of groups of people through the restriction or denial of access to dignified and meaningful participation in occupations of daily life on the basis of race, color, disability, national origin, age, gender, sexual preference, religion, political beliefs, status in society, or other characteristics. Occasioned by political forces, its systematic and pervasive social, cultural, and economic consequences jeopardize health and well-being as experienced by individuals, communities, and societies. (p. 67)

Abelenda, Kielhofner, Suarez-Balcazar, and Kielhofner (2005) point out that occupational apartheid is a form of oppression where "the resources and opportunities for choosing and engaging in occupations . . . are unevenly distributed" (p. 185) and access to occupations is denied. Stories of child survivors of the war in Kosovo (Algado, Mehta, & Kronenberg, 2002), street children in Mexico and Guatemala (Kronenberg, 2005), and mothers of children with HIV/AIDS in South Africa (Ramugondo, 2005) exemplify the role of occupational therapy practitioners who work with populations of people who suffer occupational apartheid. These examples come from a global perspective of occupational injustice.

Kronenberg and Pollard (2005) assert that "Although the terms [*occupational injustice* and *occupational apartheid*] are complimentary, occupational injustices occur within a system of occupational apartheid" (p. 66). As occupational therapy professionals explore these concepts, it is important that, instead of considering these issues to be problems seen only elsewhere in the world, they begin to examine where occupational apartheid and injustice are seen in their own client populations. An occupational justice framework can help them better understand the plight of Gulf Coast refugees (mostly poor people of color) from Hurricane

Katrina in 2005, for example, who were torn from their homes, places of employ-ment, and playgrounds.

Occupational apartheid is in place in laws and regulations that systematically deny immigrants and refugees in this country opportunities for meaningful employment. How many of the children and adults with whom occupational ther-apy practitioners work fall within the poor or working poor categories and cannot enjoy the privilege of access to meaningful employment or other occupations because the legal and social systems do not provide the support they need to move within the social hierarchy? Understanding the concepts of occupational justice and the ways they are actualized by the people and populations with whom occupation-al therapy practitioners work will broaden practitioners' thinking and approaches to intervention in a way that not only supports occupational engagement and par-ticipation for individuals and groups but also contributes to a more just society, which has been one of the tenets of the profession since its inception.

Occupational Justice and Cultural Competence

Cultural competence and occupational justice are complementary concepts. Cultural competence is necessary for sensitive, knowledgeable, and skilled interac-tions between people who have cultural differences. Many occupational therapy clients who experience occupational injustices are culturally different from the majority of occupa-tional therapy practitioners and often are socio-culturally disenfranchised. They may differ from their care providers in age, ability, sexual identity, race, class, ethnicity, religion, or political beliefs.

Cultural competence and occupational justice are complementary concepts.

Because of these differences, communication and understanding may be difficult. Unless practitioners are culturally competent, rapport, trust, and collaborative interventions may be limited or impossible. Without an open attitude and a willing-ness to learn about the lives and beliefs of the people with whom they work, occu-pational therapy practitioners cannot effectively interact with people who are cul-turally different. Without knowledge and understanding of the social systems that help maintain oppression in the United States, practitioners may not recognize occupational injustice when they see it. If they are practicing in an international context, they must understand the cultural and social dynamics of the people with whom they are working. Cultural competence is necessary for effective practice within an occupational justice framework.

True client-centered care must be culturally competent care (Black, 2005). Pro-viding an enabling approach to mitigate occupational injustices constitutes client-centered and relevant practice (Townsend & Whiteford, 2005). Thus, being cultur-ally competent is necessary to provide effective occupational therapy intervention with an occupational justice intent. Each occupational therapy practitioner has a responsibility to develop his or her cultural self-awareness, knowledge, and skills to provide the best possible practice on behalf of those who do not have access to meaningful occupations and who experience occupational injustice in this country and the world.

Reflection

1. Consider occupational injustice from a global context.

   a. Read or listen to the international news in media broadcasts, newspapers, or news magazines for the next week.

   b. Identify people or populations who are experiencing social injustice.

   c. Consider and further explore the news reports to determine if these people or populations also are experiencing occupational injustice.

   d. What external forces are maintaining these injustices?

2. Consider occupational injustice from a local context.

   a. Using the same methods as for your exploration of global occupational injustice, determine if there are people, groups, or populations in your state or community who are experiencing occupational injustice.

   b. Are there people or agencies that are attempting to alleviate these injustices?

   c. What forces are maintaining these injustices?

   d. What might you do to help alleviate these problems?

3. Plan an occupational justice project.

   a. Identify a person, group, or population in your community, health institution, or workplace that experiences occupational injustice.

   b. Consider your cultural competence in working with this group or population.

   c. Develop a community education program to raise awareness of the issues surrounding the injustice you identify.

   d. Working with community agencies (if appropriate), develop a plan to help alleviate the injustice for this person, group, or population.

   e. Implement the plan and then publish or present on the project.

References

Abelenda, J., Kielhofner, G., Suarez-Balcazar, Y., & Kielhofner, K. (2005). The Model of Human Occupation as a conceptual tool for understanding and addressing occupational apartheid. In F. Kronenberg, S. S. Algado, & N. Pollard (Eds.), *Occupational therapy without borders: Learning from the spirit of survivors* (pp. 183–196). Edinburgh, Scotland: Elsevier/Churchill Livingstone.

Algado, S. S., & Burgman, I. (2005). Occupational therapy intervention with children survivors of war. In F. Kronenberg, S. S. Algado, & N. Pollard (Eds.), *Occupational therapy without borders: Learning from the spirit of survivors* (pp. 245–260). Edinburgh, Scotland: Elsevier/Churchill Livingstone.

Algado, S. S., Mehta, N., & Kronenberg, F. (2002). Occupational therapy intervention with children survivors of war in Kosovo. *Canadian Journal of Occupational Therapy, 69*(4), 205–217.

Black, R. M. (2005). Intersections of care: An analysis of culturally competent care, client centered care, and the feminist ethic of care. *Work, 24,* 409–422.

Bryant, W., Craik, C., & McKay, E. A. (2004). Living in a glass house: Exploring occupational alienation. *Canadian Journal of Occupational Therapy, 71*(5), 282–289.

Kronenberg, F. (2003, May 25–28). *Position paper on community-based rehabilitation for the international consultation on reviewing CBR.* Paper presented at the WFOT meeting, Helsinki, Finland.

Kronenberg, F. (2005). Occupational therapy with street children. In F. Kronenberg, S. S. Algado, & N. Pollard (Eds.), *Occupational therapy without borders: Learning from the spirit of survivors* (pp. 261–276). Edinburgh, Scotland: Elsevier/Churchill Livingstone.

Kronenberg, F., Algado, S. S., & Pollard, N. (Eds.). (2005). *Occupational therapy without borders: Learning from the spirit of survivors.* Edinburgh, Scotland: Elsevier/Churchill Livingstone.

Kronenberg, F., & Pollard, N. (2005). Overcoming occupational apartheid: A preliminary exploration of the political nature of occupational therapy. In F. Kronenberg, S. S. Algado, & N. Pollard (Eds.), *Occupational therapy without borders: Learning from the spirit of survivors* (pp. 58–86). Edinburgh, Scotland: Elsevier/Churchill Livingstone.

Molineux, M. L., & Whiteford, G. E. (1999). Prisons: From occupational deprivation to occupational enrichment. *Journal of Occupational Science, 6*(3), 124–130.

Molyneaux-Smith, L., Townsend, E., & Guernsey, J. R. (2003). Occupation disrupted: Impacts, challenges, and coping strategies for farmers with disabilities. *Journal of Occupational Science, 10*(1), 14–20.

Ramugondo, E. L. (2005). Unlocking spirituality: Play as a health-promoting occupation in the context of HIV/AIDS. In F. Kronenberg, S. S. Algado, & N. Pollard (Eds.), *Occupational therapy without borders: Learning from the spirit of survivors* (pp. 313–325). Edinburgh, Scotland: Elsevier/Churchill Livingstone.

Steinberg, S. (1991, December 9). Occupational apartheid. *The Nation,* pp. 744–746.

Steinberg, S. (2001). *The ethnic myth: Race, ethnicity, and class in America.* Boston: Beacon Press.

Tenberken, S., & Kronenberg, P. (2005). The right to be blind without being disabled. In F. Kronenberg, S. S. Algado, & N. Pollard (Eds.), *Occupational therapy without borders: Learning from the spirit of survivors* (pp. 31–39). Edinburgh, Scotland: Elsevier/Churchill Livingstone.

Thibeault, R. (2005). Connecting health and social justice: A Lebanese experience. In F. Kronenberg, S. S. Algado, & N. Pollard (Eds.), *Occupational therapy without borders: Learning from the spirit of survivors* (pp. 232–244). Edinburgh, Scotland: Elsevier/ Churchill Livingstone.

Townsend, E., & Whiteford, G. (2005). A participatory occupational justice framework. In F. Kronenberg, S. S. Algado, & N. Pollard (Eds.), *Occupational therapy without borders: Learning from the spirit of survivors* (pp. 110–126). Edinburgh, Scotland: Elsevier/ Churchill Livingstone.

Townsend, E., & Wilcock, A. (2004). Occupational justice. In C. Christiansen & E. Townsend (Eds.), *Introduction to occupation: The art and science of living* (pp. 243–273). Englewood Cliffs, NJ: Prentice Hall.

Whiteford, G. E. (1995). Comment—A concrete void: Occupational deprivation and the special needs inmate. *Journal of Occupational Science: Australia, 2*(2), 80–81.

Whiteford, G. E. (1997). Occupational deprivation and incarceration. *Journal of Occupational Science: Australia, 4*(3), 126–130.

Whiteford, G. E. (2000). Occupational deprivation: Global challenge in the new millennium. *British Journal of Occupational Therapy, 63*(5), 200–204.

Whiteford, G. (2004). When people cannot participate: Occupational deprivation. In C. Christiansen & E. Townsend (Eds.), *Introduction to occupation* (pp. 221–242). Englewood Cliffs, NJ: Prentice Hall.

Whiteford, G. E. (2005). Understanding the occupational deprivation of refugees: A case study from Kosovo. *Canadian Journal of Occupational Therapy, 72*(2), 78–88.

Wilcock, A., & Townsend, E. (2000). Occupational terminology interactive dialogue. *Journal of Occupational Science, 7*(2), 84–86.

Wood, W., Hooper, B., & Womack, J. (2005). Reflections on occupational justice as a subtext of occupation-centered education. In F. Kronenberg, S. S. Algado, & N. Pollard (Eds.), *Occupational therapy without borders: Learning from the spirit of survivors* (pp. 378–389). Edinburgh, Scotland: Elsevier/Churchill Livingstone.

World Health Organization. (2001). *International classification of functioning, disability, and health.* Geneva, Switzerland: Author.

World Health Organization. (2002). ICF *as the new member in the WHO family of international classifications* [PowerPoint presentation]. Retrieved October 5, 2003, from www. who.int/classification/icf

IV

Evaluating
Cultural Competence

Research has often failed to establish the effectiveness of interventions for diverse racial, ethnic, and cultural populations.

—Stanhope, Soloman, Pernell-Arnold, Sands, and Bourjolly (2005, p. 226)

Objectives

The information in Part IV will help readers

- Understand the complexities in developing culturally relevant and appropriate research studies,

- Evaluate the validity of research studies on cultural competence,

- Identify some of the current research on cultural competence in occupational therapy and other health care disciplines,

- Recognize the need for ongoing and published research on the effectiveness of culturally competent care in occupational therapy, and

- Evaluate the effectiveness of their own ethical practice.

21

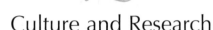

Culture and Research

*L*et's look at information as a means to make the right decisions. It can save *us a lot of time, energy, and effort.*

—Copage (1993, p. 224)

Key Points

- Research is a way to gain knowledge about others. It is essential in providing the foundation for improved health care practices and policies.

- Researcher bias and inadequate data collection instruments and research designs have shaped research in the areas of race, ethnicity, gender, language, and culture. Culturally linked research must be examined to identify problems with racial and ethnic classification, methodology associated with population sampling, interpretation of findings, and measurement instruments.

- Research models for studying culture require the use of both the *etic* (general cultural) and *emic* (culture-specific) approaches. Culture must be considered a variable in all forms and types of research. Researchers need to expand their data collection to include questions on ancestry, migration history, and language.

ALTHOUGH THERE IS A HIGH LEVEL OF INTEREST in the results of research on culturally competent intervention, several methodological challenges exist in conducting such research. Such challenges include lack of standardized definitions for interventions, of standardized evaluation measures, of culturally competent instruments, and of secondary data sources with uniform racial, ethnic, and language data. An additional challenge in this type of research is the large sample size that is required to prove that culturally competent interventions are more effective than traditional interventions alone. To reduce racism and privilege in community-based participatory research, researchers must acknowledge the diversity within racial and ethnic groups, acknowledge that race is a social construct and not a biologic determinant, and accept that outsiders cannot fully understand community and interpersonal dynamics.

Research on culture is not a new venture. Researchers' fascination with other cultures spans many decades. Generally, when the terms *culture* and *research* are used, many think of work done in faraway places. Research on culture, however, has been used to gain and discover knowledge about others in many locations, including close to home. It is essential in providing the scientific foundation for improved health care practices and policies. Unfortunately, research in the area of race, ethnicity, and nondominant cultures has been shaped by political expediency and cultural ideologies (Bhawuk & Triandis, 1996; Stanfield, 1993; Zane, Takeuchi, & Young, 1994).

Until recently, knowledge of the health status, characteristics, and behaviors of ethnic groups and women in the United States has been based on a few epidemiological activities and data that were designed with a focus not on minority groups but rather on the general population (U.S. Public Health Service, 1994; Williams, 1998; Zane et al., 1994). Minority populations and women often were inadequately or inaccurately represented in health research. Study samples either excluded them completely or included them in numbers too small to provide an understanding of the context of health and illness for these groups. For these reasons, questions have been raised about the validity and reliability of data on the health status and health-related behaviors of minority groups and women (Brooks, 1998a; Frayne, Burns, Hardt, Rosen, & Moskowitzet, 1996; McGraw, McKinlay, Crawford, Costa, & Cohen, 1992; Pinn, 1998; Williams, 1998). Advocacy groups working to improve the health of racial and ethnic minorities and women have recognized that, without data to document health problems, it is difficult to draw policymakers' attention and acquire the resources needed to tackle the problem (Carter-Pokras, 1998).

Historically, research on other cultures involved comparisons using middle-class European Americans as the standard or norm (Brookins, 1993). Researcher bias and inadequate data collection instruments, research designs, theories, and methodologies have been cited as reasons for the lack of empirical, realistic, and useful information on racial, ethnic, gender, and cultural differences (Carter-Pokras, 1998; McGraw et al., 1992; Meadow, 1998). Although improvements have been and continue to be made, data gaps and methodological issues remain in research on nondominant cultures and groups in the United States. This chapter provides a critical review of the research models and methodologies used in research on culture, gender, and health and their effect on the formation of explanations about human life, health, and policies.

Study of Culture

Emic and Etic Viewpoints

Culture is a very complex entity, and there is no one correct way to study it. In the study of culture, there are always at least two perspectives: the *emic,* which is the native's (insider) point of view and thus is culture specific, and the *etic,* which is the researcher's (outsider) view and thus is oriented to the researcher's personal or professional culture (Bhawuk & Triandis, 1996; Hughes, 1990; Stiens, 1990). The example of a Vietnamese woman who just delivered a beautiful healthy baby boy sheds light on the distinction between these perspectives; the mother's reaction puzzled the delivery nurse attendant. The new mother ignored the baby when the nurse presented him to her. On the hospital records, the nurse described the mother's response as "Bonding—0."

The nurse and mother had different views about the event. The nurse, from her etic viewpoint, observed the event as reflecting a lack of caring and appreciation for the child, whereas the mother, from her insider (emic) point of view, considered this reaction to be a form of protection. Many Asian people believe that a baby is in grave danger when first born. To recognize the child's presence by fussing over it would bring too much attention that might place the baby in jeopardy, a concept related to the evil eye (Dresser, 1996). Both the emic and etic perspectives involve tradeoffs; the emic view provides the subjective experience but limits objectivity, whereas the etic view is farther from the actual experience of the phenomenon and may be more objective but loses the insider knowledge. The culturally sensitive health care provider must become skilled at understanding both the etic and the emic perspectives.

These two words also represent two distinct approaches to studying cultures. Researchers taking the emic (culture-specific) approach believe that each culture has unique ideas, behaviors, and concepts and that this uniqueness must be the focus of the study. Anthropologists predominantly follow this approach. An emic viewpoint is essential for understanding a culture from a personal perspective, but the findings of studies cannot be generalized or used to make cultural comparisons.

Researchers using the etic (general cultural) approach believe that cultures have both specific and universal dimensions and that both dimensions should be studied. This approach is followed mainly by cross-cultural social scientists such as anthropologists, sociologists, and psychologists. *Etics* are theoretical concepts that allow generalizations about relationships among variables across cultures (Bhawuk & Triandis, 1996).

In the study of cultural similarities and differences, the etic approach starts with a construct generated in the researcher's own culture and uses it to examine another culture. This approach imposes the construct developed in the researcher's culture on another and is referred to as *pseudoetic* or *imposed etic*. It allows researchers to find out how the original construct changes in the second culture—for example, by studying the growth and development of the children of Asian refugees by comparing them to U.S. standards of height, weight, and development.

An emic approach requires that the researcher start with a theoretical construct and identify the etic and emic aspects of the construct. Researchers use focus groups and local standards to develop measurement items for both aspects, providing equivalent measures of the theoretical construct (Triandis, 1994). An emic approach and perspective protect researchers against ethnocentrism, because "using a set of behavioral standards developed according to the norms of one culture to assess a client from another culture is a culture imposition based on ethnocentricity" (Kavanagh & Kennedy, 1992, p. 32).

The methods used to study cultures depend on the research question, the investigators' knowledge, the cultural acceptability of various techniques, the sophistication of the respondents, and many other variables (Bhawuk & Triandis, 1996; McGraw, et al., 1992; Stanfield, 1993). In general, researchers should use emic approaches such as ethnographic techniques, systematic observations, and content analyses when they know relatively little about the culture and seek to obtain a holistic picture. Data collection using these strategies tends to be maximally appropriate (Bhawuk & Triandis, 1996; Facio, 1993), but "although the data have depth and are usually collected ethically, one cannot really depend upon the findings" (Bhawuk & Triandis, 1996, p. 32) to provide a full picture or explanation of the culture being studied.

Experimental designs using etic approaches such as surveys and questionnaires are useful when the researcher has limited goals, knows a great deal about the culture, and has some well-developed theory to test. However, these methods are often culturally inappropriate and obtrusive (Malpass, 1977). Even if surveys accomplish what they try to do, they often do not greatly increase the researcher's understanding of a culture (Bhawuk & Triandis, 1996; Patton, 1993). Survey analyses tend to oversimplify many of the differences among population groups and subgroups, resulting in false homogeneity within the group; all members are presumed to think alike (A. W. Smith, 1993). Bhawuk and Triandis (1996) suggest that combined etic and emic approaches are the most useful:

> Unstructured interviewing, questionnaires based on the interviews, and validation with some method are the essential elements of studies of subjective culture. The amount of work required is great, but so is the payoff in terms of understanding cultural similarities and differences. (p. 32)

Harmful Research Models

Research models that portray people from other cultures or diverse backgrounds as inferior prevent the development of appropriate, culturally sensitive, and useful intervention strategies. White, middle-class value systems often have been reflected in research regarding racial and ethnic groups. As Stanfield (1993) states it, "The act of imposing the experiences of the dominant on the subordinate as a logic for explaining their attributes and ignoring the relevance of subordinate experiences for explaining those of the dominant extend the parameters of folk racial ideologies" (p. 34). Historically, three harmful models have guided research regarding racial and ethnic groups (Sue, Arredondo, & McDavis, 1992; Sue & Sue, 1990):

1. *Inferiority or pathological model:* The basic premise is that minorities are lower on the evolutionary scale (more primitive) and are more inherently pathological.
2. *Deficiency model:* This model assumes that African Americans and other racial and ethnic minorities are deficient in desirable genes. The differences between White people and minorities are the reflection of biological and genetic inferiority.
3. *Deficiency or disadvantage model:* This model blames members of the minority culture for their problems.

These models have resulted in a data and research base that have perpetuated a view that minorities are inherently pathological, perpetuated racist research practices, and provided an excuse not to take social action to rectify inequities in the system (Katz, 1985; Stanfield & Dennis, 1993; Sue et al., 1992).

All too often, society's view of minorities emphasizes deprivation and weakness: "One of the great difficulties with formulations like culturally deprived, disadvantaged, culturally handicapped, impoverished, etc., is that they connote inadequacy, rather than present a rounded picture of the culture which would have to include strengths as well as deficiencies" (Ayers, 1967, p. i). This deficit orientation and context deny that other cultures have their own unique integrity and affix the problem within the disadvantaged person.

The U.S. health care delivery system and policies targeting minorities have historically used the harmful models, reflected in poorer outcomes of care and services. The importance of race and gender often has been downplayed or negated in health analysis, which claims that minorities experience poor health and premature death because of pathological behaviors. The blaming-the-victim approach is reminiscent of earlier justifications used to defend health care policies that denied health care to African Americans during a time when racism was sanctioned by law in a majority of states. At that time, people thought that minorities were dying because they were not seeking standard medical care or treatment, so a commitment to care for them would be wasted (Smith, 1998). Unfortunately, variations of these models and arguments continue to undergird research on race, ethnicity, gender, and culture as well as health policies.

New Research Models

New and conceptually different models of research are emerging that provide more realistic knowledge about nondominant cultures. Such models include the culturally different model (Katz, 1985), the multicultural model (Johnson, 1990), and the culturally pluralistic model (Ponterotto & Casas, 1991). These models have several premises and assumptions in common:

- To be culturally different does not equate with deviance, pathology, or inferiority.
- Racial and ethnic minorities are bicultural and function in at least two different cultural contexts.
- Biculturality is a positive and desirable quality that enriches the full range of human potential.
- Individuals are viewed in relationship to their environment and the larger social forces (e.g., racism, oppression, discrimination); the individual or minority group is not the obstacle.

Ethnographic research design uses the principles and methods of cultural anthropology to study aspects of daily life within a social group. Ethnographic research is descriptive qualitative research, and its analytic procedures are open ended. Its focus tends to be activity based, and it occurs in social settings. It requires both emic and etic descriptions and a cyclical collection and comparison of data.

Culturally linked research outcomes enable service providers to build on the strengths of the individual's culture and to use the unique resources of that culture to effect a solution. The radical demographic changes in this country and in the global society require that occupational therapists and occupational therapy assistants become proactive in establishing new models of research for the study of nondominant racial, ethnic, and gender groups to encourage refreshing and more adequate logic of inquiry.

Epistemological Issues in Research on Culture

Moving forward in research on race, ethnicity, gender, and culture requires more than the reconsideration of concepts and models. It must begin with the review, questioning, and finally creation of epistemologies to ground theories and facilitate their testing. For the purposes of research, *epistemology* includes not only the methods used to obtain knowledge but also the ethics, human values, and politics governing how researchers structure relationships with collaborators and with participants (Stanfield, 1993).

Researchers often are unaware of the racial, gender, and cultural misperceptions they bring to research. Those inaccurate perceptions and associated ethnocentric biases influence what research questions are asked, how studies are designed, which research is funded, and how results are interpreted, disseminated, and applied. In addition to ethnocentric biases, other problems associated with conducting effective research addressing race, ethnicity, gender, and culture include the questionable validity of racial and ethnic classifications, methodological errors associated with population sampling, and misinterpretation of findings. Whether researchers take a quantitative or a qualitative approach, there are certain epistemological universals such as the fallacy of homogeneity and monolithic identity in research on race, ethnicity, gender, and culture that must be considered in the design and execution of research processes.

Concepts of *Race* and *Ethnicity*

For decades, data have been collected on health care services use by racial and ethnic group (see Chapter 11). The use of such groups to categorize data assumes that standard, reliable, and valid definitions of race and ethnicity exist and that these definitions are used consistently. The validity of information provided for racial and ethnic groups in public health research and intervention often is taken for granted, and these data are routinely used with little attention to the underlying measurement problems for racial categories or the appropriateness of the ways the data will be used. In health research, race, ethnicity, and gender are rarely studied, yet they are frequently cited as a causal factor (Carter-Pokras, 1998; Centers for Disease Control and Prevention [CDC], 1993).

Race is a term often used but rarely defined. It can incorporate biological, social, and cultural characteristics. It can refer to both genetic and behavioral traits (Schulman, Rubenstein, Chesley, & Eisenberg, 1995). When race is used as a variable in research, there is a tendency to assume that the obtained results are a manifestation of the biology of racial differences. Using race as a variable implies that a genetic reason may explain differences in the incidence, severity, or outcome of medical conditions. Researchers, perhaps without intention, lead readers to assume that certain racial groups have a special predisposition, risk, or susceptibility to the condition studied. Because this assumption seldom is warranted, comparisons by racial group represent a subtle form of racism (Osborne & Feit, 1992). Many studies use race as a proxy for other socioeconomic factors not collected in the research effort. The question to ask is, Is race being used as a biogenetic variable or as a proxy variable for environmental variables?

Race is an unscientific, socially constructed taxonomy that is fluid and without boundaries (CDC, 1993; Feinleib, 1993). It is based on an ideology that views some human population groups as inherently superior to others based on external physical characteristics or geographic origin (Williams, Lavizzo-Mourey, & Warren, 1994). The concept of race is socially meaningful, but it has limited biological significance. Racial or ethnic variations in health status result primarily from exposure or vulnerability to behavioral, psychosocial, material, and environmental risk factors and resources (Scribner, 1996; Williams et al., 1994; Wray, 1992). The scientific pitfalls that stand in the way of ethnic research are formidable, because race and ethnicity are highly correlated with many social, economic, and political factors (Osborne & Feit, 1992).

> *There are ethical problems with the search for genetic reasons to explain certain types of diseases.*

There are ethical problems with the search for genetic reasons to explain certain types of diseases. Kumanyika and Golden (1991) suggest that genetic explanations of difference can play into stereotypes and may even be interpreted as reasons for not addressing environmental risk factors. Environmental explanations may be viewed as evidence of negative lifestyle practices, which are the responsibility of the individual. But environmental explanations of racial and cultural differences also may be indications of institutional racism.

If race suggests biological differences and ethnicity suggests nonbiological differences, then the value of race information in health research is limited. Ethnicity is important, but only as a marker of social, environmental, and cultural risks. A *risk factor* is an aspect of personal behavior or lifestyle, an environmental exposure, or an inborn or inherited characteristic associated with an increased occurrence of disease or other health-related event or condition. In contrast, a *risk marker* indicates the increased likelihood of the presence of a particular risk factor but is not itself related to the disease or condition. The risk factor is the true cause, whereas the risk marker is an indicator of an association but is not itself the cause (CDC, 1993). For example, the risk factor for sickle cell anemia is the presence of hemoglobin S, and a risk marker belongs to African Americans. For a relatively small number of diseases and conditions, genetic factors related to race are important (e.g., sickle cell anemia, gall bladder cancer, hepatitis B and its sequelae). For other diseases and conditions, however, race is at best a proxy measure for factors related to class, lifestyle, and socioeconomic status (Feinleib, 1993; Hahn, 1992; Osborne & Feit, 1992; Scribner, 1996; Williams et al., 1994; Wray, 1992).

Information on race and ethnicity is used in public health research for the purposes of describing health status, designing and targeting intervention programs, and ensuring equality in health status for all Americans (U.S. Public Health Service, 1994). Schulman and colleagues (1995) suggest that health services researchers focus instead on nonracial socioeconomic characteristics that might be both more informative and more useful in guiding policy formation.

Current Race and Ethnicity Categories

Because the measurement of race and ethnicity is not scientific, rules are needed to guide assignment to race categories so that the resulting statistics can be understood. Using race as a mean of classifying the population has a long statistical tradition in the United States. For more than 20 years, the Office of Management and Budget's (OMB's) Statistical Policy Directive No. 15, *Race and Ethnic Standards for Federal Statistics and Administrative Reporting,* has provided a common language for uniformity and comparability in the collection and use of data on race and ethnicity by federal agencies. Racial and ethnic categories are required in all federally sponsored data collection and reporting activities involving questions on race and ethnicity. Although most public health data and epidemiological research activities include OMB standard race and ethnicity categories, they are not universally used.

After an extensive and lengthy review process, in October 1997 the OMB revised the standards for classification of race and ethnicity in federal data. The standards have five categories for race—(a) American Indian or Alaska Native, (b) Asian, (c) Black or African American, (d) Native Hawaiian or Other Pacific Islander, and (e) White—and two categories for ethnicity—Hispanic or Latino and Not Hispanic or Latino (see Table 21.1). This classification is a sociopolitical construct designed for collecting data on the race and ethnicity of broad population groups in this country and are not anthropologically or scientifically based (OMB, 1997).

Although the OMB standard categories are valuable in promoting uniform and comparable health data, they are broad, and some encompass many subpopulations (Evinger, 1995). Use of the OMB standards may mask major differences within racial or ethnic populations (U.S. Public Health Service, 1994; Yu & Liu, 1994). For example, the National Center for Health Statistics (NCHS) collects and publishes data on births and deaths in the United States; however, ethnic identifiers for Asians and Pacific Islanders include only Japanese, Chinese, and Filipino (NCHS, 2007). No codes exist for the fastest growing and most recent Asian immigrants and refugees, such as Koreans, Vietnamese, Cambodians, Hmongs, Laotians, East Indians, Thais, Burmese, Malaysians, and Indonesians. General grouping of

Table 21.1. Office of Management and Budget Standards for the Classification of Federal Data on Race and Ethnicity

Construct	Category	Description
Race	American Indian or Alaska Native	A person having origins in any of the original peoples of North and South America (including Central America) who maintains tribal affiliation or community attachment
	Asian	A person having origins in any of the original peoples of the Far East, Southeast Asia, or the Indian subcontinent, including, for example, Cambodia, China, India, Japan, Korea, Malaysia, Pakistan, the Philippine Islands, Thailand, and Vietnam
	Black or African American	A person having origins in any of the Black racial groups of Africa. Terms such as *Haitian* or *Negro* can be used in addition to *Black* or *African American*
	Native Hawaiian or Other Pacific Islander	A person having origins in any of the original peoples of Hawaii, Guam, Samoa, or other Pacific Islands
	White	A person having origins in any of the original peoples of Europe, the Middle East, or North Africa
Ethnicity	Hispanic or Latino	A person of Cuban, Mexican, Puerto Rican, South or Central American, or Spanish culture or origin, regardless of race; the term *Spanish origin* can be used in addition to *Hispanic* or *Latino*
	Not Hispanic or Latino	

Note. From Recommendations From the Interagency Committee for the Review of the Racial and Ethnic Standards to the Office of Management and Budget Concerning Changes to the Standards for the Classification of Federal Data on Race and Ethnicity, 62 *Fed. Reg.* 36,874 (July 9, 1997).

ethnic populations does not allow researchers to identify subgroups that may be at risk, leaving their members underserved.

In addition, people of mixed racial and ethnic backgrounds have difficulty responding to the standard OMB classification. With interracial marriage, the question of how to classify people whose parents are of different races continues to be debated. Multiracial people and parents of multiracial children currently are asked to choose a single racial category. Proponents of a multiracial category argue that the current categories force people to deny the racial heritage of one parent when they must choose one race, adversely affecting self-esteem, sense of family, pride, and psychological well-being. Users of health data, however, argue that a multiracial category would result in data that are not useful in analyzing the health status of population groups historically at risk for certain diseases, such as hypertension in the African American population. Furthermore, a multiracial category with no races indicated would become increasingly problematic for the offspring of parents who are themselves multiracial. Given ongoing demographic changes, racial and ethnicity classification questions will apply to an ever-increasing proportion of the population (Evinger, 1995; Williams, 1998).

The new OMB (1997) standards recommend that self-identification be used where possible, that people be allowed to report more than one race, and that Hispanic ethnicity be asked separately from race. The OMB has developed guidelines for the implementation of the new standards for racial and ethnic data, including comparisons of data collected using the old and new standards.

Assignment of Race and Ethnicity Categories

Another problem with measuring race and ethnicity that has a significant effect on the quality of cultural data involves errors in the reporting of race and ethnicity. Race and ethnicity are assigned through either self-identification or assignment by another person based on his or her perceptions, and both methods, but particularly the latter, present risks for reliability of data. Methodological research has revealed inaccuracies in the classification and coding of race and ethnicity on vital records (U.S. Public Health Service, 1994).

Birth certificates in the United States have never listed the race of the child but instead included the race of both parents. Before 1989, the NCHS used an algorithm to determine the race of a newborn. The person completing the birth certificate was to elicit information from the parents and to provide the race of both parents. If both parents were White, the child was considered to be White. If the father was White and the mother belonged to a different race, the child was given the race of the mother. But if the father was non-White, the child was assigned the race of the father. For example, if one parent was Hawaiian and the other White, then the child was Hawaiian. Thus, unlike the assignment of race for all other racial groups, the child was White only if both parents were White.

If the race of one parent was unknown, the race of the other parent was assigned. If racial information on both parents was lacking, the child was assigned the race listed in the preceding birth record in the NCHS computer file. NCHS no longer reports vital statistics by the race of the child, instead using the mother's race. The race of the father is used only if the mother's race is unknown. However, the ethnicity of a child, both before and after 1989, is determined by the ethnicity of the mother (Hahn, 1992).

Respondent self-report is not an option on the death certificate, so officials such as funeral directors, medical examiners, and coroners who complete these forms make a decision based on their own judgment without necessarily ascertaining the race of the deceased from the next of kin. Even though consulting the next

of kin is recommended, many funeral directors consider requesting racial information to be an imposition on the family (Williams, 1998). The last name of the individual commonly is used to determine ethnicity of the person.

Williams (1998) found a discrepancy between observed and self-reported race
in a 1978 Health Interview Survey. Williams compared the racial information
reported by interviewers with that reported by respondents. Interviewers classified
as White 6% of people who reported themselves to be Black, 29% of those who
reported themselves to be Asian, 62% of those who reported themselves to be
American Indian, and 80% of those who reported themselves to be Other.

The reliability of self-identification of race and ethnicity also is questionable.
Studies have shown that people's perception of their own race and ethnicity changes
over time (CDC, 1993; LaVeist, Sellers, Brown, & Nickerson, 1997). The most dramatic evidence of change in self-identification has been among Native Americans.
Between 1960 and 1990, the self-identified American Indian population experienced a sixfold increase. This growth cannot be explained by an increase in birth
rate or international migration; according to Williams (1998), "it appears to reflect
a change in self-definition, with more adults of mixed ancestry identifying themselves as American Indian" (p. 4).

In summary, gatherers of statistical data provide different options for responses to race and ethnicity questions and use different reporting methods (self-report,
next of kin identification, and algorithms) for each data set, potentially leading to
conflicting results. Researchers must identify comparison data sets early in a
research project so that data are collected appropriately. Current approaches to race
identification for statistical purposes expect identification of one race per person,
forcing people of mixed ancestry to make a choice and increasing the number of
respondents who identify their race as Other. In addition, people may change their
reported race over time as they identify more closely with one race or the other or
when there are political, social, or economic reasons to do so.

Methodological Errors in Population Sampling

Too many studies claim to examine U.S. samples but use White populations and
provide short notes essentially explaining that the inclusion of people of color
would just complicate the analysis (Stanfield, 1993). It has been viewed as both
appropriate and normative for social researchers to select male Euro-American
populations or samples for studies with little or no regard for populations or samples made up of people of color or women.

In selecting a sample, quantitative researchers should be concerned about the
representativeness of the people they choose to interview or study. It is difficult in
epidemiological studies of racial and ethnic groups to defend the selection of
respondents using less than scientifically rigorous sampling methods and still

obtain the critical approval of statisticians who are accustomed to using conventional sampling schema. Thus, insufficient attention has been directed to improving the ability of basic health surveys and epidemiological activities to develop strategies for ensuring that sufficient numbers of minorities and women are included in study samples to support estimates (U.S. Public Health Service, 1994).

The issue of sampling from small populations is one reason that no large-scale epidemiological study has been conducted with racial or ethnic minorities. Most large-scale studies include only small samples of minority group members. Large-scale studies usually weight the data to the population figures of the community or geographic region or the nation as whole. This weighting may disguise the fact that the ethnic samples actually are quite small. Small samples do not provide sufficient statistical power to detect significant health needs or conduct complex multivariate analyses to identify high-risk subgroups. When a large sample includes Asian Americans, Hispanics, and American Indians, they often are collapsed into one category. Because these groups are quite heterogeneous, the use of a general category makes it difficult to assess needs accurately (Andersen, 1993; Stanfield, 1993; Zane et al., 1994).

According to McGraw and colleagues (1992), a valid, reliable, and efficient research study can be mounted only when researchers pay attention to the procedures used to identify and locate study subjects. Because numbers of minority group members may be limited and highly dispersed in any given geographic area, existing sampling frames can misidentify or misrepresent members of some minority groups. Census data often undercount minority populations (CDC, 1993). Commercial directories and government lists omit many dwelling units and multiple-dwelling-unit structures in low-income, urban minority communities. Some researchers have resorted to the use of telephone or ethnic directories or marketing firms to ascertain the universe of ethnic populations (Zane et al., 1994). But the accuracy and differential biases of these lists must be addressed if the surveys are to be credible.

> *Because numbers of minority group members may be limited and highly dispersed in any given geographic area, existing sampling frames can misidentify or misrepresent members of some minority groups.*

Generally in health research, the sample includes only individuals who are receiving health services. Data based on clinic populations offer insight into the health problems of the individuals who use the services but no information as to how representative the clinic population is of the ethnic community (Yu & Liu, 1994). It also is well documented that ethnic groups delay seeking professional care for their health problems (Brooks, 1998a; Ponce, 1992; Zane et al., 1994), and

because of this pattern of behavior, researchers often conclude that ethnic populations underutilize health services. Instead, they should be asking, Is the sample size
sufficient to generalize about a whole ethnic population? Why do certain groups use
or not use health services? Are there differences in need among ethnically diverse
groups? Why are services underutilized? Is there a cultural mismatch between those
in need and the service strategies used?

Frayne and colleagues (1996) reviewed original medical studies published
from 1989 to 1991 to determine how often non-English-speaking (NES) people
were excluded. They surveyed all investigators ($N = 216$) whose methodologies
involved direct interaction between researchers and participants. Of the respondents, 22% had included NES people, 16% had not considered the issue during the
study design process, and 32% thought that including NES people had affected
their study results. Among those who excluded NES people, half (51%) said they
did not think of the issue, and others cited translation issues and the difficulty of
recruiting bilingual staff. The remaining 35% indicated that no NES people were
in their study areas. Frayne and colleagues conclude that NES people often are
excluded through oversight. The exclusion of non-English-speaking people from
provider–patient communication studies greatly limits the generalizability of
the findings.

In 1987, a policy encouraging the inclusion of women and minorities was first
published, and guidelines on the inclusion of women and minorities in clinical
studies have been in place at the National Institutes of Health (NIH) since 1989
(Brooks, 1998b). Pinn (1998) describes a 1990 General Accounting Office (GAO)
investigation into the implementation of the guidelines at NIH. The results indicated that implementation of the policy was lacking, slow, and not well communicated; that gender analysis was not implemented; and that the effect of this policy
could not be determined. The GAO study also indicated that differences existed in
the implementation of the policy and that not all institutes factored adherence to
these policies into the scientific merit review.

Following the 1990 GAO report and the establishment of the Office of
Research on Women's Health (ORWH), which has a legislative mandate to ensure
that women and minorities are included in NIH-supported clinical research, the
NIH strengthened and revitalized its inclusion guidelines. The ORWH is responsible for overseeing and monitoring the implementation of the guidelines in NIH-
supported clinical trials to ensure adequate representation.

In a report of a task force on minority health data, the U.S. Public Health
Service (1994) said that "oversampling strategies may work for some populations;
but this approach is not a panacea and a multifaceted strategy is needed" (p. 40).
Other approaches involve adding minority group follow-up surveys to existing survey mechanisms and conducting special targeted surveys like the Hispanic Health

and Nutrition Examination Survey (CDC, 2007) or the survey of American Indians and Alaska Natives (U.S. Public Health Services, 1994). In large-scale registries or community-based epidemiological research studies, it may be necessary to add study sites that include adequate numbers of minority group members. For some small subpopulations, smaller scale targeted epidemiological studies may offer the best data development strategy (U.S. Public Health Service, 1994).

Researcher Bias

Another important concern is cultural similarities or disparities between the researcher and the study population. Researchers often are unaware of the racial and cultural misperceptions they bring to research. For example, in the case of research with Asian American populations, Yu and Liu (1994) described the obstacles to studies:

> At the level of the individual investigator, lack of communication between qualified mainstream and Asian Pacific American health investigators, and intense competition among trained Asian Pacific American researchers for limited resources as well as the "town-and-gown" conflict between "community advocates and "academics" on the research objectives constitute the major obstacles to studies on the health of Asian Pacific Americans. (p. 46)

Researchers who are members of dominant groups rarely reflect on the effects of their racial, ethnic, gender, and cultural identities and consciousness on what they see and interpret in their studies. By constructing what they believe to be value-neutral methods of data collection and interpretation, they unwittingly rationalize and legitimate their claims rather than acknowledge the intrusions of their life histories and cognitive styles in the research process (Andersen, 1993; Stanfield, 1993).

Study across race, class, and gender lines poses unique methodological problems for both researchers and participants. The problems inherent in doing research in ethnic communities are compounded by the social distance imposed by class and race relations when interviewers are White and middle class and interviewees are not (Andersen, 1993; Facio, 1993). Community leaders often see researchers as exploiters whose studies are divorced from real issues and real-life problems (Zane et al., 1994).

Research data also are limited by interviewer reliability. Often multiple interviewers or investigators are involved in assessments, and different interviewers create biases, especially when they must rate participants on a number of dimensions. Some investigators may be more thorough in their assessments than others, and some participants may describe their problems more openly with some researchers than with others (McGraw et al., 1992; Williams, 1998; Zane et al., 1994). Some studies note that investigators are more effective when they reside in the study neighborhoods or at least share the culture under study (Aneshensel, Becerra, Fielder, & Schuler, 1989; Salber & Beza, 1980). As McGraw and colleagues (1992) observes, "Those who study minorities can encounter problems in establishing rapport with the community, especially when the survey work is conducted over an extended period of time in a specific geographic site" (p. 284). Some have found that investigators' ethnicity had significant effects on responses to racially sensitive questions (Campbell, 1981; Cotter, Cohen, & Coulter, 1982; Schaeffer, 1980). The beliefs and values of researchers shape the answers to the questions more than any objective data that might be collected and analyzed (Duarte & Rice, 1994).

Memories of the Tuskegee Syphilis Study and the health consequences associated with the use of Diethylstibestrol (DES) and thalidomide by pregnant women have created biases and barriers against medical research for many Americans, especially members of minority populations and women (Brooks, 1998a; Pinn, 1998). Mistrust of the health system and White researchers has accounted for some of the underrepresentation of minorities in clinical trials (Meadow, 1998). According to Brooks (1998a), several studies show differences in attitude toward medical research between African Americans and White people. In "Barriers to Black Women's Participation in Cancer Clinical Trials" (Mouton, Harris, Rovi, Solorzano, & Johnson, 1997), African American women were more likely than Whites to feel that clinical research was unethical. They also were more likely to feel that the researcher did not care about them and that by participating in research, they would not have access to better care. They indicated that they would be more likely to participate in a clinical trial if the researcher also was African American. Another study found that African American men held similar attitudes (Robinson, Ashley, & Haynes, 1996); these men also lacked confidence in doctors with non-American accents.

Misinterpretation of Findings

Interpretation of differences among racial and ethnic populations can be problematic. Misinterpretation of these differences raises barriers to the development of new knowledge and more effective services. For example, results of research on race and ethnicity often overemphasize between-group differences and underemphasize within-group differences (Smith, 1993). Racial and ethnic data analysis and the interpretation of results must consider the social context of the participants studied (McGraw et al., 1992; Stanfield, 1993).

Cultural standards of data generalization are the basis of researcher presumptions about nondominant racial and ethnic and female populations. It has been the norm to assume that male Eurocentric empirical realities can be generalized to explain the realities of people of color and women. For decades, researchers using Eurocentric norms have applied Eurocentric concepts of family, deviance, social movements, psychological development, behavior, stratification, health, and even spirituality to the experiences of people of color (Stanfield, 1993), but the realities of people of color are not similarly considered as legitimate standards of generalization to Eurocentric realities:

> It is rare for mainstream scholars to select empirical observations about people of color, such as religious behaviors or female headed family structure, to explain Eurocentric realities. Yet, researchers have relabeled "deviant and pathological" patterns of the poor and of people of color and normalized such trends when they become dominant middle-class Euro-American patterns. (Stanfield, 1993, p. 28)

Inadequate Measurement Instruments

The measurement of similarities and differences across cultures relies on the development and use of standardized instruments. Medical technology can reliably detect physical disease, but cultural factors can constrain the ways individuals define and evaluate their health problems, present their problems to the physician, and seek help for their problems. Researchers, assuming that concepts and measurements of health and illness are universal, have used standardized instruments without assessing the reliability and validity of these instruments for specific ethnic, racial, or gender populations. Because cultural groups vary in their definitions of normality and abnormality, and because these variations affect models of health and illness, this assumption is unwarranted (Zane et al., 1994). Some factors that vary by culture include types and parameters of stressors, coping mechanisms, personality patterns, language systems, and expression of illness. Without proper consideration of these issues, practitioners often make errors in diagnosis, assessment, and treatment, as well as in their understanding of the group being studied.

If the study population does not speak the same primary language as the researcher or interviewer (usually English), the instrument must be translated into another language, which can introduce problems. Because of the existence of diverse languages and dialects within languages, researchers must pay attention to regional and ethnic differences in language usage when translating instruments. In one major health study, an instrument was translated from English to Spanish (Yu & Liu, 1994). In field use of the Spanish instrument, the researchers noted that respondents were scoring very low on the question, "How often do you kiss your child?" After checking and double-checking the original questionnaire, someone checked the translation and found that the translated question read, "How often do you kiss your puppy?" Attention must be given to establishing equivalency among different dialect and language versions of an instrument.

Besides translation considerations, researchers also must be concerned with conceptual, scale, and norm equivalence among instruments (McGraw et al., 1992; Zane et al., 1994). For example, do ethnic minorities and Whites think of well-being, depression, or self-esteem in the same way? Are recent immigrants or individuals not educated in the United States familiar with the practice of answering survey questions using responses on a scale from strongly agree to strongly disagree or a true–false dichotomy? Are the standards of weight and height developed among White Americans suitable for Asian Americans?

If a large proportion of the study population is bilingual or uses multiple languages, then researchers should use bilingual or multilingual interviewing staff. This strategy is preferred over conducting interviews through interpreters, a procedure that severely compromises the quality of the data (Frayne et al., 1996; McGraw et al., 1992).

Limitations in Health Data Systems

In promoting the health of the U.S. population, reliable and timely data are crucial. The U.S. Public Health Service relies on a wide variety of data sources. Yet limitations exist in current efforts to collect and provide accurate data on ethnic-minority populations and subgroups (Feinleib, 1993; McGraw et al., 1992; U.S. Public Health Service, 1994; Yu & Liu, 1994). Carter-Pokras (1998) identifies the following possible reasons for this lack of data:

- Data may not have been collected from a national data system.
- National data systems may have insufficient numbers of a particular group to allow reliable estimates.
- Puerto Rico, the U.S. Virgin Islands, and the U.S. public insular areas (i.e., U.S. Pacific territories, including American Samoa, Commonwealth of the Northern Marianas, and Guam) generally are not included in national data systems.
- Only racial and ethnic-minority groups with documented differences from the total population are included in national data surveys.

In general, national health surveys have oversampled for African American and White populations but not for others (Feinleib, 1993). Delgado and Estrada (1993) examined 21 major health data systems of the U.S. Department of Health and Human Services and found that data on Hispanics were not included in 6 of their national health data collection systems, including the Medicare statistical system. Even when collected, data on Hispanic subpopulations were found in few of the systems; only the National Vital Health Statistics system collected data for all major Hispanic subpopulations.

Routine health collection data systems tend to focus exclusively on specific diseases that are well defined in terms of pathological manifestations and clinical diagnosis. They cannot address broader concepts such as health status, health behaviors, or health utilization. These data almost are always collected in selected locations and therefore are of limited use in providing a national picture of the health status of ethnic populations. Missing data are a common problem in public records, especially data on income, occupational status, and education level, and these three variables are important in determining whether differences in health status among groups can be attributed to ethnicity or socioeconomic status. Other variables critical to understanding the health status of ethnic populations may not even be requested on health clinic forms, such as primary language, place of birth, and generation since immigration (U.S. Public Health Service, 1994; Yu & Liu, 1994). Estimates based on data systems that do not routinely use self-identification to collect racial and ethnic data (e.g., the system for mortality data) may significantly underestimate the burden of disease, disability, and death in certain racial and ethnic groups.

Racial and ethnic data are merely descriptive, however, and do not get at the underlying reasons behind the health disparities (Carter-Pokeras, 1998). Additional information on socioeconomic status, program participation, behavioral risk factors, cultural differences, birthplace and generation since immigration, and the effects of racism and discrimination are needed.

The importance of obtaining health data for understudied populations such as women and minorities was reflected in the passage of the Disadvantaged Minority Health Improvement Act of 1990 (P.L. 101-527) and the 1991 Cooperative Agreement issued by the CDC to the Asian and Pacific Islander American Health Forum and the National Coalition of Hispanic Health and Human Services Organizations to advance the understanding of the health of racial and ethnic populations and subpopulations, authorized under Section 306 (42 U.S. 242k) of the Public Health Service Act. The latter agreement provides unprecedented opportunities for researchers to analyze previously collected health data, improve existing research methodologies, and test innovative methodological techniques for gathering information on special populations.

In October 1997, the secretary of the U.S. Department of Health and Human Services issued an inclusion policy—Inclusion of Race and Ethnicity in U.S. Department of Health and Human Services' Data Collection Activities (Office of Minority Health, 2007)—that requires all data systems funded and maintained by the federal government to collect racial and ethnic data. Public hearings have been held to address the needs of Puerto Rico, Virgin Islands, and the U.S. public insular areas. The OMB and the U.S. Public Health Service have begun concerted efforts to standardize data collection, improve funding for data systems, and strengthen the quality of data to meet the objectives of *Healthy People 2010* (U.S. Department of Health & Human Services, 2000).

Moral Dilemmas

Research on race, ethnicity, and gender involves several moral dilemmas. According to Stanfield (1993), who examined the history of race and ethnicity as a field of study, the research processes used in the social sciences involve power relationships between dominant (researcher) and subordinate (participant) parties that can be studied empirically, like any other form of social inequality. Research on people of color has sometimes involved researchers asking participants embarrassing and inappropriate questions that the researcher never would answer himself or herself and certainly would not ask his or her own relatives, friends, or colleagues. Research on poor people in which participants receive services in return for participating in a research study or clinical practice takes advantage of their marginal resources and communities by developing an exploitative exchange relationship (e.g., exposure of their bodies in exchange for free access to teaching hospital clinics). Stanfield calls such abuse of participants "legal unethical behaviors."

Yu and Liu (1994) observe that new immigrants and refugees from politically oppressive regimes in Asia understandably associate surveys and research with police interrogations and punitive political actions. They may refuse to give written consent because they are unable to write their own name; others simply cannot understand why they must sign their names to answer a series of questions. Does the signature on the consent form violate the promise of anonymity and confidentiality?

Status of Research on Cultural Competence

Contrary to popular perception, research on cultural competence is ongoing and is of growing interest to the health services research community. Few studies have assessed outcomes based on culturally competent interventions, however, and research does not exist for every population or every type of culturally competent intervention. Most of this research examines the effect of language or communication barriers (Fortier & Bishop, 2004). Although a high level of interest is in the results of research on culturally competent interventions, several methodological challenges exist in conducting such research. According to Fortier and Bishop (2004), the Research Advisory Committee (a 30-member group of researchers, policymakers, and health care providers convened by the Agency for Healthcare Research and Quality [AHRQ] and the Office of Minority Health [OMH] to examine how cultural competence affects health care delivery and health outcomes) identified four major challenges in this type of research:

1. Developing standardized definitions of interventions
2. Developing standardized evaluation measures
3. Constructing culturally competent instruments
4. Establishing secondary data sources with uniform racial, ethnic, and language data.

Some of these challenges are unique to specific interventions, but most are similar to those encountered in designing empirical studies on other emerging, multifaceted health interventions. The literature on culturally competent interventions that might be correlated with improved health care delivery and health outcomes strongly highlights a lack of consistent parameters, standards, and definitions in individual activities (Health Resources and Services Administration [HRSA], 2004). This variation makes comparisons between studies and generalizability impractical and unworkable. Work, therefore, is needed on establishing theoretical models, research instruments, and data sources that define and enable the measurement of cultural competence (Fortier & Bishop, 2004).

Designing quantitative studies to explore the link between culturally competent interventions and health and health care delivery outcomes involves several concerns. What sample size would be required to compare generic clinical communication training, health promotion program, or health worker encounters with a tailored program with culturally competent elements? It is important to identify the change agent within each intervention, typically the provider of services. Thus, a researcher must have a large sample size of providers with and without training in providing culturally competent interventions to improve the power and generalizability of the study (Fortier & Bishop, 2004; HRSA, 2004; Issel, 2004). Treatment settings must be able to accommodate this type of study. Study instruments that are culturally competent represent another challenge; currently, no instruments exist to measure standard interventions, yet such tools are necessary to compare the effect of culturally sensitive programs and services with standard programs and services.

There are multiple sources of data on intervention, including health maintenance organizations, federal and state health and human services agencies, major literature databases, private and independent foundations, and health policy organizations and associations. Many of these data sets are limited in value, however, because they do not include the race, ethnicity, and language characteristics of patients (Tashiro, 2005). Many organizations and agencies do not collect this information for fear of being perceived as discriminatory, especially if prior data revealed disparities in care and outcomes (Fortier & Bishop, 2004). Because data on race, ethnicity, and language are not collected in a standardized way, comparability is often compromised (Keppel et al., 2005; Ploeg & Perrin, 2004).

Another overarching concern is the cultural appropriateness of data collection methods and the cultural competence of data collectors and interpreters. Culture, language, and ethnicity influence the development of assessment tools and the responses of individuals to survey questions and inquiries (Issel, 2004). Data collectors must clearly explain to patients the rationales for data collection activities for both administrative and research purposes. Researchers need to expand their data collection to include questions on ancestry, migration history, and language. Patients could be informed, for example, that language information is being collected to plan for and assess the availability of interpreter services: "They need to be attentive to the increasing heterogeneity of racial/ethnic groups and rethink the nature and types of research questions asked" (Chavez, Duran, Baker, Avila, & Wallerstein, 2003, p. 92).

Community representatives should be involved in the design of data collection instruments for use in program design, quality assessment, and research (Chavez et al., 2003). Their involvement may help attenuate attrition and mobility issues in long-term studies by identifying targeted populations who resist the concept of participatory research and individuals who have personal reasons for not wanting to participate in research studies (Chavez et al., 2003; Fortier & Bishop, 2004).

Researchers can use the research process and outcomes to mobilize and advocate for change to reduce health disparities and enhance race relations. Building true multicultural working relationships and, within a partnership mode, developing guidelines for data collection, analysis, publication, and dissemination of research findings can facilitate accurate and complete data gathering (Chavez et al., 2003; Minkler & Wallerstein, 2003).

The Research Advisory Committee (Fortier & Bishop, 2004) identified difficulties with funding and publication as challenges to research on cultural competence. They observed that funders and journal reviewers tended to lack familiarity with the effect of language and culture on health care delivery and that they viewed cultural competence research as being of marginal importance or involving high risk. Therefore, some funders may be unwilling to expend the amounts of money necessary to show linkages between culturally competent interventions and health outcomes, and journals may be unwilling to accept manuscripts. This committee warned researchers that cultural competence studies may be a high-risk undertaking.

Summary

One problem that contributes to service and health disparities in the United States is a lack of relevant research and data. Much of the research that has been conducted with racial and ethnic populations and women was done so without the consent, consultation, or participation of participants, and much of the resulting information never found its way back into targeted communities. The legacy of past research is not positive, and researchers' hidden agendas have challenged current researchers' ability to gain knowledge about others.

Distrust of research efforts is common in many communities. Overgeneralization from research findings has been a source of stereotyping, and classification of groups as Other in research findings is evidence of insensitivity to cultural differences. Extant research too often fails to consider culture as a variable. Funding sources historically have not been sensitive to the needs of the different cultural groups and continue to shy away from research on cultural competence.

Research methods that involve the community from planning to dissemination need to be developed and implemented. Researchers need a standardized infrastructure for the collection of data related to race, ethnicity, and language in order to promote comparability among data sets. New epistemological assumptions and methods that encourage refreshing and more adequate logic of inquiry are needed. Future research on race, ethnicity, gender, and culture must be designed and conducted on the basis of constructs identified by the people studied. Researchers need new ways of thinking and explaining the world of this century. The ability to understand the health and the people of the nation will depend on the strength and breadth of the research and data collection systems.

Reflection

- Develop a working plan for how you would involve clients from a culture other than your own in the development of a clinical research project.

- Select at least two culturally competent intervention strategies or activities. How would you compare their effectiveness in delivering culturally competent care and outcomes? What criteria would you use to measure their effectiveness?

References

Andersen, M. (1993). Studying across difference: Race, class, and gender in qualitative research. In J. Stanfield & R. Dennis (Eds.), *Race and ethnicity in research methods* (pp. 39–52). Newbury Park, CA: Sage.

Aneshensel, C. S., Becerra, R. M., Fielder, E. P., & Schuler, R. H. (1989). Participation of Mexican-American female adolescents in a longitudinal panel survey. *Public Opinion Quarterly, 47*, 567–575.

Ayers, G. E. (1967). *Rehabilitating the culturally disadvantaged*. Mankato, MN: Mankato State College.

Bhawuk, D., & Triandis, H. C. (1996). The role of culture theory in the study of culture and intercultural training. In D. Landis & R. S. Bhagat (Eds.), *Intercultural training* (2nd ed., pp. 17–34). Thousand Oaks, CA: Sage.

Brookins, G. K. (1993). Culture, ethnicity, and bicultural competence: Implications for children with chronic illness and disability. *Pediatrics, 91*, 1056–1062.

Brooks, J. (1998a, December/January). Cancer clinical trails: Barriers to African American participation. *Closing the Gap Newsletter*, p. 7.

Brooks, J. (1998b, December/January). Minority participation in clinical trials: The impact of the Tuskegee Syphilis Study. *Closing the Gap Newsletter*, p. 3.

Campbell, B. A. (1981). Race of interviewer effects among southern adolescents. *Public Opinion Quarterly, 45*, 231–244.

Carter-Pokras, O. (1998, August/September). How do we fill the data gap? *Closing the Gap Newsletter*, p. 8.

Centers for Disease Control and Prevention. (1993). *Race/ethnicity and public health statistics: An interactive case study* (Epidemiology Training Activity). Hyattsville, MD: Author.

Chavez, V., Duran, B., Baker, Q. E., Avila, M. M., & Wallerstein, N. (2003). The dance of race and privilege in community-based participatory research. In M. Minkler & N. Wallerstein (Eds.), *Community-based participatory research for health* (pp. 81–97). San Francisco: Jossey-Bass.

Copage, Eric V. (1993). *Black pearls: Daily meditations, affirmations, and inspirations for African Americans.* New York: Quill.

Cotter, P. R., Cohen, J., & Coulter P. B. (1982). Race of interviewer effects in telephone interviews. *Public Opinion Quarterly, 46,* 278–284.

Delgado, J. L., & Estrada, L. (1993). Improving data collection strategies. *Public Health Reports, 108,* 540–545.

Dresser, N. (1996). *Multicultural manners: New rules of etiquette for a changing society.* New York: Wiley.

Duarte, J. A., & Rice, B. D. (1994, October). *Cultural diversity in rehabilitation: Nineteenth Institute on Rehabilitation Issues.* University of Arkansas, Department of Rehabilitation Education and Research, Arkansas Research and Training Center in Vocational Rehabilitation, Hot Springs.

Evinger, S. (1995). How shall we measure our nation's diversity? *Chance, 8*(1), 7–14.

Facio, E. (1993). Ethnography as personal experience. In J. Stanfield & R. Dennis (Eds.), *Race and ethnicity in research methods* (pp. 75–91). Newbury Park, CA: Sage.

Feinleib, M. (1993). Data needed for improving the health of minorities. *Annals of Epidemiology, 3*(2), 199–202.

Fortier, J. P., & Bishop, D. (2004). *Setting the agenda for research on cultural competencies in health care: Final report* (C. Brach, Ed.). Rockville, MD: U.S. Department of Health and Human Services, Office of Minority Health and Agency for Healthcare Research and Quality.

Frayne, S. M., Burns, R. B., Hardt, E. J., Rosen, A. K., & Moskowitz, M. A. (1996). The exclusion of non-English-speaking persons from research. *Journal of General Internal Medicine, 11*(1), 39–43.

Hahn, R. H. (1992). The state of federal health statistics on racial and ethnic groups. *Journal of the American Medical Association, 267,* 268–271.

Health Resources and Services Administration. (2004). *Measuring cultural competence in health care settings.* Retrieved May 31, 2006, from www.hrsa.gov/culturalcompetence/measures/sectionii.htm

Hughes, C. C. (1990). Ethnopsychiatry. In T. M. Johnson & C. F. Sargent (Eds.), *Medical anthropology: A handbook of theory and methods* (pp. 132–148). New York: Greenwood.

Issel, L. M. (2004). *Health program planning and evaluation.* Boston: Jones & Bartlett.

Johnson, S. D. (1990). Toward clarifying culture, race, and ethnicity in the context of multicultural counseling. *Journal of Multicultural Counseling and Development, 18,* 41–50.

Katz, J. (1985). The sociopolitical nature of counseling. *Counseling Psychologist, 13,* 615–624.

Kavanagh, K. H., & Kennedy, P. H. (1992). *Promoting cultural diversity: Strategies for health-care professionals.* Newbury Park, CA: Sage.

Keppel, K., Pamuk, E., Lynch, J., et al. (2005). Methodological issues in measuring health disparities. National Center for Health Statistics. *Vital Health Statistics, Series 2,* No. 141.

Kumanyika, S. K., & Golden, P. M. (1991). Cross-sectional differences in health status in the U.S. racial/ethnic minority groups: Potential influence of temporal changes, disease, and life-style transitions. *Ethnicity and Disease, 1,* 50–59.

LaVeist, T. A., Sellers, R. M., Brown, K. A., & Nickerson, K. J. (1997). Extreme social isolation, use of community-based senior support services, and mortality among African American elderly women. *American Journal of Community Psychology, 25,* 721–732.

Malpass, R. S. (1977). Theory and methods in cross-cultural psychology. *American Psychologist, 32,* 1069–1079.

McGraw, S. A., McKinlay, J. B., Crawford, S. A., Costa, L. A., & Cohen, D. L. (1992). Health survey methods with minority populations: Some lessons from recent experience. *Ethnicity and Disease, 2,* 273–287.

Meadow, M. (1998, December/January). Searching for an AIDS vaccine, searching for volunteers. *Closing the Gap Newsletter,* pp. 4–5.

Minkler, M., & Wallerstein, N. (2003). Introduction to community-based participatory research. In M. Minkler & N. Wallerstein (Eds.), *Community-based participatory research for health* (pp. 3–26). San Francisco: Jossey-Bass.

Mouton, C. P., Harris, S., Rovi, S., Solorzano, P., & Johnson, M. S. (1997). Barriers to women's participation in cancer clinical trials. *Journal of the National Medical Association, 89,* 721–727.

National Center for Health Statistics. (2007). *Fast stats a to z: Health of Asian and Pacific Islander population.* [Data file]. Retrieved August 14, 2007, from www.cdc.gov/nchs/fastats/asian_health.htm

Office of Management and Budget. (1997). *Race and ethnic standards for federal statistics and administrative reporting* (Statistical Policy Directive No. 15, revised). Washington, DC: Author.

Office of Minority Health. (2007). *Policies, initiatives, and laws.* Retrieved January 22, 2007, from www.omhrc.gov/templates/browse.aspx

Osborne, N. G., & Feit, M. D. (1992). The use of race in medical research. *Journal of the American Medical Association, 267,* 275–280.

Patton, J. (1993). Psychoeducational assessment of gifted and talented African Americans. In J. H. Stanfield & R. M. Dennis (Eds.), *Race and ethnicity in research methods* (pp. 198–216). Thousand Oaks, CA: Sage.

Pinn, V. W. (1998, July). Improving the health of minority women: The role of research. *Closing the Gap Newsletter,* p. 3.

Ploeg, M., & Perrin, E. (2004). *Eliminating health disparities: Measurement and data needs* (Panel on DHHS Collection of Race and Ethnic Data). Washington, DC: National Academy of Sciences.

Ponce, N. (1992). The cultural dimensions of getting health care. In *Conference Proceedings—Partners in human service: Shaping health care and civil rights policy for Asian and Pacific Islander Americans.* Washington, DC: Office of Minority Health/Health Management Resources.

Ponterotto, J., & Casas, M. (1991). *Handbook of racial/ethnic minority counseling research.* Springfield, IL: Charles C Thomas.

Robinson, S. B., Ashley, M., & Haynes, M. A. (1996). Attitudes of African Americans regarding prostate cancer clinical trails. *Journal of Community Health, 21*(2), 77–87.

Salber, E. J., & Beza, A. G. (1980). The health interview survey and minority health. *Medical Care, 18,* 327–335.

Schaeffer, N. L. (1980). Evaluating race of interviewer effect in a national survey. *Social Methods Research, 8,* 400–419.

Schulman, K. A., Rubenstein, L. E., Chesley, F. D., & Eisenberg, J. M. (1995). The roles of race and socioeconomic factors in health services research. *Health Services Research, 30*(1, Pt. 2), 179–195.

Scribner, R. (1996). Paradox as paradigm: The health outcomes of Mexican Americans. *American Journal of Public Health, 86,* 303–305.

Smith, A. W. (1993). Survey research on African Americans: Methodological innovations. In J. H. Stanfield & R. M. Dennis (Eds.), *Race and ethnicity in research methods* (pp. 217–229). Thousand Oaks, CA: Sage.

Smith, M. B. (1998, March). Race, ethnicity, class, and culture. *Closing the Gap Newsletter,* p. 2.

Stanfield, J. H. (1993). Epistemological considerations. In J. H. Stanfield & R. M. Dennis (Eds.), *Race and ethnicity in research methods* (pp. 16–36). Thousand Oaks, CA: Sage.

Stanfield, J. H., & Dennis, R. M. (Eds.). (1993). *Race and ethnicity in research methods.* Thousand Oaks, CA: Sage.

Stanhope, V., Solomon, P., Pernell-Arnold, A., Sands, R. G., & Bourjolly, J. N. (2005). Evaluating cultural competence among behavioral health professionals. *Psychiatric Rehabilitation Journal, 28,* 225–233.

Stiens, H. F. (1990). Psychoanalytic perspectives. In T. M. Johnson & C. F. Sargent (Eds.), *Medical anthropology: A handbook of theory and methods* (pp. 73–92). New York: Greenwood Press.

Sue, D. W., Arredondo, P., & McDavis, R. J. (1992). Multicultural counseling competencies and standards: A call to the profession. *Journal of Counseling and Development, 70,* 477–485.

Sue, D. W., & Sue, D. (1990). *Counseling the culturally different: Theory and practice.* New York: Wiley.

Tashiro, C. J. (2005). Health disparities in the context of mixed race: Challenging the ideology of race. *Advances in Nursing Science, 28,* 203–211.

Triandis, H. C. (1994). *Culture and social behavior.* New York: McGraw-Hill.

U.S. Department of Health and Human Services. (2000). *Healthy People 2010.* Washington, DC: Author.

U.S. Public Health Services. (1994). *Improving minority health statistics: Report of the Public Health Task Force on Minority Health Data.* Washington, DC: U.S. Department of Health and Human Services, Office of Minority Health.

Williams, D. (1998, March). The quality of racial data. *Closing the Gap Newsletter,* p. 4.

Williams, D. R., Lavizzo-Mourey, R., & Warren, R. C. (1994). The concepts of race and health status in America. *Public Health Reports, 109*(1), 26–41.

Wray, L. A. (1992). Health policy and ethnic diversity in older Americans: Dissonance or harmony? *Western Journal of Medicine, 157,* 357–361.

Yu, E. S., & Liu, W. T. (1994). Methodological issues. In N. Zane, D. Takeuchi, & K. Young (Eds.), *Confronting critical health issues of Asian and Pacific Islander Americans* (pp. 22–50). Thousand Oaks, CA: Sage.

Zane, N., Takeuchi, D., & Young, K. (1994). *Confronting critical health issues of Asian and Pacific Islander Americans.* Thousand Oaks, CA: Sage.

22

Research Evidence for Cultural Competence and Culturally Competent Care

Class, race, gender, and ethnicity shape the process of inquiry, making research a multicultural process.

—Denzin and Lincoln (1998, p. 3)

Key Points

- Using research as evidence to support practice interventions is an important aspect of occupational therapy.
- Evidence is limited for cultural competence and culturally competent care in the occupational therapy literature; most such evidence is found in the disciplines of nursing, social work, and clinical psychology.
- Research on cultural competence has used a combination of qualitative, descriptive, and mixed methodologies.
- The published evidence on cultural competence addresses four major areas: (a) the effectiveness of education and training programs, (b) the specific attributes of cultural competence, (c) the effect of culturally competent care, and (d) client perceptions of culturally competent providers.
- A significant need exists for further research on cultural competence and culturally competent care in occupational therapy.

ALTHOUGH CULTURALLY COMPETENT CARE is not a practice intervention, it is "increasingly being seen as important to quality of care" (Chin, 2000, p. 25). Cultural competence is a necessary requirement for client-centered care; it is needed to support a climate of respect and collaboration between client and practitioner, providing the foundation for effective occupational therapy intervention. How does one know that cultural competence or client-centered care is effective? This is an important question to ask. This chapter examines the body of research evidence on cultural competence.

Many researchers emphasize how difficult it is to do effective research related to multicultural competence (for a discussion of the difficulties, see Chapter 21). Sue (1998) believes that because much of the work is related to race relations, "research into these issues will also engender many emotional responses" (p. 444). Being emotionally involved in the research certainly influences the manner in which researchers conceptualize, plan, conduct, and report their studies and often compromises any hope of objective analysis of the findings. Even if researchers feel that they have no emotional ties to the factors being studied, their unconscious and sometimes unexamined biases and worldview color the findings (Sue & Sundberg, 1996). Cauce, Coronado, and Watson (1998) state that "how one designs and conducts research is at once a scientific and sociopolitical process" (p. 305). For these reasons, researchers must use a research approach that also will allow the voice of participants to be heard most effectively. It also is vital that researchers carefully evaluate and present their own beliefs, values, and assumptions to diminish researcher bias.

Research Evidence Regarding Cultural Competence

Evidence-based practice has been discussed in the medical research literature for over 50 years (National Institute on Disability and Rehabilitation Research, 2003, cited in Bailey, Bornstein, & Ryan, 2007) and became part of the ongoing dialogue of occupational therapy in the late 1990s. *Evidence-based medicine* has been defined as "the conscientious, explicit, judicious use of current best evidence in making decisions about the care of individual patients" (Sackett, Rosenberg, Gray, Haynes, & Richardson, 1996, p. 71), and this definition is applicable to evidence-based practice in occupational therapy. At the end of 1999, the Evidenced-Based Forum became a regular column in the *American Journal of Occupational Therapy* (Bailey et al., 2007), and the importance of evidence as an integral aspect of occupational therapy practice and education is apparent in its inclusion in the latest edition of the educational standards for the profession (Accreditation Council for Occupational Therapy Education, 2007).

Much of the research on cultural competence has been done outside the field of occupational therapy, notably in the disciplines of social work, counseling psychology, and nursing. Because those fields are closely aligned with occupational therapy, the findings from these studies are easily transferable. Therefore, we will examine studies from other health and human services fields as evidence in conjunction with research from occupational therapy.

The term *cultural competence* was first seen in the U.S. occupational therapy literature in the early 1990s. Dillard, Andonian, Flores, Lai, MacRae, & Shakir (1992) described practice within a diversely populated mental health setting in San Francisco as "culturally competent care." The authors state that the purpose of the article was "to introduce the concept of cultural competence and discuss the importance of culture for occupational therapy in mental health settings" (p. 721). Many other descriptive accounts and discussions of diversity and minority issues also appeared in the 1990s (Barney, 1991; DeMars, 1992; Dyck, 1991; MacDonald, 1998; Wells, 1991), but it took a few years before research specific to cultural competence became more common. Evidential research on culturally competent care in the occupational therapy and other health professional literature addresses four major topic areas: (a) the effectiveness of education and training programs, (b) the specific attributes of cultural competence, (c) the effect of culturally competent care, and (d) client perceptions of culturally competent providers.

Education and Training Effectiveness

Education and training effectiveness is, by far, the most often researched topic in the research literature on cultural competence. Numerous training and education programs to improve cultural sensitivity and cultural competence in health professionals have been developed over the past decade. As a result, studies have been published examining the effect of these programs, most using a qualitative methodology (see Table 22.1).

Efficacy of Courses, Educational Models, and Learning Projects

Many studies have examined the effect of a particular course, educational model, or learning project (Brathwaite, 2005; Caffrey, Neander, Markle, & Stewart, 2005; Fenster & Rose, 2003; Forwell, Whiteford, & Dyck, 2001; Matzo, Sherman, Mazanec, & Virani, 2002; Moffat & Tung, 2004; Ott, Doyle, & Tarantino, 2004; Velde & Wittman, 2001; Yuen & Yau, 1999). Some of these studies are briefly described in the paragraphs that follow.

Fenster and Rose (2003), in a mixed-method study, exposed students to a curriculum focused on increasing cultural awareness, defining cultural competence and incompetence, and helping practitioners strategize and solve theoretical culturally based problems in agency settings. Their evaluation demonstrated students' increased ability to engage in critical analysis within a historical and political context

Table 22.1. Evidence Base on Cultural Competence

Topic	Studies
Education and training programs: Efficacy of programs	Brathwaite, 2005; Caffrey, Neander, Markle, & Stewart, 2005; Fenster & Rose, 2003; Forwell, Whiteford, & Dyck, 2001; Matzo, Sherman, Mazanec, & Virani, 2002; Moffat & Tung, 2004; Ott, Doyle, & Tarantino, 2004; Velde & Wittman, 2001; Yuen & Yau, 1999
Education and training programs: Evaluation of faculty skills and perceptions	Sealey, Burnett, & Johnson, 2006; Singleton, 1994
Specific attributes of cultural competence	Bassey-Jones, Genao, St. George, & Corbie-Smith, 2005; Beach et al., 2005; Black, 2000; Cui & Awa, 1992; Gray & McPherson, 2005; Martin, 1987; Olebe & Koester, 1989; Pope-Davis & Ottavi, 1994; Schim, Doorenbos, & Borse, 2006; Shapiro, Hollingshead, & Morrison, 2002; Weaver, 2004; Wiseman, Hammer, & Nishida, 1989
Client perceptions of providers	Gim, Atkinson, & Kim, 1991; Napoles-Springer, Santoyo, Houston, Perez-Stable, & Stewart, 2005; Purnell, 1999b, 2001; Rogers, 1998; Wade & Bernstein, 1991
Effect of culturally competent care	Austin, Gallop, McCay, Peternelj-Taylor, & Bayer, 1999; Karner & Hall, 2002; Schilder et al., 2001; Warda, 2000; Weaver 1999

and increased confidence in responding effectively in cross-cultural experiences compared with the control group.

Braithwaite (2005) reports similar findings in another study. Public health nurses in Ontario had improved scores on the Cultural Knowledge Scale (Campinha-Bacote, 1998) following a cultural competence educational program. In this mixed-method study, participants reported that the program increased their cultural knowledge and awareness and changed their behavior with clients. Moffat and Tung (2004) found increased scores in 84% of participants on a post-test of cultural knowledge and cultural competence following a two-day "culture-brokering" training.

In other studies in which participants had an opportunity to learn through training programs involving various levels of cross-cultural interactions, findings were again mostly positive. Using a cultural interview experience with first-year occupational therapy students, Yuen and Yau (1999) report that the participants indicated that the interview had a positive effect on their awareness of another cultural group (70%), and 45% indicated positive effects on their sensitivity and attitudes toward another culture. The authors note, however, that this exercise did not remove all ethnocentric viewpoints.

In another study, nursing students presented a 50-minute substance abuse program to racially diverse high school students in a service learning project. The nursing students had received training in cultural competence and substance abuse. Findings indicated that this direct interaction changed stereotypes held by the nursing students, helped them develop an awareness of cultural differences, and increased their own cultural self-awareness. In addition, the nursing students reported that they could begin to take action in cross-cultural experiences such as these and experienced an increased sense of advocacy.

A five-week international immersion experience proved to be much more effective than integration of cultural content in an undergraduate curriculum for nursing students in a study by Caffrey and colleagues (2005). Others (Nakanishi & Rittner, 1992; St. Clair & McKenry, 1999) note the value of immersion or experiential activities for the development of cultural competence. These results have interesting implications for occupational therapy education programs attempting to educate for the development of cultural competence.

Not all studies evaluating educational programs and projects have had only positive outcomes, however. In a pilot study, Velde and Wittman (2001) found that students immersed in a community project had improved scores on a cultural competence assessment scale, but many challenges arose as well. The authors conclude that the development of cultural competence was a lifelong process and could not be achieved with only one experience. Forwell and colleagues (2001) report similar results in their study; they conclude that curricula to help develop cultural competence are important in occupational therapy education but that "the educational goal-post for full cultural competence is just over the horizon" (p. 102). Cultural competence can be initiated, but cannot be fully achieved, through an educational program.

Evaluation of Faculty Skills and Perceptions

Another area of research related to academic programming focuses on the perceptions and skills of faculty who teach this content (Sealey, Burnett, & Johnson, 2006; Singleton, 1994; no studies of this nature can be found in the occupational therapy literature). Sealey and colleagues examined the cultural competence of nursing faculty in Louisiana using their Cultural Diversity Questionnaire for Nurse Educators. They found that only a few of the 163 faculty members had any formal preparation to teach transcultural nursing, and most had scored very low on the Cultural Knowledge variable. They also found that cross-cultural skills were low and that the majority of participants had little experience working with people from diverse backgrounds. The researchers wonder whether "the existing low levels of cultural competence among . . . students and practicing nurses is the result of erroneous approaches to teaching cultural competence" (p. 139). Although this study is not generalizable to occupational therapy educators, it is something to carefully consider.

In a qualitative, grounded theory study, Singleton (1994) reviews the comfort of social work faculty who taught content on racial oppression, one aspect of cultural competence knowledge, and concludes that many avoided, minimized, or rejected the content. If educators are not comfortable teaching the necessary content for cultural competence, the effect on students is significant. Students may feel uncomfortable with the content and avoid learning about cultural diversity, avoid people who are culturally different from themselves, and fail to apply the principles and skills of culturally competent care.

Specific Attributes of Cultural Competence

There is consensus in the health care literature that professionals who wish to become culturally competent must improve their cultural self-awareness, knowledge, and skills, and several studies have examined these attributes (Bassey-Jones, Genao, St. George, & Corbie-Smith, 2005; Beach et al., 2005; Black, 2000; Cui & Awa, 1992; Gray & McPherson, 2005; Martin, 1987; Olebe & Koester, 1989; Pope-Davis & Ottavi, 1994; Schim et al., 2006; Shapiro et al., 2002; Weaver, 2004; Wiseman et al., 1989).

In a study that examined the relationships among intercultural communication competence, knowledge of the host culture, and cross-cultural attitudes, Wiseman and colleagues (1989) found that the degree of ethnocentrism a person exhibited was the strongest predictor of competence in culture-specific communication. Another study investigated the relationship between previous intercultural experience and self-perceived intercultural competence (Martin, 1987). Not surprisingly, participants with the most intercultural experience rated themselves higher in cultural self-awareness and the ability to facilitate communication. Olebe and Koester (1989) found that the three most important predictors of intercultural effectiveness were task roles, empathy, and respect.

These studies suggest that there may not be general agreement on which attributes provide an unequivocal basis for cultural competence. Nevertheless, later studies have continued to focus on the three major attributes or characteristics the previous studies identified: awareness or attitude, knowledge, and skills.

Schim and colleagues (2006) examined cultural competence among hospice nurses and found a "significant association between higher education and cultural awareness and sensitivity, as well as an association between diversity training and self-reported cultural competence behaviors" (p. 302). In an occupational therapy study focusing on practitioner attitudes, Gray and McPherson (2005) found generational differences in attitudes, "older-generation therapists having greater attitudinal change than that [of] the younger-generation therapists" (p. 39). They also found that personal experiences, including direct contact with people from other cultures, the amount and distance they had traveled, and personal experiences of being discriminated against, were an important factor in attitudinal change.

A study examining skill in cross-cultural communication (Shapiro et al., 2002) used focus groups with primary care residents, faculty, and patients to explore the meaning of, barriers to, and approaches to overcoming barriers to cross-cultural communication. The researchers found that medical residents were skeptical about training that included components of self-awareness and sensitivity; they wanted to learn practical tools but had little patience for examining larger, contextual cross-cultural issues. In contrast, the faculty participants favored the teaching of the latter issues.

Weaver (2004) conducted a survey of Native American social workers, nurses, and psychologists that "provided preliminary information about what kinds of knowledge, skills, and values/attitudes are associated with culturally competent helping with Native Americans" (p. 30). The most significant finding was the importance of being open and nonjudgmental.

Finally, Beach and her colleagues (2005) performed a systematic literature review and analysis of interventions that improved cultural competence in health professionals. They examined 34 studies and found "excellent evidence that culturally competent training improved the knowledge of health professionals and good evidence that it improves the attitudes and skills of health professionals" (p. 356).

Effect of Culturally Competent Care

Although much of the literature on culturally competent care is written in a generalized, theoretical manner (Chin, 2000) or describes culturally competent care in interventions with specific groups of people, including African Americans (Giger, 2000), Appalachians (Purnell, 1999a), and sexual minorities (Gonser, 2000), research is limited about the results or outcomes of culturally competent care with specific groups of people (Austin et al., 1999; Karner & Hall, 2002; Schilder et al., 2001; Warda, 2000; Weaver, 1999). A Canadian study examined culturally competent care provided by 1,700 psychiatric nurses working with culturally diverse clients with a history of sexual abuse (Austin et al., 1999). On the survey question that asked the nurses to rate their ability to provide culturally competent care, four overall themes emerged:

1. *Culture is not the problem.* Some nurses felt incompetent working with the diagnostic problem, regardless of the client's culture.
2. *Culture is not an issue.* Some nurses did not acknowledge any implications of cultural differences. Interestingly, these nurses rated themselves at the highest level of cultural competence (5 on a scale of 1 to 5).
3. *Culture influences perspective and responses.* Many respondents believed that culture is always an issue and that it shapes perceptions and affects clients and treatment regardless of the presenting problem. Many of these nurses rated themselves at the midpoint (3) in cultural competence.
4. *Culturally specific competence may be distinguishable from cultural competence.* Some nurses felt more competent with specific cultures than they did with others (Austin et al., 1999).

Overall, only 4.6% of the respondents saw themselves as very culturally competent. Austin and her colleagues conclude that the nurses surveyed recognized the importance of culturally competent care but needed more knowledge and understanding of cultural norms and practices to provide that kind of care.

A qualitative study found similar results concerning the need for increased cultural knowledge for effective and culturally competent care (Schilder et al., 2001). Forty-seven HIV-positive men were interviewed and participated in focus groups that elicited information about their health care experiences. Participants reported that many health care providers neither recognized homosexual and transgender culture nor attempted to learn more about it. Positive experiences occurred only with a few culturally competent providers who could "identify and include the social and sexual identity of their patients and were aware of inherent cultural values and beliefs" (p. 1657).

Karner and Hall (2002) conducted 50 interviews with staff members who had been successful in working with Latino and African American families who had a family member with Alzheimer's disease. The authors sought the perceptions and insights of staff members to inform the development of culturally appropriate services for diverse populations. They discovered that building trust, addressing language and cultural issues, and providing clear expectations and consistency in service delivery were all vital aspects of culturally competent care and that successful "providers tailored and individualized services to better meet the unique needs and concerns of their client populations" (p. 129).

Finally, Weaver (1999) reports the results of a study of culturally competent helping practices with Native Americans. Sixty-two Native American social workers and social work students completed a survey on attributes necessary to provide culturally competent care to Native clients. Within the attribute of knowledge, respondents cited as necessary the need to understand the diversity, history, culture, and contemporary realities of Native American populations. Necessary skills included general skills such as communication and problem solving and containment skills, which require staff to refrain from speaking. Necessary values included helper wellness and self-awareness, humility and willingness to learn, respect, open-mindedness and a nonjudgmental attitude, and social justice. Results of this study help answer the question of what knowledge, skills, and values are necessary for culturally competent care for this population. Because of the continuing dearth of outcomes measures for culturally competent care, we agree with Weaver that researchers must find a way to measure cultural competence to better serve clients from a variety of backgrounds.

Client Perceptions of Culturally Competent Providers

Although it is important to assess the effectiveness of culturally competent care and of training and practice as measured by practitioners, a more important assessment of these behaviors is how care recipients view their effectiveness. How do clients recognize and evaluate culturally competent care? Again, not enough research has been done in this area, but a few investigative studies have been done (Gim, Atkinson, & Kim, 1991; Napoles-Springer, Santoyo, Houston, Perez-Stable, & Stewart, 2005; Purnell, 1999b, 2001; Rogers, 1998; Wade & Bernstein, 1991).

> *Although it is important to assess the effectiveness of culturally competent care and of training and practice as measured by practitioners, a more important assessment of these behaviors is how care recipients view their effectiveness.*

In two related studies, Purnell examined the health practices of Panamanians (1999b) and Guatemalans (2001) and explored their perceptions of health care practitioners. He found in both studies that respect was a vital and valued practitioner characteristic, and both groups defined respect and nonrespect in both verbal and nonverbal communication. Interestingly, in both studies, participants used more phrases to describe nonrespectful behaviors despite the findings that respect was identified as the more valued behavior. It is more common for people to use more phrases to describe something of value rather than something that is not valued, yet these two studies found the opposite to be true.

Napoles-Springer and colleagues (2005) used focus group interviews with 163 ethnically and linguistically diverse patients to examine their perceptions of cultural factors that affected the quality of their medical encounters. Patients from all groups identified the following influential factors as negatively affecting quality: (a) lack of sensitivity to complementary or alternative medicine, (b) health insurance–based discrimination, (c) social class–based discrimination, (d) ethnic discordance between physician and patient, and (e) age-based discrimination. Patients reported the following factors as positively influencing medical encounters:

- Positive values, beliefs, and attitudes
- Effective communication skills
- Patient- and family-centered decision making
- Respect for privacy and modesty
- Openness to immigration
- Nutritional awareness
- Language and ethnic concordance
- Lack of discrimination
- Promotion of empowerment
- Complementary and alternative medicine
- Respect for spirituality (p. 14).

Other studies have focused on the racial and ethnic match between provider and client. Wade and Bernstein (1991) examined the perceptions and satisfaction of 80 African American female clients regarding their counselors' skills and characteristics after the counselors had engaged in sensitivity training; they also looked at these clients' attrition rates. At the end of the first three counseling sessions, the clients were asked to complete three instruments to assess their perceptions of their counselors' skills. The clients whose counselors had completed sensitivity training rated them more positively and had lower attrition rates. Another important finding was that clients' perceptions were more positively affected by the counselor's sensitivity than by the counselor's race.

Rogers (1998) found that consultants who engaged in race-sensitive verbal behavior were consistently seen by participants as being more culturally competent and sensitive. Consultants who were able to talk openly about racial issues were seen as being more credible regardless of racial match, although racial match also was an influencing factor. Similarly, Gim and colleagues (1991) found that Asian American participants rated counselors as more credible and competent when the counselors exhibited culture-sensitive behaviors and when they were Asian American.

In summary, clients were able to identify and name the aspects of cultural competence that were important to them. Although most rated caregivers who exhibited culturally competent skills more highly, the racial or ethnic match of the provider with the client resulted in varied responses. As Sue (1998) observes,

Individual differences in the effects of [therapist–client] match appear to be very important, so that [racial or ethnic] match is neither a necessary nor sufficient condition for positive treatment outcomes. In other words, match may be important for some, but not for all clients. (p. 444)

Although research has addressed ethnic and racial match between client and provider, we found no studies in the literature that examined any other matching characteristic, such as gender, age, socioeconomic class, or sexual identity, yet in our experience these characteristics are very important to both clients and providers.

Summary

The research literature provides evidence of the effectiveness of culturally competent awareness and attitudes, knowledge, and skills; of culturally competent care; and of educational programs that address cultural competence. This literature, however, is limited, and few studies have been done in occupational therapy. Although occupational therapists and occupational therapy assistants, students, and educators can learn from the research described in this chapter, most of these studies are not generalizable to the occupational therapy field. Many occupational therapy educators are including content in their courses to move students further along the cultural competence continuum, and practitioners are taking more steps to provide culturally competent care. Research for evidence of the efficacy of these efforts continues to be necessary.

Reflection

1. Identify current research in occupational therapy about cultural competence.

   a. Use multiple databases to search the literature.

   b. Explore the occupational therapy literature outside the United States as well.

   c. Add new citations to the cultural competence evidence chart in Table 22.1.

2. Develop a research study that evaluates the outcomes of culturally competent care.

   a. Locate an intervention program that works with a diverse population.

   b. Using a survey format, determine the extent of cultural competence training or experience of the occupational therapy staff and management at your organization.

   c. Interview or survey clients to determine their perceptions of the cultural competence of the staff of your organization.

3. Determine another way to evaluate for culturally competent care.

References

Accreditation Council for Occupational Therpay Education. (2007). Accreditation Council for Occupational Therapy Education (ACOTE) standards and interpretive guidelines. *American Journal of Occupational Therapy, 61.*

Austin, W., Gallop, R., McCay, E., Peternelj-Taylor, C., & Bayer, M. (1999). Culturally competent care for psychiatric clients who have a history of sexual abuse. *Clinical Nursing Research, 8*(1), 5–25.

Bailey, D. M., Bornstein, J., & Ryan, S. (2007). A case report of evidence-based practice: From academia to clinic. *American Journal of Occupational Therapy, 61*, 85–91.

Barney, K. F. (1991). From Ellis Island to assisted living: Meeting the needs of older adults from diverse cultures. *American Journal of Occupational Therapy, 45*, 586–593.

Bassey-Jones, J., Genao, I., St. George, D. M., & Corbie-Smith, G. (2005). Knowledge of cultural competence among third-year medical students. *Journal of the National Medical Association, 97*, 1272–1276.

Beach, M. C., Price, E. G., Gary, T. L., Robinson, K. A., Gozu, A., Palacio, A., Smarth, C., et al. (2005). Cultural competence: A systematic review of health care provider educational interventions. *Medical Care, 43*, 356–373.

Black, R. M. (2000). *The essence of cultural competence: Listening to the voices of occupational therapy students.* Unpublished doctoral dissertation, Lesley University, Cambridge, MA.

Braithwaite, A. C. (2005). Evaluation of a cultural competence course. *Journal of Transcultural Nursing, 16*, 361–369.

Caffrey, R. A., Neander, W., Markle, D., & Stewart, B. (2005). Improving the cultural competence of nursing students: Results of integrating cultural content in the curriculum and an international immersion experience. *Journal of Nursing Education, 44*, 234–240.

Campinha-Bacote, J. (1998). Cultural diversity in nursing education: Issues and concerns. *Journal of Nursing Education, 37*(1), 3–4.

Cauce, A. M., Coronado, N., & Watson, J. (1998). Conceptual, methodological, and statistical issues in culturally competent research. In M. Hernandez & M. R. Isaacs (Eds.), *Promoting cultural competence in children's mental health services* (pp. 305–329). Baltimore: Paul H. Brookes.

Chin, J. L. (2000, January–February). Culturally competent health care. *Public Health Reports, 115*, 25–33.

Cui, G., & Awa, J. E. (1992). Measuring intercultural effectiveness: An integrating approach. *International Journal of Intercultural Relations, 16*, 311–328.

DeMars, P. A. (1992). An occupational therapy life skills curriculum model for a Native American tribe: A health promotion program based on ethnographic field research. *American Journal of Occupational Therapy, 46*, 745–750.

Denzin, N. K., & Lincoln, Y. S. (1998). Entering the field of qualitative research. In N. K. Denzin & Y. S. Lincoln (Eds.), *The landscape of qualitative research: Theories and issues* (pp. 1–34). Thousand Oaks, CA: Sage.

Dillard, M., Andonian, L., Flores, O., Lai, I., MacRae, A., & Shakir, J. (1992). Culturally competent occupational therapy in a diversely populated mental health setting. *American Journal of Occupational Therapy, 46*, 721–726.

Dyck, I. (1991). Multiculturalism and occupational therapy: Sharing the challenge—National Perspective. *Canadian Journal of Occupational Therapy, 58*(5), 224–226.

Fenster, J., & Rose, L. (2003). Testing a curriculum to teach cultural competence to nonmainstream college students interning in mainstream agencies. *Journal of Teaching in Social Work, 23*(3/4), 127–142.

Forwell, S. J., Whiteford, G., & Dyck, I. (2001). Cultural competence in New Zealand and Canada: Occupational therapy students' reflections on class and fieldwork curriculum. *Canadian Journal of Occupational Therapy, 68*(2), 90–103.

Giger, J. N. (2000). Developing culturally competent care techniques to assist African-Americans to survive in the 21st century. *Journal of National Black Nurses Association, 11*(1), vii–viii.

Gim, R. H., Atkinson, D. R., & Kim, S. J. (1991). Asian-American acculturation, counselor ethnicity and cultural sensitivity, and ratings of counselors. *Journal of Counseling Psychology, 38*(1), 57–62.

Gonser, P. A. (2000). Culturally competent care for members of sexual minorities. *Journal of Cultural Diversity, 7*(3), 72–75.

Gray, M., & McPherson, K. (2005). Cultural safety and professional practice in occupational therapy: A New Zealand perspective. *Australian Occupational Therapy Journal, 52,* 34–42.

Karner, T. X., & Hall, L. C. (2002). Successful strategies for serving diverse populations. In R. J. V. Montgomery (Ed.), *A new look at community-based respite programs* (pp. 107–131). New York: Haworth Press.

MacDonald, J. (1998). What is cultural competency? *British Journal of Occupational Therapy, 61,* 325–328.

Martin, R. M. (1987). *A study of Black preschool children's performance on the Miller Assessment for Preschoolers.* Richmond, VA: Chesterfield County School System.

Matzo, L. M., Sherman, D. W., Mazanec, P., & Virani, R. (2002). Teaching cultural considerations at the end of life: End-of-life nursing education consortium program recommendations. *Journal of Continuing Education in Nursing, 33*(6), 270–278.

Moffat, J., & Tung, J.-T. (2004). Evaluating the effectiveness of culture brokering training to enhance cultural competence of independent living center staff. *Journal of Vocational Rehabilitation, 20,* 59–69.

Nakanshi, M., & Rittner, B. (1992). The inclusionary cultural model. *Journal of Social Work Education, 28*(1), 27–35.

Napoles-Springer, A. M., Santoyo, S., Houston, K., Perez-Stable, E. J., & Stewart, A. L. (2005). Patients' perceptions of cultural factors affecting the quality of their medical encounters. *Health Expectations, 8*(1), 4–17.

Olebe, M., & Koester, J. (1989). Exploring the cross-cultural equivalence of the Behavior Assessment Scale for Intercultural Communication. *International Journal of Intercultural Relations, 17,* 355–379.

Ott, C. H., Doyle, L. H., & Tarantino, S.-L. (2004). The impact of an urban outreach teaching project: Developing cultural competence. *International Journal of Nursing Education Scholarship, 1*(1). Retrieved on May 16, 2007, from www.bepress.com/ijnes/vol1/iss1/art22

Pope-Davis, D. B., & Ottavi, T. M. (1994). Examining the association between self-reported multicultural counseling competencies and demographic variables among counselors. *Journal of Counseling and Development, 72,* 651–654.

Purnell, L. (1999a, November/December). Culturally competent care for traditional Appalachians. *Imprint,* pp. 56–59.

Purnell, L. (1999b). Panamanians' practices for health promotion and the meaning of respect afforded them by health care providers. *Journal of Transcultural Nursing, 10,* 331–339.

Purnell, L. (2001). Guatemalans' practices for health promotion and the meaning of respect afforded them by health care providers. *Journal of Transcultural Nursing, 12,* 40–47.

Rogers, M. R. (1998). The influence of race and consultant verbal behavior on perceptions of consultant competence and multicultural sensitivity. *School Psychology Quarterly, 13,* 265–280.

Sackett, D., Rosenberg, W., Gray, J., Haynes, R., & Richardson, W. (1996). Evidence-based medicine: What it is and what it isn't. *British Medical Journal, 312*(7023), 71–72.

Schilder, A. J., Kennedy, C., Goldstone, I. L., Ogden, R. D., Hogg, R. S., & O'Shaughnessy, M. V. (2001). "Being dealt with as a whole person": Care seeking and adherence: The benefits of culturally competent care. *Social Science and Medicine, 52,* 1643–1659.

Schim, S. M., Doorenbos, A. Z., & Borse, N. N. (2006). Cultural competence among hospice nurses. *Journal of Hospice and Palliative Nursing, 8*(5), 302–307.

Sealey, L. J., Burnett, J., & Johnson, G. (2006). Cultural competence of baccalaureate nursing faculty: Are we up to the task? *Journal of Cultural Diversity, 13*(3), 131–140.

Shapiro, J., Hollingshead, J., & Morrison, E. H. (2002). Primary care resident, faculty, and patient views of barriers to cultural competence, and the skills needed to overcome them. *Medical Education, 36,* 749–759.

Singleton, S. M. (1994). Faculty personal comfort and the teaching of content on racial oppression. In P. R. Keys (Ed.), *School social workers in the multicultural environment: New roles, responsibilities, and educational enrichment* (pp. 5–16). New York: Haworth Press.

St. Clair, A., & McKenry, L. (1999). Preparing culturally competent practitioners. *Journal of Nursing Education, 38*(5), 228–234.

Sue, D. W. (1998). *Multicultural counseling competencies: Individual and organizational development.* Thousand Oaks, CA: Sage.

Sue, D. W., & Sundberg, N. D. (1996). Research and research hypotheses about effectiveness in intercultural counseling. In P. D. Pedersen, J. G. Draguns, W. J. Lonner, & J. E. Trimble (Eds.), *Counseling across cultures* (4th ed.). Thousand Oaks, CA: Sage.

Velde, B. P., & Wittman, P. P. (2001). Helping occupational therapy students and faculty develop cultural competence. *Occupational Therapy in Health Care, 13*(3/4), 23–32.

Wade, P., & Bernstein, B. L. (1991). Cultural sensitivity training and counselor's race: Effects on Black female clients' perceptions and attrition. *Journal of Counseling Psychology, 38*(1), 9–15.

Warda, M. R. (2000). Mexican Americans' perceptions of culturally competent care. *Western Journal of Nursing Research, 22,* 203–224.

Weaver, H. (1999). Indigenous people and the social work profession: Defining culturally competent services. *Social Work, 44,* 217–225.

Weaver, H. (2004). The elements of cultural competence: Applications with Native American clients. *Journal of Ethnic and Cultural Diversity in Social Work, 13*(1), 19–35.

Wells, S. A. (1991). Clinical considerations in treating minority women who are disabled. *Occupational Therapy Practice, 2*(4), 13–22.

Wiseman, R. L., Hammer, M. R., & Nishida, H. (1989). Predictors of intercultural communication competence. *International Journal of Intercultural Relations, 13,* 349–370.

Yuen, H. K., & Yau, M. K. (1999). Cross-cultural awareness and occupational therapy education. *Occupational Therapy International, 6*(1), 24–34.

23

Ethical Practice and
Cultural Competence

It is not the color of the skin that makes the man, but the principles formed within the soul.

—MARIA W. STEWART (CITED IN JOHNSON, 1995, P. 102)

Key Points

- *Ethics* involve principles of conduct that help govern human behaviors. Society uses ethics to determine which acts are right and which are wrong and to evaluate the behaviors of individuals and groups. All moral and ethical choices involve values and beliefs that are culturally sensitive, contextually defined, and dependent on a network of sociocultural relationships that provide meaning and significance.

- Contemporary ethical decision-making approaches used by occupational therapists and occupational therapy assistants are based on bioethical concepts that assume that all societies share common moral values and that reasonable people will reach the same conclusions when faced with an ethical problem, issue, or dilemma. In multicultural settings, patients and their families, as well as providers, hold many cultural models of morality and moral reasoning. The constant overlapping and interaction of cultures create daily conflicts and dilemmas in providing health care services.

- The concepts of moral deliberation are based on four ethical principles: *autonomy, beneficence, nonmaleficence,* and *justice.* Autonomy often is at the center of ethical decisions or conflicts, especially those dealing with truth telling, advance directives, and informed consent, in health care contexts.

- Professional codes of ethics provide a moral framework for and define the ideal standard of practice. They and associated documents provide practitioners with guidelines and standards for resolving ethical conflicts, dilemmas, and issues.

- The values of ethical relativism and pluralism hold that practitioners respect the moral choices patients make in light of their cultural or religious beliefs. Acceptance of these values increases learning opportunities and facilitates cultural competency. The ethic of diversity matrix offers practitioners an opportunity to extend human knowledge by finding wisdom in dissimilar cultural practices.

ETHICAL DILEMMAS HAVE ASSUMED MAJOR IMPORTANCE in health care as advances in medical technology and rising health care costs have forced providers to deal with difficult ethical choices surrounding life-and-death issues, allocation of resources, and provider–client relationships (Ferguson, 1994). Every health provider constantly makes ethical choices. Sometimes those choices are dramatic, life-and-death decisions, but often they are more subtle, less conspicuous, and yet very important.

The increasingly multicultural composition of the U.S. population has produced new and often unforeseen ethical dilemmas and choices in current practices. Cultural pluralism poses challenges for both health care providers and patients from diverse backgrounds. The moral consequences of not respecting differences in a multicultural society are complex and are raising difficult questions for ethicists and policymakers as well as researchers and clinicians (Davis & Koening, 1996).

In the presence of cultural differences, health practitioners frequently find themselves confronting choices that depend more on moral and ethical values than on medical knowledge. Religious, cultural, and family values can greatly influence the clinical decision-making process. For example, many Asian cultures are reverent toward people in positions of authority (e.g., health professionals, therapists); families from those cultures may be open to discussing their medical condition and treatment options, but they may expect the professional to know what is best and to tell them what to do. In contrast, many Native Americans believe that any discussion of negative possibilities about their health will negatively influence treatment outcomes. This cultural value system conflicts with the generally accepted U.S. medical practice of providing clients with information and allowing them to make informed decisions about their own care. Whose cultural values and morals should be followed?

This chapter examines how culture influences the ethics of health care decision making and policy. It also examines the ethical responsibilities of practitioners and the rights of the client and family.

Types of Ethics

Ethics are the study of moral decision making and are concerned with the concepts of right and wrong. The term comes from the Greek word *ethos,* meaning "cultural custom or habit." The word *moral,* which often is used interchangeably with the term *ethical,* also means "customs." The identification of ethics and morality with cultural norms or customs reflects the fact that most adults tend to identify morality with cultural customs (Boss, 1998). The dictionary defines *ethics* as

A system of moral principles: the ethics of a culture; the rules of conduct recognized in respect to a particular class of human actions or particular group, culture, etc.: medical ethics, Christian ethics; moral principles, as of an individual: His ethics forbade betrayal of a confidence; the branch of philosophy dealing with values related to human conduct, with respect to the rightness and wrongness of certain motives and ends of such actions. (*Random House College Dictionary*, 1988)

In this chapter we define *ethics* as principles of conduct that help govern the behaviors of individuals and groups. It involves the study of the values and guidelines by which people live, as well as the justification of these values and guidelines. Ethics refer to "a set of standards of right and wrong established by a particular group and imposed on members of that group as a means of regulating and setting limits on their behavior" (Boss, 1998, p. 5). It represents what ought to be.

Ethics affect all levels of life. Normative ethics involve practical guidelines or norms that one can apply to real-life situations, such as "do not lie" or "do no harm." Individuals use personal ethics in cultivating a virtuous character and developing proper self-esteem. Interpersonal ethics deal with the rightness and wrongness of particular actions, the nature of obligations toward others, and obligations to oneself. Social ethics focus on policies that affect the wider community, the protection of the community, and the treatment of each member of the community. Environmental ethics, or one's moral obligation toward the environment, are becoming increasingly important (Boss, 1998). Ethics and lifestyle are intertwined. What we do or fail to do often affects not only us and those close to us but also people all over the world.

Theoretical ethics (also called *theoretical morality*) operate at a more fundamental level. Morality, like culture, is different for different people. It can vary from time to time and from person to person. Behavioral standards or moral values that are accepted by virtually all societies or can apply to all humans—for example, human rights—may be referred to as *universalistic*. *Particularistic*, or culture-specific, ethics involve moral norms adhered to by a given cultural community but not by others—for example, ancestor worship. Ethics come into play in situations when a shared universal or cultural standard does not automatically apply and decisions are a function of the specific circumstances (e.g., telling "white lies"; Becker, 1995; Boss, 1998; Howell, 1981; Paige & Martin, 1996). *Clinical ethics* refer to the day-to-day moral decision making of practitioners caring for patients (D. Callahan, 1995).

Moral Principles

What ethical standards should be used to determine what kinds of acts are right or which conduct is correct? In approaching moral decisions, it is important to recognize the moral principles that facilitate wise or correct choices. Philosophical tradition has placed an emphasis on *principilism*—the value of particular moral principles—in the making of decisions (Beauchamp & Childress, 1989; Childress, 1989).

Moral principles are rules used by society to evaluate the behavior of individuals and groups. These principles are universally binding and fundamentally transcultural (Boss, 1998), affecting all people regardless of their personal desires, culture, or religion. Both individual interests and cultural customs can influence how particular moral principles are carried out. Moral principles are abstract criteria for evaluating human behavior in its entirety (see Table 23.1 for a list of moral principles). A moral principle is "a duty to perform certain actions—such as keeping promises and repaying favors—irrespective of our motives" (Boss, 1998, p. 325).

Moral rules have plausibility because they are supported by universal standards. Without moral principles or standards, choices would be left to whim, to circumstances, and to the strongest desire of the individual (Buford, 1984). No one principle stands by itself. Each is a necessary condition for morally correct conduct, and collectively they are sufficient for determining the correctness of any conduct. Yet people are not compelled to engage them.

The advantage of moral principles is that, in varying ways and to different degrees, they protect individuals against harm and highlight the good in people. Moral principles are grounded in broad theories of ethics. Historically, two theories of justification of conduct have dominated: utilitarianism and deontology.

The *utilitarian approach* asks which choice, action, or policy would promote the best possible outcome (Boss, 1998). In other words, moral conduct is evaluated in terms of the consequences of behaviors. Phrases such as "the end justifies the means" and "the greatest good for the greatest number" are consistent with this approach. A utilitarian approach to health care rationing, for instance, would emphasize the collective social benefit rather than individual gains (Buford, 1984; D. Callahan, 1995).

Deontological theory holds that moral conduct must be evaluated in terms of standards alone and that the consequences of conduct are not germane to the evaluation of that conduct. Deontology focuses on determining which choices most respect the worth and value, and particularly the fundamental rights, of individuals (Boss, 1998; Buford, 1984). The question of one's basic obligation to other individuals is central. Good consequences may on occasion have to be set aside to respect inalienable human rights. For example, that it is wrong to subject a human being to dangerous medical research without the person's consent, even if the consequences of doing so might include saving the lives of many others, is a deontological belief (Buford, 1984; D. Callahan, 1995).

Ethical Decision Making

Good intentions alone are insufficient to guide moral decision making. Consequences matter when applying moral principles and making a judgment. According to D. Callahan (1995), good individual moral decision making encompasses

Table 23.1. Principles for Evaluating Moral Choices

Principle	Duty Involved
Consistency	To choose consistently or logically
Self-improvement	To improve one's knowledge and virtue
Equality	To treat all humans equally
Justice	To give each person equal and fair consideration
Beneficence	To do good acts and to promote well-being
Autonomy	To respect each individual's right to self-determination
Veracity	To tell the truth
Fidelity	To keep promises (e.g., confidentiality), to be loyal
Nonmaleficence	To do no harm
Axiology	To make consistent, harmonious, and coherent choices
Consequences	To consider foreseeable consequences of actions
Altruism	To respect all people and cooperate with others in the production and enjoyment of shared values

Note. Data from *Ethics for life: An interdisciplinary and multicultural introduction,* J. A. Boss, 1998, Mountain View, CA: Mayfield; *Personal philosophy: The art of living,* T. O. Buford, 1994, New York: CBS College; *In good conscience: Reason and emotion in moral decision making,* S. C. Callahan, 1991, San Francisco: Harper; *Case studies in allied health ethics,* R. M. Veatch and H. E. Flack, 1997, Upper Saddle River, NJ: Prentice-Hall.

three elements: (a) self-knowledge, (b) knowledge of moral theories and tradition, and (c) cultural perception. Self-knowledge is fundamental because one's feelings, motives, inclinations, and interests both enlighten and obscure moral understanding. Moral theories, traditions, and principles by themselves are not necessarily absolute or always the right ones to follow in every situation. People are social beings and reflect a particular society at a particular time. Their social embeddedness shapes the way they understand themselves, the moral problems they encounter, and what they take to be plausible and feasible responses to these problems (Boss, 1998; S. C. Callahan, 1991; D. Callahan, 1995).

What are practitioners' duties and obligations to other individuals whose lives and well-being may be affected by their actions? What do they owe to the common good, or the public interest, in their lives as members of society? These questions are general to all people and can be asked in any moral situation or context. When these ethical questions are posed in health care decisions, two views arise. One holds that a moral decision in health care involves the application of good moral thinking in general to the specific domain of health care; a medical component does not make the decision a different kind of moral problem, so general moral values or principles apply (Clouser, 1978).

A more traditional viewpoint is that ethical decision making in health care is different from general ethical decision making, because the domain of medicine is different from other areas of human life and because medicine has it own moral approaches and traditions. Proponents of this view argue that making a decision in a medical context requires a detailed and sensitive appreciation of the characteristics of health care practice and the unique features of sick and dying people (Pellegrino & Thomasma, 1981). It is not that the ethical principles and virtues of medicine are different from the more general principles of ethics; it is the context of health care that requires special consideration.

Moral Conflicts

Moral choices involve questions about what is objectively good in itself and for all people, what makes life worth living, and what is considered a good life (Fower & Richardson, 1996). There are moral rights and duties that are dependent on race or culture, tradition, or form of government. These rights and duties define, in terms of practice and action, human beings as human beings and as citizens of this or that society (Becker, 1995). All choices involve values. A choice occurs whenever value options conflict. All values are culturally sensitive, because they are contextually defined and dependent on a network of sociocultural relationships that provide meaning and significance (Buford, 1984).

When two values present themselves, and people choose one over another, they are saying, based on their cultural context and beliefs, that one option is more valuable than the other. For example, respect for patient autonomy that stresses the right of competent patients to make their own choices based on their cultural context can conflict with the principle of beneficence if patients' choices may be harmful.

There is no set formula for determining which action to take in a moral dilemma or conflict. One must carefully weigh the moral principles, decide the most compelling ones for that particular situation, and try to honor as many of the principles as possible. One must use creativity and reason to make a judgment. More important, however, moral decision making requires that one personally enter into the process. In the end, individual selves, alone with their thoughts and private lives, must wrestle with moral problems. And once a decision is made, one must act on it. A decision of conscience blends moral judgment and the will to act on that judgment (S. C. Callahan, 1991). Good moral decision making, therefore, requires moving back and forth among the necessary elements: the reflective self, the interpreted culture, and the contributions of moral theory.

Codes and Other Ethical Directives

When confronted with a moral conflict, choice, or decision, health care professionals may turn to their professional code of ethics or to other ethical directives such as oaths, prayers, and bills of rights. *Codes of ethics* articulate minimal standards of character and conduct and basic ethical principles relevant to professional practice. They often relate general moral values, duties, and virtues to the unique situations encountered in health care practice. Oaths, prayers, and bills of rights are collective summaries of moral ideals and conduct (Spicer, 1995; Veatch & Flack, 1997).

Professional codes of ethics serve a dual purpose: (a) to promote the integrity and reputation of the profession by maintaining specific standards of practice and (b) to serve society's well-being by protecting clients from incompetent practice. Professional ethics documents provide a moral framework for professional practice and define an ideal standard of practice at which to aim. At the center of professional ethics codes and other ethical directives lay the values held by the profession. Some organizations focus on general values such as benefits, well-being, or the greatest good of consumers or clients as the fundamental value to be pursued (Spicer, 1995).

The moral duties articulated in ethics documents may be broad, such as respecting the dignity and self-determination of individuals, or specific, such as maintaining client confidentiality or not engaging in sexual relations with a client. The more general duties permit a certain amount of interpretation in their implementation by the individual practitioner, whereas the more specific ones establish minimum standards for professional behavior. Many groups also provide accompanying guides for professional conduct that elaborate behaviors consistent with their selected principles and virtues.

Professional ethics documents inform and guide practitioners as they seek to engage in ethical practice. Moral guidelines may focus on the character of the individual, with the assumption that moral behavior will flow naturally from a moral person. Professional codes of ethics and other ethical directives ideally serve as something to aspire to. The ethical principles of the *Occupational Therapy Code of Ethics* (American Occupational Therapy Association [AOTA], 2005) that are relevant to cultural competence are as follows:

- *Principle 1:* Occupational therapy personnel shall demonstrate a concern for the safety and well-being of the recipients of their services. (*Beneficence*) (p. 639)
- *Principle 4:* Occupational therapy personnel shall achieve and continually maintain high standards of competence. (*Duty*) (p. 640)
- *Principle 7:* Occupational therapy personnel shall treat colleagues and other professionals with respect, fairness, discretion, and integrity. (*Fidelity*) (p. 641)

The *Guidelines to the Occupational Therapy Code of Ethics* (AOTA, 1998) specifically state,

> Occupational therapy personnel shall develop an understanding and appreciation for different cultures in order to be able to provide culturally competent service. Culturally competent practitioners are aware of how service delivery can be affected by economic, ethnic, racial,

geographic, gender, religious and political factors, as well as marital status, sexual orientation, and disability. [4.3] . . . In areas where the ability to communicate with the client is limited (aphasia, different language, literacy), occupational therapy personnel shall take appropriate steps to facilitate meaningful communication and comprehension. [4.4]

Under the *Core Values and Attitudes of Occupational Therapy Practice* (AOTA, 1993), the concepts that are related to cultural competence are equality, justice, dignity, and truth. The *Occupational Therapy Code of Ethics* (AOTA, 2005) recognizes that culture may influence how individuals cope with problems and interact with each other. The ways in which occupational therapy services are planned and implemented need to be culturally sensitive to be culturally effective. The code of ethics clearly shows that occupational therapists and occupational therapy assistants have an ethical responsibility to be culturally competent practitioners.

Bioethics

Bioethics is a specific term that refers both to the intersection of ethics and the life sciences and to an academic discipline. Bioethics has become a political force in medicine, biology, and environmental studies and a cultural perspective of some consequence (D. Callahan, 1995). Bioethics ranges from the private and individual dilemmas health care workers face (e.g., What should I do here and now?) to the societal choices citizens and legislators face as they try to devise equitable health or environmental policies (e.g., What should we together do as citizens and fellow human beings?). As the field has developed, four general areas of inquiry have emerged that in practice often overlap: health care ethics, theoretical bioethics, regulatory or policy bioethics, and cultural bioethics.

Health care ethics focus on "the delivery of health care, on patient obligations and rights, and on the ethics of the providing professions, including medicine, nursing, dentistry, and allied health" (Anderson & Glesnes-Anderson, 1987, p. 3). Its approach to decision making has been governed by tradition, values, and emotion. Health care ethics involve questioning the ways human beings are treated in medicine, rehabilitation, and other related fields in light of personal and universal moral principles, rights, and values. Because of its context, health care ethics focus on the individual case, seeking to determine what has to be done here and now with specific patients.

Theoretical bioethics deals with the intellectual foundations of the field of medicine, including its moral roots and the ethical warrant for moral judgments in the name of bioethics. *Regulatory or policy bioethics* involves the development of legal or clinical rules and procedures applied to medical cases or general practices. Examples of issues falling into this area include the use of fetal tissue in research, the definition of death, guidelines for do-not-resuscitate orders in hospitals, euthanasia, cloning, and the rationing of health care resources This area seeks to provide legal and policy solutions to pressing societal problems that are ethically defensible and clinically sensible and feasible.

Cultural bioethics refer to ethical questions in relation to the historical, ideological, cultural, and social contexts in which bioethical principles are expressed. How do trends within bioethics reflect the larger culture of which they are a part? What ideological leanings do the moral theories undergirding bioethics openly or implicitly reflect?

Bioethics involve moral principles that cause conflicts, ethical dilemmas, or moral choices in health care. It involves seeking answers to questions, such as the following:

- What is the most just way to distribute scarce resources such as health care technology?
- What is society's and individual practitioners' obligation in providing health care to disadvantaged people?
- What obligation do health care providers have to treat clients in ethically acceptable ways?

Bioethics thus deal with the daily moral dilemmas and ethical puzzles that are a part of contemporary health care practice and environmental stewardship. It helps shape the social context in which those dilemmas and puzzles play themselves out. And it moves between the concreteness of individual and policy decisions and the broad notions and dynamic of the human situation.

Ethical Issues in Pluralistic Settings

Ethical dilemmas and conflicts arise frequently in culturally pluralistic settings. Most questions center on whether health care providers are obligated to act in accordance with what contemporary U.S. medical ethics dictate or to respect the cultural identity of each patient and act according to the family's wishes (Kaufert & Putsch, 1997; Macklin, 1998). Problems arise when the participants in the health care encounter have different interpretations of illness and treatment, hold disparate values in relation to death and dying, and use language or decision-making frameworks differently.

Autonomy and Individual Rights

Mainstream U.S. culture views the "good life" as one that includes a large measure of individual autonomy and mastery, rewarding associations with family and chosen friends, financial success, and personal happiness (Fower & Richardson, 1996). Health care ethics in the United States operate mainly within a modern Western philosophical framework that also emphasizes autonomy and individual rights (Becker, 1995; Longmore, 1995; Macklin, 1998; Yesley, 1995). Bioethics principles reflect Western notions of the sovereignty of the individual and of individual life (Kaufert & Putsch, 1997). Renee Fox (1990), an American sociologist, said, "From the outset, the conceptual framework of bioethics has accorded paramount status to the value-complex of individualism, underscoring the principles of individual rights, autonomy, self-determination, and their legal expression in the jurisprudential notion of privacy" (p. 206).

The ethos of autonomy and individual rights, however, can be at odds with the values of different cultures and religions. The moral principle of autonomy holds that an action or practice is morally wrong insofar as it attempts to control the actions of "substantially autonomous" persons on the basis of a concern for their own welfare. In other words, this principle says that individuals have a right to be self-determined insofar as their actions affect only themselves (Veatch & Flack, 1997). The importance attached to individual rights and respect for persons in consent laws assumes the existence of autonomous decision makers (Gostin, 1995). Currently, the principle of autonomy is at the center of medical decision making, especially as related to truth telling, advance directives, and informed consent (Macklin, 1998; Murphy et al., 1996).

> ... the principle of autonomy is at the center of medical decision making, especially as related to truth telling, advance directives, and informed consent.

Yet much of the world, if not most, embraces a value system that places the family, the community, or the society as a whole above the individual. The good or primacy of the family or community may take precedence over the autonomy of the individual (Kaufert & Koolage, 1984; Kaufert & Putsch, 1997; Macklin, 1998). Solidarity, rather than autonomy, is their highest value (Fox, 1990). A *monistic* (principle of one) focus on the individual may cut patients off from their families, religious practices, or cultural values.

For example, a 52-year-old Nigerian immigrant with an abiding fear of cancer visited his doctor because of a small growth on his lip. The pair had a long-standing physician–patient relationship, and the doctor was aware of the patient's fear. When the biopsy was completed, the doctor informed the patient's son and daughter of the patient's diagnosis and terminal prognosis. The son and daughter asked that all information be withheld from the patient and one of their sisters. They reported a strong cultural prohibition against the telling of bad news and explained that disclosure would abate hope and might hasten the patient's death. They also expressed the fear that if their sister learned of the prognosis, it would place her unborn child at risk.

Did this physician have an obligation to inform the patient of the diagnosis, placing autonomy above all other values? Or was the physician obligated to follow the family's wishes, thereby respecting their cultural custom? The patient and family were immigrants from a culture in which health care providers normally inform the family rather than the patient of a diagnosis. The family's perspective clearly prohibited communication of a terminal prognosis, a perspective that appeared to reflect their cultural values. But perhaps the conflict is not as insuperable as it seems. Patients from all cultures want and need the support of their families, and recognition of the culturally important role that families play when a loved one is ill demonstrates respect for individual values and wishes, thus supporting the principle of autonomy.

According to Gostin (1995), research in this area has raised questions about whether principles of autonomy and individual rights are "truly respectful of all people in all cultures" (p. 844). A heavy emphasis on the moral principle of autonomy and self-determination reflects the political and ideological bias of culturally individualistic societies. Other societies—for example, in central and eastern Europe, Asia, and Africa—give societal rather than individual concerns a more pronounced priority (Fox, 1990). "Countries with strong paternalistic traditions may not consider it necessary to consult with patients about some kinds of decisions; they will not see the issue at all—yet they may have a far livelier dedication to equality of access to health care" (D. Callahan, 1995, p. 251).

Beliefs and reactions related to illness cannot be ascertained on the basis of language, education, class, or ethnicity. Just as important are issues of autonomy and individual rights, ethical and cultural value systems, and family processes, which influence the positions and assumptions that patients and health care providers carry into, and throughout, the delivery of health care.

Truth Telling

Truth telling is central to communication between the patient and the health care provider in clinical practice. It is not about the disclosure of a unilateral truth from the provider to the patient; it is about an ongoing process of communication with patient (Fallowfield, 2004; Surbone & Zwitter, 2000). Cross-cultural differences in truth-telling attitudes and practices have become a major source of debate among bioethicists, who interpreted it as the interplay between autonomy and beneficence under the influence of cultural variables. The debate surrounds not only the ethical justifications for truth telling or withholding but also entail how and when to share information with patients (Anderlik, Pentz, & Hess, 2000; Carrese & Rhodes, 1995; Fallowfield & Jenkins, 2004; Surbone & Zwitter, 2000).

The predominant practice in the United States of disclosing a diagnosis of serious illness to the patient is not considered appropriate by members of some ethnic and religious cultures. Among many cultural groups, truth telling is influenced by four major social–cultural and ethical factors: (a) family as a key player in medical-related decision making, (b) harmony as an essential value for both the individual and family, (c) taboos about discussing death and related issues, and (d) ethical concerns in truth telling—the predominant value of *nonmaleficence* (do no harm) leads to not telling the truth (Lai, 2006). In a study by Murphy and colleagues (1996), Korean Americans tended to have negative attitudes toward telling a patient the truth about a diagnosis and prognosis. They believed that the family, not the patient, should make important health care decisions and that the family, not the patient, should be told the truth about the patient's diagnosis and prognosis. Many Mexican Americans endorse the view that doctors should not discuss death and dying with patients because doing so could be harmful to the patients, and this population also tends to place emphasis on family-centered decision-making styles.

Murphy and colleagues (1996) cite data from other countries that indicate a similar gap between the autonomy model and the family-centered model prevalent in Europe, Asia, and Africa. They conclude that health care providers should ask patients if they want to receive information and make decisions regarding treatment or whether they prefer that their families handle such matters. Imposing the truth on an unprepared patient whose cultural expectation is to be shielded from painful medical truths is not necessarily an act of respect for autonomy.

Informed Consent

Disclosing risks during an informed consent discussion and offering patients the opportunity to make advance directives can pose problems for adherents of traditional cultural beliefs. Carrese and Rhodes (1995) found that Western biomedical and bioethical concepts and principles conflicted with traditional Navajo values and ways of thinking. The traditional Navajo belief is that health is maintained and restored through positive ritual language. When health care providers disclose the risks of a treatment in an informed consent discussion, they speak in a negative way, thereby violating the Navajo value of thinking and speaking in a positive way. The Navajo traditionally have believed that thought and language have the power to shape and control events. Therefore, advance care planning and discussions of end-of-life treatment are considered a dangerous violation of traditional Navajo values. Should providers adhere to the ethical and legal standards pertaining to informed consent as accepted in the United States and risk harming their Navajo patients by talking in a negative way? Or should they behave consistent with the Navajo belief system, avoid doing harm to their patient but violating the ethical requirement of disclosing potential risk?

Disparate Views

Patients and health care providers often come from different educational, cultural, or class backgrounds, and providers and clients may not agree on a common set of cultural values. What may be regarded as morally wrong in one culture may be morally praiseworthy in another. For example, the sick role in occupational therapy is viewed as an active role; the client is expected to achieve an optimal level of functioning through active participation in treatment. In other societies, however, the sick role is a passive one. In Chinese society, for example, it sometimes is believed that a person is chronically ill because of sins committed by family members. Thus, family members may try to do everything for the sick person, encouraging maximum dependence (Jang, 1995). Is it unethical to deny practices or treatments that are clearly unacceptable by the standards of Western culture but are clearly acceptable by the standards of other culture of origin?

Power Issues

Ethical dilemmas and conflicts can be complicated by the unequal distribution of power between client and provider. In the provider–client relationship, the provider has the ultimate responsibility for developing conclusions and proposing treatment alternatives. Providers often reframe human realities according to their own learned practices, rules, and guidelines and thus often are influenced by their own biases (Kaufert & Putsch, 1997). Clients faced with medical decisions may be either over-influenced or underinfluenced by the health care system and its codes of ethics, which can change the relationship power distribution. Power issues can influence decisions, which can range from how to maximize independent function in keeping with the individual's potential to whether to begin invasive or aggressive treatment therapies (Wilson, 1998).

Issues such as autonomy, individual rights, truth telling, informed consent, and advance directives raise questions about whether the principles of autonomy and veracity are respectful of all cultures. Sometimes the institution or health care provider must decide whether to accede to the family's wishes or withdraw care. It is not the cultural tradition that should determine whether disclosure to a patient is ethically appropriate, however, but rather the patient's wish to communicate directly with the provider, to leave communication to the family, or something in between. To ask patients how much they want to be involved in decision making shows respect for their autonomy (Macklin, 1998; Veatch & Flack, 1997): "Negotiation does not, and should not, always lead to acquiescence to Western views of informed consent, truth-telling, or patient's autonomy" (Kaufert & Putsch, 1997, p. 84).

Unilateral decision making by health care providers without consulting the patient and failure to respect the wishes of people regardless of religious or cultural beliefs shows disrespect for people at a fundamental level. When a belief can cause harm to others, attempts to prevent harmful consequences are justifiable. For example, the use of coin rubbing, a traditional Asian folk practice believed to cure a cold or flu commonly used on children, can leave round red or blister burn marks, scars, or disfigurements on the individual's back or abdomen. Respect for autonomy grants patients who have been properly informed in a manner appropriate to the patient's beliefs and understanding the right to refuse a proposed medical treatment. Western medicine does not have all the answers. Some traditional healing practices not only are not harmful but may be as beneficial as those of Western medicine: Health care providers "ought to able to respect cultural diversity without having to accept every single feature embedded in traditional beliefs and rituals" (Macklin, 1998, p. 19).

Ethical Clinical Practice

In every clinical encounter, occupational therapists and occupational therapy assistants are speaking across cultural gaps. The interaction of clients and practitioners embodies a form of multiculturalism in which several cultures—the health care profession, institution, family, community, and traditional culture—are merged (Genao, Bussey-Jones, Brady, Branch, & Corbie-Smith, 2003). To genuinely understand a client, practitioners should consider each therapeutic exchange to be a cross-cultural event. The challenge in providing ethical and culturally competent care is in the diversity of meanings that can be applied to similar concepts and principles (Iwama, 2003). The meanings people assign to ideas and concepts are culturally based and culturally driven.

Culture shapes people's views of illness and well-being in both the physical and spiritual realms and affects their perceptions of health care and the outcome of treatment (Carrese, 1993). Some practitioners may be comfortable with the idea of respecting cultural difference when the patient is a competent adult, but when children are involved they may be unwilling to tolerate decisions that result in what they perceive to be compromised care or harm, even when these decisions make sense in the context of a particular culture (Carrese, 1993; Catherwood, 2000; Pooser, 2002). Cultural competence is key to making sound, ethical, culturally, appropriate decisions.

The literature has demonstrated that beliefs and values serve as a basis for moral decision making and do indeed vary by culture. Ethics are greatly influenced by the cultural framework in which an interpersonal encounter takes place. Practitioners need to be aware of the value assumptions embodied in biomedical approaches and in the culture, power, and ethics of medicine to identify how they play out in clinical practice (Coward & Hartick, 2000). Patients and their families, as well as health care providers, bring many different cultural models of morality and moral reasoning to the clinical setting. It is the constant overlapping and interaction of cultures that create daily conflicts and dilemmas in providing health care services.

Because present bioethical concepts of moral deliberation offer little insight into how to develop meaningful responses to deal with cultural pluralism, religious diversity, and norm conflicts, Wells (2005) proposes an ethic of diversity matrix with moral principles and rules of human conduct for finding resolutions in a pluralistic environment (see Table 23.2). This matrix—which includes the principles of understanding, tolerance, standing up to evil, fallibility, respect, cultural competence, justice, and care—provides occupational therapists and occupational therapy assistants and students with a framework and moral construct to guide decisions when conflicts arise within a multicultural setting without sacrificing equality, justice, or respect. The ethic of diversity helps therapists and students engage in moral reasoning and test their moral opinions against those of others. It supports the expectation of differences in all clinical interactions.

The values of ethical relativism and pluralism hold that practitioners respect the moral choices patients make in light of their cultural or religious beliefs (Haddad, 2001). Embracing these values increases learning opportunities and facilitates cultural competence (Coward & Hartick, 2000; Erlen, 1998). Using an ethic of diversity as a guideline offers practitioners an opportunity to extend human knowl-

Table 23.2. An Ethic of Diversity Matrix

Principle	Definition
Understanding	We seek to understand other cultures before we pass judgment on them.
Tolerance	We recognize that there are important areas in which intelligent people of good will in fact differ.
Standing up to evil	We recognize that, at some point, we must stand up against evil, even when it is outside of our own bodies.
Fallibility	We recognize that, even with the best of intentions, our judgment may be flawed and mistaken.
Respect	We recognize that all human beings are worthy of respect simply because they are human.
Cultural competence	We seek self-exploration, knowledge, and skills to interact effectively and humanely with people different from ourselves.
Justice	We seek to deal with everyone fairly and equitably in the distribution of goods and services.
Care	We recognize that the needs of others play a part in all ethical decision making.

Note. These principles can be used to protect individuals against harm and to help identify the good in people. These principles collectively assist practitioners in acknowledging difference as the norm.

Source: Data from Wells, S. A. (2005). *An ethic of diversity.* In R. B. Purtilo, G. M. Jensen, & C. B. Royeen (Eds.), *Educating for moral action: A sourcebook in health and rehabilitation ethics* (pp. 31–41). Philadelphia: F. A. Davis.

edge by finding wisdom in dissimilar cultural practices and allows them to teach patients what, from a medical point of view, may damage health and to learn more about the rationale for and techniques of many traditional practices. It assists therapists in discovering ways to give care to people who have different values and lifestyles.

A cross-cultural ethical conflict may not have a single, ethically correct resolution but rather many possible resolutions, each with ethical costs and advantages. Which resolution ultimately is chosen will depend on which voices are included in the moral dialogue. A sound moral decision requires practitioners to reflect on their own values and biases, interpret the cultures involved, and acknowledge the contributions and principles of moral reasoning.

Larger Ethical Responsibilities

As health care providers, do occupational therapists and occupational therapy assistants have a moral obligation or social responsibility to ensure the just distribution of access to health care to all people? The state of health care in the United States is insufficient for poor people, ethnic groups, and women. For many members of these groups, it is a continuous struggle to obtain adequate health care, to make copayments, and to receive the same dignity and respect that more affluent, educated, or politically informed patients demand and receive (Dula & Goering, 1994). Access to health care is related to the status of having a full-time job or to the social merit of having served in the armed forces. It can be diminished by divorce. Children have access to health care in direct proportion to the status of their parents rather than in proportion to their needs. Medicare for elders is the only exception to statutes-based access to health care (Dowling, 1994; Miles, 1994). Health status differences between poor and nonpoor people, White people and people of color, and adults and children can be linked to differences in available services, the nature and quality of those services, and the ways people who are helped use them.

The United States has long recognized the specialness of health care and articulated the idea of a right to health care. Dowling (1994) observes that these ideas have been supported by generous public funding for medical education, special programs for medically needy people and, in the past, the insulation of health professionals from market pressure. According to Dowling, this specialness is the foundation for creating a public moral obligation for health care providers to practice in poor areas. Professional health care ethics involve more than an obligation to individual patients and other appropriate constituencies; they include an obligation to the public as a whole (Jennings, Callahan, & Wolf, 1987). Health professionals have an obligation and responsibility to control the cost of their services, to maintain (or allow for) an adequate supply of professionals, and to cultivate a professional culture that promotes service to others over self-interest.

Edmund Pellegrino (1987), a medical ethicist and professor of medical ethics at Georgetown University Medical Center, believes that health professionals have an ethical responsibility to ensure that all segments of the population have access to health care. He states that each provider must establish some hierarchy of values and priorities that will define his or her individual and social ethical responsibility. The provider's first priority is moral integrity in dealing with the clients he or she treats. A second-order responsibility is to help shape policies that bear directly on the health of the larger community.

Ferguson (1994) asks how physicians can provide medical care to "people whose language, culture, sexual orientation, and socioeconomic status are different from their own" (p. 123). He explains that this question places physicians in an ethical quagmire: how to serve the poor and get paid at the same time. He infers that not only the lack of economic incentive to work with the poor but also cultural differences were to blame for this shortage of medical providers. Some of the physicians he interviewed felt inadequate in dealing with clients who speak another language or have different views about compliance. Others cited the bureaucratic tangle of dealing with Medicaid and Medicare for reimbursement. Others complained about clients' lack of incentive to meet scheduled appointments.

Health care providers must take responsibility for understanding the attitudes and values that shape their delivery of health care. Personal views about racially and ethnically diverse groups either can maintain or reduce the distance between provider and client. To resolve questions of ethical responsibility, practitioners must weigh their own rights against those of society. On one hand, providers in the United States have a right to serve and work where they please and should not be subject to national and societal needs. On the other hand, poor people, people of color, and children have a right to basic health care, which is necessary for equality of opportunity.

Dowling (1994) asks, "Do [health care providers] have a micro responsibility to provide care to some individuals, or do they, in fact, have a macro or societal obligation as gatekeepers for the social good that is a prerequisite for equal opportunity?" (p. 138). In other words, does the health care provider's moral obligation to do no harm to clients on an individual level translate into a societal obligation to ensure access and just distribution of care to all, because the absence of care does harm? The moral challenge to health providers, according to McTernan (1989), is to remember that they exist to serve the health care needs of the community and that those needs do not exist to provide them with opportunities for achieving wealth and status.

Why should health care professionals address the needs of various ethnic, cultural, and poor groups? The answer is simple: Because all people are members of the human community, regardless of their different identities. Racism, social injustice, insensitivity, and irresponsibility on the part of society and the medical profession have given members of ethnic minorities and other diverse groups a different perspective and outlook on life. To understand the morality and the real-life effects of unfair access and services, providers need to look at the health experiences of real people and different populations. They must be concerned with more than what they can see in hospitals or clinics; they also must address the wider social issues that affect not only health but also decisions about health.

Summary

If health care providers' views on the ethical principles that govern decision making are in conflict with the values held by their patients and their patients' families or communities, disagreement over cultural values may lead to confrontation. Conflicts based on cultural differences can be mediated using strategies that allow both the patient and the provider the opportunity to clarify their values (Jecker, Carrese, & Pearlman, 1995). Negotiation does not, and should not, always lead to acquiescence to Western views about informed consent, truth telling, or patient autonomy.

When working with a client from a different background, practitioners must explore the cultural context as well as the cultural effect of their advice and intervention. They should openly discuss their personal views and the sources of those views. Such discussions help clients better understand their options and help provide answers to frequent ethical dilemmas. Further, dialogue with patients can help practitioners develop health approaches, systems, and policies that fully recognize and include the effects of the practitioner's and society's culture on the ethics of medical decisions (Dula & Goering, 1994; Stanfield, 1993; Wilson, 1998).

Openness to personal bias will stimulate practitioners to critically examine the cultural norms of their own practice. By embracing the principles outlined in the ethic of diversity matrix in Table 23.2, occupational therapists and occupational therapy assistants will have a framework to guide decision making when conflicts arise. Increasing their personal self-exploration, knowledge, and skills (including cultural competence) will enhance practitioners' ability to engage in ethical decision making that is (a) guided by the ability to communicate appropriately and effectively, (b) culturally framed while remaining aware of individual variances, and (c) based on sound principles of moral reasoning.

Medical ethicists need to discuss health care providers' obligation to treat clients in ethically acceptable ways and reassure the communities that while there are good reasons for distrust, suspicion must not stand in the way of beneficial treatments (Miles, 1994). Health care providers must "embody an ethic of caring and respect for all groups, a responsibility to condemn unjust medical practices, and a humility and an empathy regarding human suffering, which in the end transcends all cultural and racial prejudices and differences" (Dula & Goering, 1994, p. 8). The U.S. health care system must ensure that all people receive ethical preventive and curative care and that the widening disparities affecting ethnic and cultural minorities, women, and poor people are reduced and ultimately eliminated.

Reflection

1. Write a personal code of ethics that includes principles to guide your interaction with culturally diverse individuals.

2. Discuss in writing or with a colleague whether occupational therapists have an ethical responsibility to ensure that all people have access to occupational therapy services regardless of racial or ethnical background, socioeconomic status, religious beliefs, cultural backgrounds, or health status.

References

American Occupational Therapy Association. (1993). Core values and attitudes of occupational therapy practice. *American Journal of Occupational Therapy, 47,* 1085–1086.

American Occupational Therapy Association. (1998). Guidelines to the occupational therapy code of ethics. *American Journal of Occupational Therapy, 52,* 881–884.

American Occupational Therapy Association. (2005). Occupational therapy code of ethics. (2005). *American Journal of Occupational Therapy, 59,* 639–642.

Anderlik, M. R., Pentz, R. D., & Hess, K. R. (2000). Revisiting the truth telling debate: A study of disclosure practices at a major cancer center. *Journal of Clinical Ethics, 11,* 251–259.

Anderson, G. R., & Glesnes-Anderson, V. A. (1987). *Health care ethics: A guide for decision makers.* Rockville, MD: Aspen Systems.

Beauchamp, T. L., & Childress, J. F. (1989). *Principles of biomedical ethics* (3rd ed.). New York: Oxford University Press.

Becker, G. K. (1995). Asian and Western ethics: Some remarks on a productive tension. *Eubios Journal of Asian and International Bioethics, 5,* 31–33.

Boss, J. A. (1998). *Ethics for life: An interdisciplinary and multicultural introduction.* Mountain View, CA: Mayfield.

Buford, T. O. (1984). *Personal philosophy: The art of living.* New York: CBS College.

Callahan, D. (1995). History of bioethics. In W. T. Reich (Ed.), *Encyclopedia of bioethics* (rev. ed., Vol. 1, pp. 248–256). New York: Macmillan.

Callahan, S. C. (1991). *In good conscience: Reason and emotion in moral decision making.* San Francisco: Harper.

Carrese, J. (1993). Commentary (on culture, healing, and professional obligations). *Hastings Center Report, 23*(4), 16.

Carrese, J. A., & Rhodes, L. A. (1995). Western bioethics on the Navajo reservation: Benefit or harm? *Journal of the American Medical Association, 274,* 826–829.

Catherwood, J. F. (2000). An argument for intolerance. *Journal of Medical Ethics, 26,* 427–443.

Childress, J. (1989). The normative principles of medical ethics. In R. Veatch (Ed.), *Medical ethics* (pp. 27–48). Boston: Jones & Bartlett.

Clouser, K. D. (1978). Bioethics. In W. T. Reich (Ed.), *Encyclopedia of bioethics* (Vol. 1, pp. 115–127). New York: Free Press.

Coward, H., & Hartick, G. (2000). Perspectives on health and cultural pluralism: Ethics in medical education. *Clinical Investigations in Medicine, 23,* 261–266.

Davis, A. J., & Koening, B. A. (1996). A question of policy: Bioethics in a multicultural society. *Nursing Policy Forum, 2*(1), 6–11.

Dowling, P. (1994). Access to medical care: Do physicians and academic medical centers have a societal responsibility? In A. Dula & S. Goering (Eds.), *"It just ain't fair": The ethics of health care for African Americans* (pp. 134–142). Westport, CT: Praeger.

Dula, A., & Goering, S. (Eds.). (1994). *"It just ain't fair": The ethics of health care for African Americans.* Westport, CT: Praeger.

Erlen, J. (1998). Culture, ethics, and respect: The bottom line in understanding. *Orthopedic Nursing, 17*(6), 79–85.

Fallowfield, L., & Jenkins, V. (2004). Communicating sad, bad, difficult new medicine. *Lancet, 363,* 312–319.

Ferguson, W. J. (1994). The physician's responsibility to medically underserved poor people. In A. Dula & S. Goering (Eds.), *"It just ain't fair": The ethics of health care for African Americans* (pp. 123–133). Westport CT: Praeger.

Fower, B. J., & Richardson, F. C. (1996). Why is multiculturalism good? *American Psychologist, 51,* 609–621.

Fox, R. C. (1990). The evolution of American bioethics: A sociological perspective. In G. Weisz (Ed.), *Social science perspectives on medical ethics* (pp. 201–220). Philadelphia: University of Pennsylvania Press.

Genao, I., Bussey-Jones, J., Brady, D., Branch, W. T., & Corbie-Smith, G. (2003). Building the case for cultural competence. *American Journal of the Medical Sciences, 326,* 136–140.

Gostin, L. O. (1995). Informed consent, cultural sensitivity, and respect for persons. *Journal of the American Medical Association, 274,* 844–845.

Haddad, A. (2001). Ethics in action. *RN Journal, 64*(3), 21–24.

Howell, W. S. (1981, November). *Ethics of intercultural communication.* Paper presented to the Speech Communication Association, Anaheim, CA.

Iwama, M. (2003). Toward culturally relevant epistemologies in occupational therapy. *American Journal of Occupational Therapy, 57,* 582–588.

Jang, Y. (1995). Chinese culture and occupational therapy. *British Journal of Occupational Therapy, 58,* 103–106.

Jecker, N. S., Carrese, J. A., & Pearlman, R. A. (1995). Caring for patients in cross-cultural settings. *Hastings Center Report, 25*(1), 6–14.

Jennings, B., Callahan, D., & Wolf, S. M. (1987, February). The professions: Public interest and common good. *Hastings Center Report, 17*(Special Suppl.), 3–10.

Johnson, V. (1995). *Heart full of grace: A thousand years of Black wisdom.* New York: Simon & Schuster.

Kaufert, J. M., & Koolage, W. W. (1984). Role conflict among culture brokers: The experiences of Native Canadian medical interpreters. *Social Science and Medicine, 18,* 283–286.

Kaufert, J. M., & Putsch, R. W. (1997). Communication through interpreters in health care: Ethical dilemmas arising from differences in class, cultures, language, and power. *Journal of Clinical Ethics, 8*(1), 71–87.

Lai, Y.-H. (2006). Views from Asia: Truth-telling in cancer diagnosis and prognosis in Taiwan. UICC World Cancer Congress 2006, Washington, DC. Retrieved on August 3, 2007, from http://2006.confex.com/uicc/uicc/techprogram/P10430.htm

Longmore, P. K. (1995). Medical decision making and people with disabilities: A clash of cultures. *Journal of Law, Medicine and Ethics, 32,* 82–87.

Macklin, R. (1998). Ethical relativism in a multicultural society. *Kennedy Institute of Ethics Journals, 8*(1), 1–22.

McTernan, E. J. (1989). *Action in affirmation: Toward an unambiguous profession of nursing.* New York: McGraw-Hill.

Miles, S. (1994). Commentary. In A. Dula & S. Goering (Eds.), *"It just ain't fair": The ethics of health care for African Americans* (pp. 143). Westport, CT: Praeger.

Murphy, S. T., Palmer, J. M., Azen, S., Frank, G., Michel, V., & Blackhall, L. J. (1996). Ethnicity and advance care directives. *Journal of Law, Medicine, and Ethics, 24,* 108–117.

Paige, R. M., & Martin, J. N. (1996). Ethics in intercultural training. In D. Landis & R. S. Bhagat (Eds.), *Handbook of intercultural training* (2nd ed., pp. 35–60). Thousand Oaks, CA: Sage.

Pellegrino, E. D. (1987). Toward an expanded medical ethics: The Hippocratic ethic revisited. In J. B. Rogers (Ed.), *In search of the modern Hippocratic* (pp. 45–64). Iowa City: University of Iowa.

Pellegrino, E. D., & Thomasma, D. C. (1981). *A philosophical basis of medical practice: Toward a philosophy and ethic of the healing professions.* New York: Oxford University Press.

Pooser, P. (2002). When clinician and parent disagree (Ethics). *ASHA Leader, 7*(21), 9.

Random House College Dictionary (rev. ed.). (1988). Ethics. New York: Random House.

Spicer, C. M. (1995). Nature and role of codes and other ethics directives. In W. T. Reich (Ed.), *Encyclopedia of bioethics* (rev. ed., Vol. 1, pp. 260–261). New York: Macmillan.

Stanfield, J. H. (1993). Epistemological considerations. In J. Stanfield & D. Rutledge (Eds.), *Race and ethnicity in research methods* (pp. 16–36). Newbury Park, CA: Sage.

Surbone, A., & Zwitter, M. (2000). Communication with the cancer patient: Information and truth. In *Annals of the New York Academy of Sciences* (2nd ed., pp. 109–118). New York: John Hopkins University.

Veatch, R. M., & Flack, H. E. (1997). *Case studies in allied health ethics.* Upper Saddle River, NJ: Prentice-Hall.

Wells, S. A. (2005). An ethic of diversity. In R. B. Purtilo, G. M. Jensen, & C. B. Royeen (Eds.), *Educating for moral action: A sourcebook in health and rehabilitation ethics* (pp. 31–41). Philadelphia: F. A. Davis.

Wilson, G. (1998). *Medical ethics and culture: Whose ethics should we follow?* (Contemporary Issues, Cleveland Clinic Foundation, Department of Bioethics). Retrieved March 20, 1999, from www.ccf.org/ed/bioethic/biocon11.htm

Yesley, M. S. (1995). Diversity in bioethics. *Eubios Journal of Asian and International Bioethics, 5,* 87.

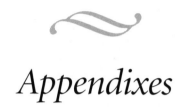

Appendixes

A

National Standards for Culturally and Linguistically Appropriate Services (CLAS) in Health Care

Standard 1

Health care organizations should ensure that patients/consumers receive from all staff members effective, understandable, and respectful care that is provided in a manner compatible with their cultural health beliefs and practices and preferred language.

Standard 2

Health care organizations should implement strategies to recruit, retain, and promote at all levels of the organization a diverse staff and leadership that are representative of the demographic characteristics of the service area.

Standard 3

Health care organizations should ensure that staff at all levels and across all disciplines receive ongoing education and training in culturally and linguistically appropriate service delivery.

Standard 4

Health care organizations must offer and provide language assistance services, including bilingual staff and interpreter services, at no cost to each patient/con-

Note: From *National standards for culturally and linguistically appropriate services in health care. Executive summary,* Office of Minority Health, U.S. Public Health Service, 2001, Washington, DC: U.S. Department of Health and Human Services.

sumer with limited English proficiency at all points of contact, in a timely manner during all hours of operation.

Standard 5

Health care organizations must provide to patients/consumers in their preferred language both verbal offers and written notices informing them of their right to receive language assistance services.

Standard 6

Health care organizations must assure the competence of language assistance provided to limited English proficient patients/consumers by interpreters and bilingual staff. Family and friends should not be used to provide interpretation services (except on request by the patient/consumer).

Standard 7

Health care organizations must make available easily understood patient-related materials and post signage in the languages of the commonly encountered groups and/or groups represented in the service area.

Standard 8

Health care organizations should develop, implement, and promote a written strategic plan that outlines clear goals, policies, operational plans, and management accountability/oversight mechanisms to provide culturally and linguistically appropriate services.

Standard 9

Health care organizations should conduct initial and ongoing self-assessments of CLAS-related activities and are encouraged to integrate cultural and linguistic competence-related measures into their internal audits, performance improvement programs, patient satisfaction assessments, and outcomes-based evaluations.

Standard 10

Health care organizations should ensure that data on the individual patient's/consumer's race, ethnicity, and spoken and written language are collected in health records, integrated into the organization's management information systems, and periodically updated.

Standard 11

Health care organizations should maintain a current demographic, cultural, and epidemiological profile of the community as well as a needs assessment to accurately plan for and implement services that respond to the cultural and linguistic characteristics of the service area.

Standard 12

Health care organizations should develop participatory, collaborative partnerships with communities and utilize a variety of formal and informal mechanisms to facilitate community and patient/consumer involvement in designing and implementing CLAS-related activities.

B

Electronic Resources for Cultural Competence and Related Topics

American Association of University Professors (AAUP) diversity bibliography: http://aaup.org/AAUP/issuesed/diversity/Diversitybib.htm.

Afrol News (gender, women): www.afrol.com/categories/gender_women/news

Boston Center for Refugee Health and Human Rights: www.glphr.org/refugee/library.htm

California Endowment Program (cultural competence): www.calendow.org/program_areas/cultural_competence_recent_publications.stm

Center for Cross-Cultural Health: www.crosshealth.com

Cultural Competence Resources: www.med.yale.edu/library/education/culturalcomp

Cultural Competence Resources for Health Care Providers: http://hrsa.gov/culturalcompetence

Cultural Competency Web Page: http://cecp.air.org/cultural/default.htm

Cultured Med at the Peter J.Cayan Library, State University of New York Institute of Technology: http://culturedmed.sunyit.edu

DiversityRx: www.DiversityRx.org/HTML/ESLANG.htm

Gay, Lesbian, and Straight Education Network: http://www.glsen.org

Global Health Source: www.globalhealth.gov

Issues in Hispanic Health: www.uic.edu/depts/lib/lhs/resources/hispanichealth

Migration Information Source: www.migrationinformation.org

Minority Health Concerns and Cultural Competence Resources
(National Network of Libraries of Medicine, Midcontinental Region):
http://nnlm.gov/mcr/resources/community/competency.html

National Center for Cultural Competence: http://www11.georgetown.edu/
research/gucchd/nccc

National Guide for Interpreting in Health Care: http://ncihc.org

Office of Minority Health: www.omhrc.gov/templates/browse.aspx?lvl=1&lvlID=3

Provider's Guide to Quality and Culture: http://erc.msh.org/qualityandculture

U.S. Department of Health and Human Services, Office of Minority Health:
www.omhrc.gov

C

Assessment Tools Used to Measure Cultural Competence

The majority of the tools in the list are from the field of behavioral health. Two weaknesses of these tools are their reliance on self-report measures and their focus on race and ethnicity and neglect of other cultural factors (Stanhope, Solomon, Pernell-Arnold, Sands, & Bourjolly, 2005).

- Cross-Cultural Adaptability Inventory (CCAI; Kelley & Meyers, 1992)
- Cross-Cultural Counseling Inventory–Revised (CCCI–R; LaFromboise, Coleman, & Hernandez, 1991)
- Multicultural Knowledge-and-Skills Survey (MAKSS; Andrea, Daniels, & Heck, 1991)
- Multicultural Counseling Inventory (MCI; Sodowsky, Taffe, Gutkin, & Wise, 1994)
- Multiultural Counseling Knowledge and Awareness Scale (MCKAS; Ponterotto et al., 1996).

References

D'Andrea, M., Daniels, J., & Heck, R. (1991). Evaluating the impact of multicultural counselor training. *Journal of Counseling and Development, 70,* 143–150.

Kelley, C., & Meyers, J. (1999). The cross-cultural adaptability inventory. In S. Fowler and M. Mumford (Eds.), *Intercultural sourcebook: Cross-cultural training methods,* (Vol. 2, pp. 53–70). Yarmouth, ME: Intercultural.

LaFramboise, T. D., Coleman, H. L. K., & Hernandez, A. (1991). Development and factor structure of the Cross-Cultural Counseling Inventory—Revised. *Professional Psychology: Research and Practice, 22,* 380–388.

Ponterottok, J. G., & Alexander, C. M. (1996). Assessing the multicultural competence of counselors and clinicians. In L. A. Suzuki, P. J. Meller, & J. G. Ponterotto (Eds.), *Handbook of multicultural assessment: Clinical, psychological, and educational applications* (pp. 651–672). San Francisco: Jossey-Bass.

Sodowsky, G. R., Taffe, R. C., Gutkin, T. B., & Wise, S. L. (1994). Multicultural counseling inventory (MCI): A self-report measure of multicultural counseling competencies. *Journal of Counseling Psychology, 41,* 137–148.

Stanhope, V., Solomon, P., Pernell-Arnold, A., Sands, R. G., & Bourjolly, J. N. (2005). Evaluating cultural competence among behavioral health professionals. *Psychiatric Rehabilitation Journal, 28,* 225–233.

D

AOTA Position Paper:
Complementary and Alternative Medicine

Purpose of Paper

The American Occupational Therapy Association, Inc. (AOTA) asserts that complementary and alternative medicine (CAM) may be used by occupational therapists and occupational therapy assistants as part of a comprehensive approach to enhance engagement in occupation (Giese, Parker, Lech-Boura, Burkhardt, & Cook, 2003). Because the use of CAMs is expanding in various health care practices, the purpose of this paper is to define the appropriate use of complementary and alternative medicine within the scope of occupational therapy practice.

Explanation of CAMs

The National Center for Complementary and Alternative Medicine (NCCAM) of the National Institutes of Health has identified five domains of CAM practice and defines *complementary and alternative medicine* as "a group of diverse medical and health care systems, practices, and products that are not presently considered to be part of conventional medicine" (NCCAM, 2002). The five domains of CAM practice are (1) alternative medical systems, (2) mind–body interventions, (3) biologically based treatments, (4) manipulative and body-based methods, and (5) energy therapies. Though the terms *complementary* and *alternative* often are interchanged, the commonly accepted distinction between them is that alternative medicine is practiced *in place of* conventional medicine, while complementary practices are accessed *in conjunction with* allopathic medical practices. The newer terms *integrative medicine* and *blended medicine* also are used to reference complementary medicine. The definition of complementary and alternative medicine is, by its very nature, dynamic. Practices contained within the definition of CAMs change as some become adopted into conventional health, and new ones emerge (Giese et al., 2003).

CAM services, though often paid for privately, increasingly are covered by insurance companies and health maintenance organizations (Astin, Pelletier, Marie, & Haskell, 2000; Cleary-Guida, Okvat, Oz, & Ting, 2001; Wolsko, Eisenberg, Davis, Ettner, & Phillips, 2002). Factors that compel third-party payers to include selected CAMs in health care policies include cost-effectiveness, consumer demand, demonstrated clinical efficacy, and state mandate (Pelletier & Astin, 2002; Pelletier, Astin, & Haskell, 1999). Further support for the use of CAMs is provided by the funding for research and training of CAM practices by the NCCAM.

Research is important to determine the efficacy and effectiveness of CAM practices in health and wellness arenas. The current number of outcomes studies for any specific CAM method is small. Research that does exist generally has limited and nonrandomized sample sizes and inconsistently defined terms, thereby reducing the power of the evidence and the ability to generalize results. Results that do exist show mixed evidence on the efficacy of CAM practices. These findings suggest the need for more studies to validate the efficacy of specific CAM practices with scientific evidence using randomized, controlled trials.

Use of CAMs Within Occupational Therapy Practice

Occupational therapists and occupational therapy assistants have used various CAM techniques in the delivery of occupational therapy services. CAMs may be used within the scope of occupational therapy practice when they are used as preparatory methods or purposeful activities to facilitate the ability of clients to engage in their daily life occupations.

Occupational therapy values engagement in occupations and has as its core mission to support participation in context (AOTA, 2002). Occupations are "activities . . . of everyday life, named, organized, and given value and meaning by individuals and a culture" (Law, Polatajko, Baptiste, & Townsend, 1997). Occupations encompass activities of daily living, instrumental activities of daily living, education, leisure skills, play, social participation, and work (AOTA, 2002). The occupational therapist is responsible for all aspects of occupational therapy service delivery and is accountable for the safety and effectiveness of the occupational therapy service delivery process. The occupational therapy assistant is responsible for providing safe and effective occupational therapy services under the supervision of and in partnership with the occupational therapist (AOTA, 2004b).

To determine whether to use CAMs in the delivery of occupational therapy services, occupational therapists and occupational therapy assistants must evaluate the client, develop an intervention based on the client's needs and priorities, and conduct outcomes measurement. The evaluation enables the occupational therapist and the occupational therapy assistant to gain an understanding of the client's strengths, priorities, and current limitations in carrying out daily occupations.

Evaluation and intervention address factors that influence the client's occupational performance, including how the client performs the daily life occupations, the demands of those occupations, and the environments where those occupations are performed. As part of the evaluation and the intervention, the occupational therapist and the occupational therapy assistant must determine whether the use of CAMs is consistent with the client's cultural practices, priorities, and needs; is safe to use; and is an appropriate approach to facilitate the ability of the client to participate in daily life occupations. Outcomes are measured to determine the effectiveness of occupational therapy services and future therapeutic interventions with the client. The occupational therapist and the occupational therapy assistant must measure whether the use of CAMs resulted in positive outcomes.

Some CAM techniques currently being utilized in occupational therapy include guided imagery, massage, myofascial release, meditation, yoga, and behavioral relaxation training (Lindsay, Fee, Michie, & Heap, 1994; Scott, 1999). Because individuals receiving occupational therapy services are embedded in their cultures and because some CAM practices are embedded within particular cultures, occupational therapists and occupational therapy assistants need to understand how those cultures influence where and when to use CAM techniques. Outcome studies continue to need to be conducted to determine the efficacy and effectiveness of using CAM techniques during occupational therapy intervention to enable individuals to engage in their daily life occupations.

The *Occupational Therapy Code of Ethics* (AOTA, 2000) mandates safe and competent practice, holding occupational therapy professionals responsible for the maintenance of high standards of competence. CAM techniques used within the scope of occupational therapy practice may require additional training, competency examinations, certification, and regulatory knowledge. The use of specific CAM techniques may be subject to federal, state, and often local municipal regulations that govern practice, advertising, ethics, professional terminology, and training. It is the responsibility of the occupational therapist and the occupational therapy assistant to know and comply with applicable laws and regulations associated with CAM techniques as well as those mandated for the occupational therapy profession. Occupational therapists and occupational therapy assistants must abide by state regulations when billing for occupational therapy services that incorporate the use of CAMs. They must distinguish between when they are using CAMs within the scope of occupational therapy practice and when they are using CAMs as a primary approach beyond the scope of occupational therapy practice (AOTA, 2002, 2004a).

Issues of client safety and health care worker safety are salient to all areas of occupational therapy practice. The use of CAMs requires attention to client safety in consumer decision making, client interventions, and professional education and training. The risks and benefits of CAMs used in occupational therapy should be communicated to clients as standard practice in a client-centered, evidence-based approach to care.

Summary

Occupational therapy professionals facilitate proficient and satisfying engagement in the significant tasks and meaningful activities of life. Complementary and alternative medical practices, systems, and products may be appropriately incorporated into occupational therapy practice as a way to encourage a client's engagement in meaningful occupations. Scientific studies are needed to validate the safety and efficacy of CAM methods within occupational therapy practice. Advanced-level training and continuing education are important to acquire the knowledge and skill to utilize CAM methods, to address the concerns for patient safety and informed consent, and to meet the rigors of regulatory requirements.

References

American Occupational Therapy Association. (2000). Occupational therapy code of ethics (2000). *American Journal of Occupational Therapy, 54,* 614–616.

American Occupational Therapy Association. (2002). Occupational therapy practice framework: Domain and process. *American Journal of Occupational Therapy, 56,* 609–639.

American Occupational Therapy Association. (2004a). *Definition of occupational therapy practice for the AOTA Model Practice Act.* (Available from the State Affairs Group, American Occupational Therapy Association, 4720 Montgomery Lane, Bethesda, MD 20814)

American Occupational Therapy Association. (2004b). Guidelines for supervision, roles, and responsibilities during the delivery of occupational therapy services. *American Journal of Occupational Therapy, 58,* 663–667.

Astin, J. A., Pelletier, K. R., Marie, A., & Haskell, W. L. (2000). Complementary and alternative medicine use among elderly persons: One-year analysis of a Blue Shield Medicare supplement. *Journals of Gerontology, Series A, Biological Sciences and Medical Sciences, 55*(1), M4–M9.

Cleary-Guida, M. B., Okvat, H. A., Oz, M. C., & Ting, W. (2001). A regional survey of health insurance coverage for complementary and alternative medicine: Current status and future ramifications. *Journal of Alternative and Complementary Medicine, 7,* 269–273.

Giese, T., Parker, J. A., Lech-Boura, J., Burkhardt, A., & Cook, A. (2003). *The role of occupational therapy in complementary and alternative medicine* [White Paper]. Adopted by the AOTA Board of Directors 6-22-03. (Available from American Occupational Therapy Association, 4720 Montgomery Lane, Bethesda, MD 20814.)

Law, M., Polatajko, H., Baptiste, W., & Townsend, E. (1997). Core concepts of occupational therapy. In E. Townsend (Ed.), *Enabling occupation: An occupational therapy perspective* (pp. 29–56). Ottawa, ON: Canadian Association of Occupational Therapists.

Lindsay, W. R., Fee, M., Michie, A., & Heap, I. (1994). The effects of cue control relaxation on adults with severe mental retardation. *Research in Developmental Disabilities, 15,* 425–437.

National Center for Complementary and Alternative Medicine. (2002). What is complementary and alternative medicine? Retrieved July 14, 2002, from http://www.nccam.nih.gov/health/whatiscam/.

Pelletier, K. R., & Astin, J. A. (2002). Integration and reimbursement of complementary and alternative medicine by managed care and insurance providers: 2000 update and cohort analysis. *Alternative Therapies in Health and Medicine, 8*(1), 38–39, 42, 44.

Pelletier, K. R., Astin, J. A., & Haskell, W. L. (1999). Current trends in the integration and reimbursement of complementary and alternative medicine by managed care organizations (MCOs) and insurance providers: 1998 update and cohort analysis. *American Journal of Health Promotion, 4,* 125–133.

Scott, A. H. (1999). Wellness works: Community service health promotion groups led by occupational therapy students. *American Journal of Occupational Therapy, 53,* 566–574.

Wolsko, P. M., Eisenberg, D. M., Davis, R. B., Ettner, S. L., & Phillips, R. S. (2002). Insurance coverage, medical conditions, and visits to alternative medicine providers: Results of a national survey. *Archives of Internal Medicine, 162,* 281–287.

Additional Reading

Bausell, R. B., Lee, W. L., & Berman, B. M. (2001). Demographic and health-related correlates to visits to complementary and alternative medical providers. *Medical Care, 9,* 190–196.

Burkhardt, A., & Parker, J. (1998, November 26). OT perspective: Complementary care survey results. *OT Week, 12*(48), 4.

Carlson, J. (2003). *Complementary therapies and wellness: Practice essentials for holistic healthcare.* Upper Saddle River, NJ: Prentice Hall.

Eisenberg, D. M., Davis, R. B., Ettner, S. L., Appel, S., Wilkey, S., Van Rompay, M., et al. (1998). Trends in alternative medicine use in the United States, 1990–1997: Results of a follow-up national survey. *Journal of the American Medical Association, 280,* 1569–1575.

Eisenberg, D. M., Kessler, R. C., Van Rompay, M. I., Kaptchuk, T. J., Wilkey, S. A., Appel, S., et al. (2001). Perceptions about complementary therapies relative to conventional therapies among adults who use both: Results from a national survey. *Annals of Internal Medicine, 135,* 344–351.

Kaboli, P. J., Doebbeling, B. N., Saag, K. G., & Rosenthal, G. E. (2001). Use of complementary and alternative medicine by older patients with arthritis: A population-based study. *Arthritis and Rheumatology, 45,* 398–403.

Ni, H., Simile, C., & Hardy, A. M. (2002). Utilization of complementary and alternative medicine by United States adults: Results from the 1999 national health interview survey. *Med Care, 40,* 353–358.

Author

Terry Giese, MBA, OT/L, FAOTA

for

The Commission on Practice
Sara Jane Brayman, PhD, OTR/L, FAOTA, *Chairperson*

Adopted by the Representative Assembly 2005C217

Note: This document replaces the 2003 AOTA White Paper "Complementary and Alternative Medicine."

E

~

AOTA Position Paper:
Occupational Therapy's Commitment
to Nondiscrimination and Inclusion

The occupational therapy profession affirms the right of every individual to access and full participation within society. This paper states the profession's stance on nondiscrimination and inclusion.

Nondiscrimination exists when we accept and treat all people equally. In doing so, we avoid differentiating between people because of biases or prejudices. We value individuals and respect their culture, ethnicity, race, age, religion, gender, sexual orientation, and capacities. Nondiscrimination is a necessary prerequisite for inclusion. Inclusion requires that we ensure not only that everyone is treated fairly and equitably but also that all individuals have the same opportunities to participate in the naturally occurring activities of society, such as attending social events, having access to public transportation, and participating in professional organizations. We also believe that when we do not discriminate against others and when we include all members of society in our daily lives, we reap the benefits of being with individuals who have different perspectives, opinions, and talents from our own.

We support nondiscrimination and inclusion throughout our profession. Our concerns are twofold—for the persons who receive occupational therapy services and for our professional colleagues. In professional practice, our evaluations and interventions are designed to facilitate our clients' engagement in occupations to support participation in the various contexts of their lives, including their social and cultural contexts. As occupational therapists and occupational therapy assistants, we assume a collaborative partnership with clients and their significant others to support the individual's right to self-direction.

We believe that inclusion is achieved through the combined efforts of clients, their families, and significant others; health, education, and social service professionals; legislators; community members; and others. We support all individuals and their significant others' rights to fully participate in making decisions that concern their daily occupations: activities of daily living, instrumental activities of daily living, work, education, play, leisure, and social participation.

The American Occupational Therapy Association and its members recognize the legal mandates concerning nondiscriminatory practices. However, the concept of nondiscrimination is not limited to that which is dictated by law. This professional association, through its members, boards, commissions, committees, officers, and staff, supports the belief that all members of the occupational therapy professional community are entitled to maximum opportunities to develop and use their abilities. These individuals also have the right to achieve productive and satisfying professional and personal lives.

We are committed to nondiscrimination and inclusion as an affirmation of our belief that the interests of all members of the profession are best served when the inherent worth of every individual is recognized and valued. We maintain that society has an obligation to provide the reasonable accommodations necessary to allow individuals access to social, educational, recreational, and vocational opportunities. By embracing the concepts of nondiscrimination and inclusion, we will all benefit from the opportunities afforded in a diverse society.

Authors

Ruth H. Hansen, PhD, FAOTA
Jim Hinojosa, PhD, OT, FAOTA

for

The Commission on Practice
Mary Jane Youngstrom, MS, OTR, *Chairperson*

Adopted by the Representative Assembly 1999M4

Edited by the Commission on Practice 2004

Received by the Representative Assembly 2004C28

Note: This document replaces the 1995 Position Paper *Occupational Therapy: A Profession in Support of Full Inclusion,* the accompanying 1996 White Paper *The Role of the Occupational Therapy Practitioner in the Implementation of Full Inclusion,* and the 1999 Position Paper *Occupational Therapy's Commitment to Nondiscrimination and Inclusion.*

F

AOTA's Statement on Health Disparities

It is widely recognized that disparities in health status and the availability of health and social services exist in the United States. The Trans-National Institutes of Health (NIH) Work Group on Health Disparities defined the term *health disparities* as "the difference in the incidence, prevalence, morbidity, mortality, and burden of diseases and other adverse health conditions that exist among specific population groups" (NIH, 1999).

As noted by the NIH Work Group, experts assert that "health disparities arise from a complex combination of social and economic factors, the physical environments, cultural beliefs and values, educational level, personal behaviors, and genetic susceptibilities" (NIH, 1999). Occupational therapy is well positioned to intervene with individuals and communities to limit the effects of health disparities on participation in meaningful occupations because of practitioners' knowledge and skills in evaluating and intervening with persons who face physical, social, emotional, or cultural challenges to participation. Further, the American Occupational Therapy Association (AOTA) supports advocacy to increase access to health services for persons in need, and efforts to lessen or eliminate health disparities are consistent with the *Core Values* and the *Code of Ethics* for the profession of occupational therapy (AOTA, 1993, 2005).

References

American Occupational Therapy Association. (1993). Core values and attitudes of occupational therapy practice. *American Journal of Occupational Therapy, 47*, 1085–1086.

American Occupational Therapy Association. (2005). Occupational therapy code of ethics (2005). *American Journal of Occupational Therapy, 59*, 639–642.

National Institutes of Health. (1999). Trans-NIH Work Group on Health Disparities. Retrieved January 30, 2006, from http://www.nidcr.nih.gov/Research/HealthDisparities/TransWorkGroup.htm

Author

Brent Braveman, PhD, OTR/L, FAOTA

for

The Representative Assembly Coordinating Council (RACC)
Janet Raisor, OTR, *Chairperson*
Brent Braveman, PhD, OTR/L, FAOTA
Linda Fazio, PhD, OTR/L, LPC, FAOTA
Wendy C. Hildenbrand, MPH, OTR/L, FAOTA
Penelope Moyers, EdD, OTR, FAOTA
S. Maggie Reitz, PhD, OTR/L, FAOTA
Susanne Smith Roley, MS, OTR/L, FAOTA
Carol H. Gwin, OT/L, *Staff Liaison*

Adopted by the Representative Assembly 2006C360

Subject Index

Page numbers followed by an *f* indicate a figure and *t* indicate an exhibit or table.

A

Access to health care disparities, 135–137
Accommodation theory, 57
Accreditation Council for Occupational
    Therapy Education, 12, 25–26, 110
Acquired immune deficiency syndrome,
    135, 143
Active engagement, 207–208
Adjustment behavior, 253
Affective classroom, 281–283
Affective domain, 42
Affective learning, 282
African Americans
    Black English and, 216–218
    classification standards for, 344*t*
    clinical trial bias of, 350
    culturally competent care and, 369
    demographics of, 20
    health disparities in, 134–135
    health indicators for, 163–164
    treatment implications for, 265
    White guilt and, 98
Alaska Natives
    classification standards for, 344*t*
    demographics of, 20
    health indicators for, 164
    treatment implications for, 265

Alcohol abuse, 144
Alternative medicine, 408–411
American cultural myths, 19
American Occupational Therapy
    Association, 25, 110, 202
Asians
    classification standards for, 344*t*
    demographics of, 20
    general cultural knowledge on, 259
    health disparities in, 134–135
    health indicators for, 164
    treatment implications for, 265
Assessment of community. See
    Community assessment methods
Assessment process, 255–259
Assessment process case study, 259–262
Assessment tools
    bias in, 252–253
    in cultural competence measure-
        ment, 406
    measurement inadequacy of,
        351–352
Asset mapping, 308
Assimilation of students, 274–275
Association for Supervision and
    Curriculum Development Multicultural
    Education Commission, 58
Asthma, 137
At-risk groups, 142–145
Autonomy, 377, 385–387

Citation Index

A

Abdi, A., 178, 179

Abdi, M., 178, 179

Abdullahi, M.D., 172, 173, 175, 176, 178

Abelenda, J., 327

Accreditation Council for Occupational
Therapy Education, 12, 25, 102, 110,
232, 276, 363

Acosta, T.P., 193

Adams, A., 185, 310

Adams, W., 189, 190, 191

Adams, P.F., 163, 164

Aday, L.A., 142, 143, 144, 145, 296

Aden, A.H., 173

Adler, M., 307

Agency for Healthcare Research and
Quality, 65, 66, 136, 137, 150, 162, 165

Ahmed, B., 177, 178, 179, 180

Ahmed, O., 177

Alarcon, G., 147

Alexander, C.M., 406

Alexander, R.G., 61

Algado, S.S., xiii, 7, 321, 322, 327

Allison, H., 123

Allport, G.W., 90

Allsup, C., 220

Althaus, F.A., 178

American Medical Student Association,
138, 149, 233

American Occupational Therapy
Association, xiii, 8, 10, 11, 25, 33, 37, 48,
110, 202, 232, 248, 250, 266, 273, 383,
384, 409, 410, 415

American Psychological Association, 214

American Public Health Association, 139,
140

Ananeh-Firempong, O., 139

Anderlik, M.R., 387

Anders, E., 191

Andersen, M., 347, 349

Anderson, G.R., 384

Anderson, R.N., 162, 163, 164

Andonian, L., 41, 64, 364

Aneshensel, C.S., 350

Arkansas Research and Training Center in
Vocational Rehabilitation, 65, 66

Arredondo, P., 41, 339

Asbury, C.A., 147

Ashley, M., 350

Astin, J.A., 409

Atkinson, D.R., 370, 371

Augoustinos, M., 90

Austin, W., 368, 369

Avenant, C., 120

Avila, M.M., 310, 356

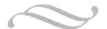

About the Authors

Roxie M. Black, PhD, OTR/L, FAOTA, has been an occupational therapist for almost 40 years, 25 of them as an educator. She is the Director of the Master of Occupational Therapy Program at the University of Southern Maine at Lewiston–Auburn and also is an invited adjunct teacher at the University of Indianapolis. Black's scholarly work has focused on curricular issues and diversity, particularly in the area of cultural competence, and in these areas she has presented regionally, nationally, and internationally in these areas as well as published many articles and book chapters, including co-authoring *Cultural Competency for Health Professionals* (2000). She currently is researching issues of occupational justice with Somali women.

Shirley A. Wells, MPH, OTR, FAOTA, has practiced occupational therapy for 28 years, working 8 years as an educator. She has worked with several diverse populations across the United States, addressing issues facing women living with chronic pain. She served as the manager of the Multicultural Affairs Program of the American Occupational Therapy Association. Wells's scholarly work includes many national and international presentations as well as books and articles on culture, diversity, and ethics, including *Cultural Competency for Health Professionals* (2000) and *A Guide to Reasonable Accommodation for Practitioners With Disabilities: Fieldwork and Environment* (1998). She currently is a doctoral candidate for a DrPH in community health from the School of Public Health, University of Texas Health Sciences Center at Houston, where her research focus is on health literacy and occupational performance among Mexican Americans with end-stage renal failure living on hemodialysis.